Short Bowel Syndrome in Adults

Anca Trifan • Carol Stanciu
Liana Gheorghe
Editors

Short Bowel Syndrome in Adults

From Basic Concepts to Future Prospects in Clinical Practice

Springer

Editors
Anca Trifan
Gastroenterology Department
Grigore T. Popa University of Medicine
and Pharmacy
Iaşi, Romania

Institute of Gastroenterology and Hepatology
St. Spiridon Emergency Hospital
Iaşi, Romania

Carol Stanciu
Gastroenterology Department
Grigore T. Popa University of Medicine
and Pharmacy
Iaşi, Romania

Institute of Gastroenterology and Hepatology
St. Spiridon Emergency Hospital
Iaşi, Romania

Liana Gheorghe
Carol Davila University of Medicine
and Pharmacy
Bucharest, Romania

Center for Digestive Diseases
and Liver Transplant
Fundeni Clinical Institute
Bucharest, Romania

ISBN 978-3-031-95847-2 ISBN 978-3-031-95848-9 (eBook)
https://doi.org/10.1007/978-3-031-95848-9

This Springer imprint is published by the registered company Springer Nature Switzerland AG
The registered company address is: Gewerbestrasse 11, 6330 Cham, Switzerland

Contents

1 Definition and Classification of Short Bowel Syndrome

Cristian Gheorghe and Roxana Vadan

1.1 Definition

The role of the gut is to digest and absorb nutrients and fluids; different parts of the gut have specific roles in this process. Reduction of functional intestinal area and transit time by surgically removing parts of the bowel impairs digestion and can lead to various degrees of malabsorption, resulting in chronic diarrhoea, steatorrhoea, macro- and micronutrient deficiencies, fluid losses, and electrolyte imbalances.

Chronic intestinal failure (CIF) was recently defined by the European Society for Parenteral and Enteral Nutrition (ESPEN) [1] as "persistent reduction of the gut function below the minimum necessary for the absorption of macronutrients and/or water and electrolytes, such that intravenous supplementation (IVS) is required to maintain health and/or growth, in a patient who is metabolically stable," whereas the term "intestinal insufficiency" (or "intestinal deficiency" for those languages where "insufficiency" and "failure" have the same meaning) describes the cases in which although the gut function is affected there is no need for IVS because the patient can compensate for the missing bowel length by various mechanisms (hyperphagia, dietary counselling, and nutritional, pharmacological, or surgical interventions).

CIF is classified into five pathophysiological conditions, namely short bowel syndrome, intestinal fistula, intestinal dysmotility, mechanical obstruction, and extensive small bowel mucosal disease [1].

Short bowel syndrome (SBS) is a clinical condition that results from extensive surgical resection of the small bowel, with residual small bowel in continuity being less than 200 cm and is the primary cause of chronic intestinal failure—64.4% of cases [2].

C. Gheorghe · R. Vadan (✉)
Carol Davila University of Medicine and Pharmacy, Bucharest, Romania

Center for Digestive Diseases and Liver Transplant, Fundeni Clinical Institute, Bucharest, Romania

A. Trifan et al. (eds.), *Short Bowel Syndrome in Adults*,
https://doi.org/10.1007/978-3-031-95848-9_1

1.2 Classification of Short Bowel Syndrome

The length of small bowel is variable in adults, ranging from 3 to 8 m so after surgical resection is of utmost importance for the surgeon to record not the length of resected bowel but the length of remaining small intestine, measured along the antimesenteric border of unstretched bowel distal to the Treitz angle (duodenojejunal flexure). In the absence of surgical reports on the remaining bowel, the length can be estimated using computed tomography enteroclysis ("virtual enteroscopy") or barium contrast small bowel series.

Typically, in SBS, the length of the remaining small bowel in continuity is less than 150–200 cm, but the severity of SBS-associated intestinal failure (IF) depends on other factors such as the part of the small bowel remaining (jejunum or ileum) and the presence or absence of ileocecal valve and colon.

Based on anatomy and length of the remaining bowel, SBS can be classified as follows:

1. SBS type 1: End jejunostomy, results from resection of both ileum and colon.
2. SBS type 2: Jejunocolonic anastomosis (no ileocecal valve, most of the ileum is resected, jejunum in continuity with part of the colon).
3. SBS type 3: Jejunoileocolonic anastomosis with at least 10 cm of terminal ileum and ileocecal valve preserved, with colon in continuity.

Based on the major impact of the presence or absence of colon on the severity of intestinal failure in SBS, not only due to colon's role in absorptive function but also for its role in hormone secretion and energy production (through short chain fatty acids) another, pathophysiological, classification of SBS was proposed [3]:

1. SBS without colon in continuity (corresponding to anatomical type 1).
2. SBS with colon in continuity (corresponding to anatomical types 2 and 3).

Based on the time elapsed from the surgical resection, SBS has three phases:

1. Acute, early phase that last 3–4 weeks, characterized by high intestinal fluid losses, electrolyte, and acid–base imbalances.
2. Adaptive phase that lasts a variable time, generally between 1 and 2 to 3 years, when structural and functional changes gradually occur and the absorptive capacity of the bowel increases, reducing the need for IVS.
3. Chronic, maintenance phase, in which the need of IVS is stabilized.

The early phase starts immediately after the surgical intervention; patients are metabolically unstable, having high intestinal losses, which puts them at risk of dehydration and acute renal failure; they need intensive care and specialized, multidisciplinary team management. After the acute phase, a chronic intestinal failure phase follows, and a progressive process of intestinal adaptation occurs. ESPEN recommends that with the aim to maximize the opportunity of weaning off parenteral nutrition, these patients should be referred early to IF/rehabilitation centres with expertise in CIF management where medical and/or surgical intestinal rehabilitation programmes are available and optimal timing of intestinal transplantation can be established [1]. With various interventions such as dietary counselling and pharmacological treatment (aimed at reducing the fluid losses by inhibiting digestive secretions or at prolonging intestinal transit time or by the use of drugs that enhance the adaptation process) and also by specialised surgical procedures, between 20 and 80% of adult patients with CIF can be weaned off from parenteral nutrition. Weaning is more likely to occur in patients with partially or totally preserved colon [2, 3]. Patients with CIF that are still dependent on home parenteral nutrition (HPN) 3 years after the last surgery are unlikely to be weaned for HPN at a later date and will need lifelong parenteral nutritional support.

Based on the grade of the residual gut function, SBS can be classified into:

1. SBS with intestinal failure.
2. SBS with intestinal insufficiency/deficiency.

According to ESPEN recommendations, the severity of intestinal failure can be graded based on two parameters: the volume of IVS and the type of IVS (only fluids and electrolytes [FE] or parenteral nutrition [PN]) required to maintain health (1). Eight categories emerged (Table 1.1) that have prognostic significance [4]. In general, patients requiring supplementation with FE alone have better prognosis than those requiring PN (hence energy). The categories are independently associated with the odds of weaning of HPN (higher for PN1 than for FE or any of PN 2, 3, or 4), are associated with mortality (lower for any volume of FE and higher for PN dependent patients), and also correlate with complications such as intestinal-associated liver disease (cholestasis, liver failure) or catheter-related blood stream infections: FE (any volume) = PN1, PN4 > PN3 > PN2 > PN1 (the larger the PN volume, the worse the prognosis).

SBS patients with intestinal insufficiency do not require IV nutrition or fluids but necessitate oral/enteral or intramuscular supplementation (nutrients, micronutrients) to maintain optimal nutritional status.

Table 1.1 Categories of nutritional interventions and their significance

Volume[a] infused daily (ml)	Fluid and electrolytes	Parenteral nutrition	Prognostic significance
<1000	FE1	PN1	Weaning off HPN:
1001–2000	FE2	PN2	PN1 > FE = PN2 = PN3 = PN4
2001–3000	FE3	PN3	Death:
>3000	FE4	PN4	FE1,2,3,4 < PN1,2,3,4 Complications (liver disease, catheter): FE (any volume) = PN1, PN4 > PN3 > PN2 > PN1

[a]The value is the mean of the total volume infused in a week divided by seven

The term "functional short bowel" describes the surgical cases that have more than 200 cm of small bowel left but due to diseased mucosa in the remnant intestine (inflammatory bowel disease, radiation enteritis) or due to an accelerated intestinal transit develop nutritional deficiencies and need the same management as typical SBS patients.

References

1. Pironi L, Cuerda C, Jeppesen PB, Joly F, Jonkers C, Krznarić Ž, Lal S, Lamprecht G, Lichota M, Mundi MS, Schneider SM, Szczepanek K, Van Gossum A, Wanten G, Wheatley C, Weimann A. ESPEN guideline on chronic intestinal failure in adults—update 2023. Clin Nutr. 2023;42(10):1940–2021. https://doi.org/10.1016/j.clnu.2023.07.019. Epub 2023 Jul 29
2. Pironi L, Konrad D, Brandt C, Joly F, Wanten G, Agostini F, et al. Clinical classification of adult patients with chronic intestinal failure due to benign disease: an international multicenter cross-sectional survey. Clin Nutr. 2018;37(2):728e38. https://doi.org/10.1016/j.clnu.2017.04.013. Epub 2017 Apr 19
3. Pironi L. Definition, classification, and causes of short bowel syndrome. Nutr Clin Pract. 2023;38:S9–S16. https://doi.org/10.1002/ncp.10955.
4. Pironi L, Steiger E, Joly F, Wanten GJA, Chambrier C, Aimasso U, et al. Intravenous supplementation type and volume are associated with 1-year outcome and major complications in patients with chronic intestinal failure. Gut. 2020;69(10):1787e95. https://doi.org/10.1136/gutjnl-2018-318172. Epub 2020 Jan 21

Epidemiology and Survival of Short Bowel Syndrome

2

Cristian Gheorghe and Roxana Vadan

Short bowel syndrome (SBS) is a rare disease, being included in the Orphanet (the portal for rare diseases and orphan drugs) as ORPHA:95427 with prevalence unknown. The prevalence is difficult to estimate accurately, data are limited globally, and estimates are variable depending on geographic region.

The epidemiological difficulties reside from the heterogeneity of the SBS patients, due to different etiology and variations in definition, in the clinical classifications, and in healthcare data collection (most studies relying on retrospective analysis of medical records or prescriptions). Based on the fact that the only constant characteristic of SBS is the dependency at least at some point in its natural history on parenteral nutrition (PN), which is a life supportive treatment in acute settings and in chronic SBS-intestinal failure (IF) cases, most published data regarding the incidence and prevalence of SBS are derived from those of intestinal failure, which can be estimated by the utilization of home parenteral nutrition (HPN). In this approach, the cases that can be classified as SBS but without IF (weaned off HPN at that time point or with various grades of intestinal insufficiencies that do not need IV supplementation) cannot be estimated.

SBS is the most frequent indication for HPN. An international multicentric survey conducted in 30 adult intestinal failure centers (the majority having around 100 patients and one-third with over 200 patients) revealed that SBS was the cause of IF in median 50% of cases (ranging from 20 to 80%) [1].

The historical (1992) reports from the USA that utilized the North American Medicare Home Parenteral Nutrition Registry estimated the annual prevalence of HPN to about 120 per million population (40,000 patients) from which SBS

C. Gheorghe · R. Vadan (✉)
Carol Davila University of Medicine and Pharmacy, Bucharest, Romania

Center for Digestive Diseases and Liver Transplant, Fundeni Clinical Institute, Bucharest, Romania

A. Trifan et al. (eds.), *Short Bowel Syndrome in Adults*,
https://doi.org/10.1007/978-3-031-95848-9_2

represented approximately 25%, so about 30 per million [2]. More recent reports show a decline in the prevalence of patients receiving HPN in the USA to 79 patients per million (25,000 patients) in 2013 study that used data from Medicare [3] and a comparable figure of 75 patients per million in 2020 based on PN prescriptions: approximately 24,000 patients receiving HPN between 2012 and 2020 [4].

Compared with the USA, European incidence and prevalence figures are much lower. Data for 13 European countries were collected retrospectively using a questionnaire designed by the members of the European Society for Parenteral and Enteral Nutrition (ESPEN)-Home Artificial Nutrition Working Group; two retrospective surveys on HPN use were realized in 1993 and 1997 [5, 6]. In more recent years, the use of HPN in Europe has increased. No new multicentric data were published but several single-center reports confirm the increased number of patients receiving HPN. Prevalence data are available for Great Britain (prevalence of 36.1per million in 2015, compared with 15 per million in 2008) [7], Italy (prevalence of 45 per million in 2012) [8], Spain (prevalence of 5.9 per million in 2018) [9], Czech Republic (55.0 per million in 2024) [10], and Poland (threefold increase of prevalence from 2010 to 53.26 per million in 2020) [11] (Table 2.1).

From other parts of the globe, data are scarce: Incidence of SBS-IF was reported in Argentina (data from the multicenter prospective impRovE underSTanding of short bOwel syndRomE in Argentina (RESTORE) registry) as 19.6 new cases per year [12].

Based on the peculiarities of home artificial nutrition coverage in France, the number of beneficiaries is accessible in an anonymized open database for the entire country, per year. Also, the demographic statistic for the French population is annually updated and is precise, so reliable prevalence data can be calculated for home artificial nutrition, enteral and parenteral. Using these advantages, Buhl et al. [13] carried out an epidemiological study on the entire adult French population (50.881.948 inhabitants) in 2019. The average incidence of HPN was 2.2/1.000.000 inhabitants/year, and the overall prevalence was 2.53/1.000.000 inhabitants/year (12,859 patients). The prevalence of long-term (over 12 weeks) HPN was 0.62/1.000.000 inhabitants (3122 patients). Both incidence and prevalence were variable according to age and sex, being higher after 60 years and higher in men. The figures reported by the authors are reliable, since they could accurately identify all patients with prescriptions for home artificial nutrition. But the real prevalence and incidence are probably higher since in the analysis, two categories of patients could not be included: the medical services for poly-pathological patients with home hospitalization and the residents of medical institutions, both of which are differently reimbursed in France. No data about the indication for home nutrition were available so the percentage of patients with SBS is unknown.

Results from the ESPEN international multicenter cross-sectional survey describe the characteristics of the SBS population. In the survey 65 centers from 22 countries participated. A large cohort of 1880 adult SBS-IF patients were evaluated. The data collected showed that 60% of patients had SBS-I (with jejunostomy), 30.9% SBS-II (jejunocolic), and 9.1% SBS-III (jejunoileocolic). So, the most prevalent type of SBS was type I, especially in countries like United Kingdom and

Table 2.1 Incidence and prevalence of HPN use in Europe during time

	Incidence patients/million/year		Prevalence patients/million inhabitants								
Country	1993	1997	1993	1997	2008	2010	2012	2015	2018	2020	2024
Belgium	0.24	2.6	2.2	3.0		11					
Denmark	4.6	2.8	12.2	12.7		66					
France	2.4	2.9	2.3	3.6		6					
Poland	0.2	0.36	0.5	1.1		18				53.26	
Spain	0.3	0.7	0.3	0.65					5.9		
Italy	2.2	–	1.7	–			45				
United Kingdom	0.8	1.2	2.6	3.7	15			36.1			
The Netherlands	1.0	3.0	2.4	3.7							
Czech Republic											55.0

Denmark where it accounted for over 75% of cases but was also frequently encountered (50–60%) in the rest of the countries that participate to the survey. The etiology of SBS was in almost two-thirds of cases either Crohn's disease (27.1%) or mesenteric ischemia (26.7%). Surgical complications were the next most frequent cause of SBS, accounting for 16.7% of cases. Radiation enteritis (6.3%) and volvulus (3.7%) were not very frequent, while adhesions, chronic intestinal pseudo-obstruction, polyposis, trauma, and ulcerative colitis each accounted for less than 2% of cases. Crohn's disease was more prevalent in SBS type I, while mesenteric ischemia in type II SBS and surgical complications and mesenteric ischemia in type III SBS. All types of SBS were more frequently encountered in women (female to male ratio of 2:1) presumably due to a shorter intestinal length in females correlated with the smaller height and weight in female sex. Regarding etiology, differences were observed between countries. Crohn's disease was the first cause of SBS cases from the USA (48%), the United Kingdom (35.4%), the Netherlands, and Denmark, whereas mesenteric ischemia was more frequent in SBS patients from France, Italy, and Poland. The differences probably derive from the variability in treatment protocols for the originating disease and in the management of IF and HPN between participating countries [14]. In the prospective multicentric observational registry from Latin America (RESTORE), SBS etiology was as follows: surgical complications in 42%, intestinal ischemia 28%, abdominal trauma 9%, volvulus 5%, and others 16%, being different from North America and European data by a very low proportion of inflammatory bowel disease cases [15]. Data from Japan (a real-world observational study including 393 patients) showed similarities with the Western population; the most frequent causes of SBS-IF were ileus (31.8%), Crohn's disease (20.1%), and mesenteric ischemia (16.0%) [16].

Regarding prognosis, apart from the influence of primary disease (which caused the intestinal resection that led to intestinal failure), and of preexisting comorbidities, the outcome of patients with SBS is mainly determined by the consequences of malabsorption: diarrhea, steatorrhea, weight loss, malnutrition, dehydration, electrolyte imbalance (hyponatremia, hypokalemia, hypomagnesemia), vitamin deficiencies, renal complications (renal failure, calcium oxalate kidney stones), liver complications (intestinal failure-associated liver disease, cholestasis, gallstones), bacterial overgrowth, and D-lactic acidosis. Patients with SBS have an increased risk of sepsis due to the presence of malnutrition, due to surgical-related infections (surgical site infections, anastomotic leaks, fistulas, and intraabdominal abscesses) and, specifically for HPN, catheter-associated sepsis which is the most frequent complication of home nutrition and an indicator of quality of care [17].

Few studies compare survival of HPN patients with that of general population. A cohort study carried out in an UK national reference center between 1978 and 2018 included 840 patients with nonmalignant IF observed for 7344 patient-years. The probability of survival was 91.8% at 1 year, 69.3% at 5 years, 54.3% at 10 years, 29.8% at 20 years, and 16.7% at 30 years. Compared with the UK general population, patients with SBS had a 6.82-fold higher mortality rate and a life expectancy of 17 years [18]. Survival data are variable; multiple factors contributing to the prognosis of SBS patients as follows: the anatomical characteristics of SBS (length of the residual intestine, presence of colon, the severity of IF), the primary disease that lead to the intestinal resection (malignant or nonmalignant), and the time period from which the data are collected, recent advances in SBS therapy having their impact on prognosis. There is a general agreement in the literature that anatomical type of SBS is the most important factor for prognosis. Type I (jejunostomy) has the worst prognosis because it more frequently necessitates long-term PN, while in type III, weaning of PN can be achieved in most cases. In PN-dependent cases, the volume of nutrition is also larger for patients with type I SBS: 14.2 L/week, 6.1 days/week; for type II, 11.2 L/week, 5.5 days/week; and for type III, 9.8 L/week, 5.2 days/week [19]. In the long-term SBS survival study reported by Messing et al. [15] after the multivariate analysis, the only parameters that remained significantly associated with decreased survival rate were type I digestive circuit (end jejunostomy), bowel length of <50 cm, and mesenteric infarction as a cause of SBS (PN dependence and age of the patient over 60 years lost statistical significance). The causes of death were directly related to PN only in 22% of cases (septicemia and liver failure); the majority (78%) were consequence of the primary disease (mostly due to vascular disease), comorbidities (diabetes, malignancy, respiratory failure), or secondary to malnutrition (cachexia, hypokalemia, sepsis not related to catheter) [20].

Survival is always better in HPN-independent patients. In a long-term follow-up (mean 4.4 years, range 0.3-24 years) of SBS patients from France, the dependence on PN was 74%, 64%, and 48% at 1, 2, and 5 years [21]. The favorable prognostic factors for PN autonomy were a remnant small bowel length over 75 cm, more than >57% remaining colon in continuity, and early (<6 months) plasma citrulline concentration > 20 μmol/l. The time needed to achieve autonomy was 1 year for 54.5% of cases, between 1 and 2 years for 19%, and over 2 years for 26.5% of cases.

Regarding hospitalizations and mortality of SBS patients, relevant data emerged from a report [22] that utilized the largest hospitalization database in the USA National Institutes of Health (NIH) and its records between 2005 and 2014 and identified a large sample size of 53,000 patients hospitalized with SBS, with the mean age of 56.6 ± 15.8 years, more than two-thirds (67.8%) being women. The study showed that an increase of 55% in the number of annual hospitalizations occurred during the 10-year observation period presumably because of the increased frequency of the diseases that lead to intestinal resection (inflammatory bowel disease, vascular diseases, neoplasms) and also due to increased utilization of HPN and increased survival of SBS patients. The primary causes for hospitalization in the US report, occurring in approximately half of the patients, were fluid and electrolyte disturbances (mostly hypokalemia and hyponatremia). The overall rate of hospital mortality was 3.8%, with a steady and statistically significant decline in time. The independent risk factors associated with in hospital mortality were as follows: age > 65 years (aOR3.49; 95%CI2.68–4.56, $p < 0.001$), sepsis (aOR3.38, 95%CI 3.02–3.78, $p < 0.001$), concurrent congestive heart failure (aOR2.64, $p < 0.001$), concurrent liver disease (aOR2.36; $p < 0.001$), severe malnutrition (aOR1.64, $p < 0.001$), and metastatic cancer (aOR1.53, $p < 0.001$).

Over time, HPN became available in many countries, experience with its use increased, standards of practice were established, specialized high volume intestinal failure centers with a multidisciplinary approach for SBS care were organized and all these factors are premises for a better prognosis and increased survival of SBS patients. Other new developments may contribute to longer lifespan of SBS patients, such as hormonal new developments with glucagon-like peptide 2 (GLP-2) analogs: teduglutide, approved for use, apraglutide, long acting, under clinical development in phase III studies. Also, various new surgical techniques designed to lengthen the bowel (such as serial transverse enteroplasty) and the availability of intestinal transplant have their impact on the prognosis of patients with SBS.

In conclusion, SBS is a rare and complex disease with potentially adverse outcomes. Identifying its true incidence and prevalence is difficult. Morbidity and mortality are high compared to general population but special care in dedicated centers by multidisciplinary teams with state-of-the-art approach has the potential to improve the outcomes of SBS patients.

Bibliography

1. Lakananurak N, Moccia L, Wall E, Herlitz J, Catron H, Lozano E, Delgado A, Vanuytsel T, Mercer D, Pevny S, Berner-Hansen M, Gramlich L. Characteristics of adult intestinal failure centers: an international multicenter survey. Nutr Clin Pract. 2023;38(3):657–63. https://doi.org/10.1002/ncp.10926. Epub 2022 Oct 29
2. Howard L, Ament M, Fleming CR, Shike M, Steiger E. Current use and clinical outcome of home parenteral and enteral nutrition therapies in the United States. Gastroenterology. 1995;109(2):355–65. https://doi.org/10.1016/0016-5085(95)90321-6.
3. Mundi MS, Pattinson A, McMahon MT, Davidson J, Hurt RT. Prevalence of home parenteral and enteral nutrition in the United States. Nutr Clin Pract. 2017;32(6):799–805.
4. Mundi MS, Mercer DF, Iyer K, Pfeffer D, Zimmermann LB, Berner-Hansen M, Bishop J, Seidner DL. Characteristics of chronic intestinal failure in the USA based on analysis of claims data. JPEN J Parenter Enteral Nutr. 2022;46(7):1614–22. https://doi.org/10.1002/jpen.2426. Epub 2022 Jul 24. PMID: 35726729
5. Van Gossum A, Bakker H, De Francesco A, Ladefoged K, Leon-Sanz M, Messing B, et al. ESPEN-Home Artificial Nutrition Working Group. Home parenteral nutrition in adults: a multicentre survey in Europe in 1993. Clin Nutr. 1996;15(2):53e9.
6. Bakker H, Bozzetti F, Staun M, Leon-Sanz M, Hebuterne X, Pertkiewicz M, et al. Home parenteral nutrition in adults: a European multicentre survey in 1997. ESPEN-Home Artificial Nutrition Working Group. Clin Nutr. 1999;18(3):135e40.
7. Naghibi M, Toskas A, Willsmore J, Smith T, Hughes SJ, Gabe S, the British Artificial Nutrition Survey Committee. United Kingdom artificial nutrition database: the changing landscape of adult home parenteral support. JPEN J Parenter Enteral Nutr. 2023;47(5):635–45. https://doi.org/10.1002/jpen.2504. Epub 2023 May 3
8. Pironi L, Regional Coordinators of SINPE. Development of home artificial nutrition in Italy over a seven year period: 2005–2012. BMCNutr. 2017;3(6):2–8. https://doi.org/10.1186/s40795-016-0118-y644.
9. Arhip L, Serrano-Moreno C, Romero I, Camblor M, Cuerda C. The economic costs of home parenteral nutrition: systematic review of partial and full economic evaluations. Clin Nutr. 2021;40(2):339–49. https://doi.org/10.1016/j.clnu.2020.06.010.
10. Koudelková K, Waldauf P, Wohl P, Šenkyřík M, Beneš P, Kohout P, Vejmelka J, Maňák J, Těšínský P, Novák F, Meisnerová E, Fencl F, Gojda J. The Czech Home Parenteral Nutrition Registry REDNUP: comprehensive analysis of adult patients' data. Ann Nutr Metab. 2024;80(3):143–52. https://doi.org/10.1159/000538232. Epub 2024 Mar 12. Erratum in:

Ann Nutr Metab. 2024;80(6):354. doi: 10.1159/000542030. PMID: 38471467; PMCID: PMC11152004

11. Folwarski M, Kłęk S, Szlagatys-Sidorkiewicz A, Wyszomirski A, Brzeziński M, Skotnicka M. Trend observations in home parenteral nutrition. Prevalence, hospitalizations and costs: results from a nationwide analysis of health care provider data. Nutrients. 2021;13(10):3465. https://doi.org/10.3390/nu13103465. PMID: 34684466; PMCID: PMC8539115
12. Gondolesi GE, Ortega ML, Doeyo M, et al. First registry of adult patients with chronic intestinal failure due to short bowel syndrome in Argentina: the RESTORE project. J Parenter Enter Nutr. 2022;46:1623–31. https://doi.org/10.1002/jpen.2387.
13. Buhl ND, Bourry J, Seguy D, Lescut D. Epidemiology of home enteral and parenteral nutrition in adults: Comprehensive national data. Clin Nutr ESPEN. 2024;60:79–85. https://doi.org/10.1016/j.clnesp.2024.01.010. Epub 2024 Jan 18
14. Pironi L. Definition, classification, and causes of short bowel syndrome. Nutr Clin Pract. 2023;38(Suppl 1):S9–S16. https://doi.org/10.1002/ncp.10955.
15. Rumbo C, Solar H, Ortega M, Busoni V, de Barrio S, Martinuzzi A, Martínez MI, Plata C, Donnadio L, Aurora SZ, Saure C, Perez C, Tanzi MN, Consuelo A, Becerra A, Manzur A, Moya DA, Rudi L, Moreira E, Buncuga M, Hodgson MI, Clariá RS, Fernandez A, Gondolesi G. Short bowel syndrome related intestinal failure outcomes in Latin America: Insights from the RESTORE Registry. JPEN J Parenter Enteral Nutr. 2024;48(8):956–64. https://doi.org/10.1002/jpen.2693. Epub 2024 Oct 5
16. Mizushima T, Udagawa E, Hasegawa M, et al. Etiologies and treatments of chronic intestinal failure-short bowel syndrome (SBS) in Japanese adults: a real-world observational study. Surg Today. 2022;52:1350–7. https://doi.org/10.1007/s00595-022-02469-9.
17. Dreesen M, Pironi L, Wanten G, et al. Outcome indicators for home parenteral nutrition care: point of view from adult patients with benign disease. JPEN J Parenter Enteral Nutr. 2015;39(7):828–36. [PubMed: 24917517]
18. Kopczynska M, Hvas CL, Jepsen P, et al. Standardised survival and excess Life Years Lost in patients with type 3 intestinal failure. Clin Nutr. 2022;41(11):2446–54. https://doi.org/10.1016/j.clnu.2022.09.010.
19. Pironi L, Steiger E, Joly F, et al. Characteristics of adult patients with chronic intestinal failure due to short bowel syndrome: an international multicenter survey. Clin Nutr ESPEN. 2021;45:433–41. https://doi.org/10.1016/j.clnesp.2021.07.004.
20. Messing B, Crenn P, Beau P, Boutron-Ruault MC, Rambaud JC, Matuchansky C. Long-term survival and parenteral nutrition dependence in adult patients with the short bowel syndrome. Gastroenterology. 1999;117(5):1043–50. https://doi.org/10.1016/s0016-5085(99)70388-4.
21. Amiot A, Messing B, Corcos O, Panis Y, Joly F. Determinants of home parenteral nutrition dependence and survival of 268 patients with non-malignant short bowel syndrome. Clin Nutr. 2013;32(3):368–74. https://doi.org/10.1016/j.clnu.2012.08.007. Epub 2012 Aug 23
22. Siddiqui MT, Al-Yaman W, Singh A, Kirby DF. Short-Bowel syndrome: epidemiology, hospitalization trends, in-hospital mortality, and healthcare utilization. JPEN J Parenter Enteral Nutr. 2021;45(7):1441–55. https://doi.org/10.1002/jpen.2051. Epub 2020 Dec 17. PMID: 33233017; PMCID: PMC9254738

Pathophysiology and Anatomical Considerations in Short Bowel Syndrome

3

Cristian Gheorghe and Roxana Vadan

3.1 Pathophysiology in Short Bowel Syndrome

The primary mechanism of chronic intestinal failure in short bowel syndrome (SBS) is the loss of absorptive surface secondary to intestinal resection. The accelerated intestinal transit time also contributes to the effectiveness of the digestion and absorption processes, but the length of the intestine is the main driving factor for the occurrence and for the severity of intestinal failure.

From a pathophysiological point of view, it is of utmost importance to know the exact length of the remaining bowel. Though, in many cases, after intestinal resections, surgical reports give information only on the length of the resected intestine. This is not useful because the length of the normal small bowel is very variable (in adults, it was reported to be between 300 and 800 cm), and thus, the length of the remaining bowel cannot be calculated by simply subtracting the resected part [1, 2]. Historically, the length of the intestine was measured ex vivo, on cadavers, a method that was shown to underestimate the real bowel length. More accurate measurements are those done in vivo, during surgery, when the intestine is relaxed, and its real extent can be appreciated. This underscores once more the importance of a precise surgical report. In the absence of such a report, the remaining bowel can be measured radiologically. The newly available technology: Computed tomography (CT) or small bowel barium follow through (classic SBFT) can be applied in the evaluation of intestinal length in humans. The measurement of small bowel length from the X-ray films of a barium meal follow-through can be done by using an opisometer (device used for measuring distances on maps), but can be difficult when overlapping of the bowel loops occurs [3]. Reports show that three-dimensional CT

C. Gheorghe · R. Vadan (✉)
Carol Davila University of Medicine and Pharmacy, Bucharest, Romania

Center for Digestive Diseases and Liver Transplant, Fundeni Clinical Institute, Bucharest, Romania

A. Trifan et al. (eds.), *Short Bowel Syndrome in Adults*,
https://doi.org/10.1007/978-3-031-95848-9_3

enterography has a better correlation to surgical measurements as compared with SBFT [4].

Once the length and type of the remaining bowel are accurately established and its absorptive capacity (normal mucosa or abnormal mucosa due to the primary disease) is known, the specific nutritional consequences can be anticipated. The most important part of the absorption process occurs in the first 100-150 cm of the jejunum, where the specific transporters are located. Here, most of the digested protein, carbohydrates, and water-soluble vitamins are absorbed. Lipids are absorbed over a larger portion of the small bowel.

Specific nutrient digestion sites, absorption sites, and specific mediator (hormones and neurotransmitters) synthesis sites along the digestive tract are represented in Table 3.1.

The type and severity of SBS symptoms depend also on the time elapsed from the surgery, since the physiological process of adaptation starts immediately after resection. As mentioned in the previous chapter (definitions and classification of SBS), an acute phase of SBS (first 3–4 weeks) is followed by an adaptive phase (lasting generally 1–2 years, sometimes up to 3 years) in which the maximal adaptation capacity of the remaining intestine is reached, which is followed by a chronic, stable phase. In the acute phase, after large enterectomies, temporary (lasting for up to 12 months) gastric hypergastrinemia and gastric acid hypersecretion occur. The mechanism involved is considered to be the loss of the parts of bowel responsible for the secretion of regulatory hormones (gastric inhibitory peptide [GIP] and vasoactive intestinal peptide [VIP]). Consequently, a larger volume of acidic secretions enters the remaining small bowel, diluting and, by changing the luminal pH to an acidic value, inactivating the digestive enzymes. Subsequently, maldigestion occurs, enhancing malabsorption and loss of nutrients which, by osmosis, attract more water into the lumen, therefore significantly increasing the fluid and electrolyte losses (diarrhea). Dehydration, hyponatremia, hypokalemia, hypocalcemia, and hypomagnesemia need correction through intravenous (IV) infusions early after surgical intervention in these patients. Also, potentially severe peptic complications can occur, and proton pump inhibitor use is important.

In both acute and chronic phases, malabsorption is characteristic for SBS patients. The physiological process of digestion and absorption has a proximal-to-distal anatomical absorptive gradient [5]. The duodenum is approximately 25–30 cm long, jejunum corresponds to the proximal two-fifths of the small intestine (approximately 160–200 cm), while the distal three-fifths corresponds to the ileum [6]. Most nutrient absorption (proteins, carbohydrates, and vitamins) normally occurs in the first 100–150 cm of the jejunum, and lipids are absorbed on larger parts of the small intestine. This is due to the specific structural characteristics of the proximal jejunum which confer a maximal surface area and hence a maximal absorption capacity: Jejunal diameter is bigger, the circular folds are larger, and the villi and the microvilli are longer compared with the more distal parts of the small intestine. The maximal concentration of the nutrients occurs in the lumen of the proximal jejunum; also, the maximal absorption capacity is encountered here. It is long known that the presence of nutrients, in particular complex nutrients, in the intestine have

Table 3.1 Nutrient digestion, absorption, and mediator synthesis according to anatomical regions of the digestive system

Anatomical region	Digestion	Absorption	Secretion
Stomach	Pepsin breaks down proteins to polypeptides	Water Ethyl alcohol Iodine Fluoride Molybdenum	Gastrin Ghrelin Intrinsic factor
Duodenum and proximal jejunum	Triglycerides are digested into monoglycerides and fatty acids (most part) Carbohydrates are digested to disaccharides (most part). Proteins are digested into oligopeptides and amino acids (most part)	Peptide/amino acids Carbohydrates Lipids Iron Folate Calcium Magnesium phosphorus Copper Water-soluble vitamins Fat-soluble vitamins Water	Cholecystokinin Secretin VIP GIP
Jejunum and ileum	Triglycerides are digested into monoglycerides and fatty acids Carbohydrates are digested to disaccharides Proteins are digested into oligopeptides and amino acids	Peptide/amino acids Carbohydrates Lipids Lactose Calcium Manganese Molybdenum Water-soluble vitamins Fat-soluble vitamins Water	Neurotensin
Distal ileum		Bile acids Vitamin B12 Intrinsic factor SCFA	Peptide YY GLP-1 GLP-2
Colon	Carbohydrate fermentation	Water Amino acids SCFA Minerals: Sodium, chloride, potassium Vitamin K Bile acids (small amount)	Peptide YY GLP-1 GLP-2

VIP vasoactive intestinal peptide; *GIP* glucose-dependent insulinotropic peptide, *GLP* glucagon-like peptide, *SCFA* short-chain fatty acid

a trophic effect on the intestinal mucosa and determines increased villus height [7]. This explains the abovementioned characteristics of the proximal jejunum which adapted fully to the presence of a multitude of luminal digestive enzymes and digestion products. In contrast, the absence of nutrients in the lumen is associated with reduced villus height and mitotic index [8]. Proximal jejunum synthesizes cholecystokinin (CCK), secretin, which regulate the pancreatic and biliary secretion, which are generally preserved in patients with SBS.

3.2 Site-Specific Effects of Intestinal Resection

3.2.1 End Jejunostomy

Intestinal resections that involve less than 50% of intestinal length are well tolerated, without significant nutritional consequences. Resections that involve more than 70–75% of the intestine determine a global malabsorption of nutrients, which results directly from the reduced absorptive surface and leads to various grades of malnutrition and deficiencies in vitamins and minerals [6].

Generally, parenteral nutritional support is needed in type I SBS (end jejunostomy) when jejunal length is less than 100 cm [9].

Apart from absorption of nutrients, throughout the small and especially large bowel, absorption of water and electrolytes takes place. Daily approximately 4 L of intestinal secretions are produced: 0.5 L of saliva, 2 L of gastric acid, and 1.5 L of pancreaticobiliary secretions, which are added to the volume of ingested liquids.

The absorption of water is passive, accompanying the active transport of nutrients and electrolytes. The jejunal epithelial cells have between them relatively large intercellular junctions [5], so in this part of the small bowel, the absorption of fluids is not very efficient.

The absorption of the sodium in the jejunum is an active process occurring against a concentration gradient, coupled with glucose, but sodium can diffuse back easily, passively, into the lumen through the loose junctions between jejunal epithelial cells. So, in type I SBS (end jejunostomy), a significant loss of water and electrolytes occurs, and variable volumes of IV fluids are needed to avoid dehydration. In each liter of jejunostomy output, about 100 mEq of sodium is lost, which makes sodium deficiency common. Not always serum sodium levels reflect sodium depletion, a useful diagnostic tool being a random urinary sodium concentration of less than 10 mEq/L. Magnesium is also lost by reduced absorption (resection of the specific absorption sites—magnesium is absorbed normally in the distal small intestine and colon—also lost due to its binding by the malabsorbed fatty acids) and by increased urinary losses (in cases of sodium depletion). Magnesium deficiency is common in patients with an end jejunostomy. If less than 100 cm of jejunum is remaining, the patients can become "net secretors," and the stomal output of fluid and electrolytes exceeds the fluid intake because the gastric and intestinal secretions are lost, not absorbed. It has been shown that in the healthy subjects, jejunal motility is more intense with more migrating clustered contractions, higher velocity, and longer propagation distance comparative with the ileal motility. The rapid physiological transit time of nutrients through the jejunum does not favor nutrient absorption [10]. The removal of distal ileum and colon also determines the loss of enteroendocrine hormone-producing L cells (source of PYY, GLP-1, and GLP-2, responsible for the ileal "brake," vide infra), another contributor to the accelerated gastric emptying and accelerated intestinal transit time in end jejunostomy patients, increasing the stomal fluid loss [11]. Also, due to the loss of the distal ileum, parenteral supplementation of vitamin B12 is required.

For end jejunostomy, we can anticipate that parenteral nutrition is needed to meet the energy requirements; sodium and fluid supplementation and magnesium and vitamin B12 supplementation are also necessary.

It was shown that depending on the length of the residual jejunum, the required parenteral support is as follows: For jejunum length < 85 cm, both parenteral nutrition and IV fluids (saline) are needed. For jejunum length between 85 and 100 cm, IV saline is needed but parenteral nutrition is not always required. For jejunal length between 101 and 150 cm, enteral or oral nutrition is sufficient, and fluid requirements are met by using enteral or oral glucose/saline solution. For jejunal length between 151 and 200 cm, only oral glucose/saline solution is required [12].

3.2.2 Jejunoileostomy

At the ileal level, the intercellular junctions are tighter, water is following the active transport of sodium and does not diffuse back and so the intestinal content can be concentrated.

Regarding nutrient absorption, the ileum (as opposed to the jejunum) can undergo a complex process of adaptation. Intestinal adaptation is an innate compensatory process that starts after large resections of the small bowel; it is highly variable and usually reaches its maximum after 2, sometimes 3, years. In this process, the remaining bowel suffers anatomical and physiological changes that lead to increased digestive and absorptive capacity.

The most important stimulus for this process is the presence of nutrients in the intestinal lumen.

For the duodenum, studies in children with SBS showed the lack of adaptative hyperplasia and only molecular signs of altered mucosal function with enhanced, facilitative glucose transport [13]. The jejunum is already structurally at its maximum absorptive capacity, so it adapts little, mostly functionally, by some increase in enzyme production. So, if jejunum alone is removed, malabsorption and energy malnutrition do not occur because the ileum can undertake all jejunum functions. By removing the jejunum, the loss of CCK and secretin can impair the feedback inhibition of gastrin and gastric acid secretion with acid hypersecretion and low pH in the proximal intestine which can potentially alter digestion, but the effect is transient. The ileum can suffer massive structural adaptative changes in all its layers. At mucosal level, a so-called jejunization process occurs, by which the ileum progressively resembles more and more with the jejunum. An increase in villus and microvilli length takes place, with associated increase in crypt depth, and an increase in enterocyte number (epithelial hyperplasia). Also enhanced proliferation rate and more rapid migration of newly formed enterocytes to the tip of the villi occurs. The estimated increase in villus height can reach 70–75% [14], while crypts can elongate by 35% [15]. All the layers of the intestine grow. The muscular layer is hypertrophied. At macroscopic level, enlargement of the mucosal folds, elongation, and dilation of the bowel are seen, with increased bowel weight. Also, functional changes occur at ileal level: The synthetic capacity of the enterocytes increases with more brush border enzymes (disaccharidases and peptidases), more protein cotransporters (sodium, glucose, and amino acid transporters) and more receptors (for calcium, cobalamin, and biliary acids). The enterocytes are more efficient, mature more quickly, and reach earlier fully functional capacity, and the density of transporter proteins implicated in absorption of nutrients, water, and electrolytes is increased [16]. Due to ileal adaptation, generally resections that involve the proximal bowel (duodenum and jejunum) are better tolerated. The transit time is slow to ensure a longer contact between the intestinal content and the brush border and, subsequently, a better absorption of nutrients. Various parts of the intestine secrete specific hormones. The endocrine L cells located in the distal ileum (and proximal colon) are responsive for the jejunal, ileal, and colonic "brake" due to the hormones produced. Glucagon-like peptides 1 and 2, neurotensin, and peptide YY have important motility-modulating properties [7], controlling the transit time through the gastrointestinal tract (slowing gastric emptying and intestinal transit) and optimizing in this way the nutrient digestion and absorption.

The distal ileum has a specific absorptive role in the absorption of bile salts and vitamin B12, role that cannot be replaced. After distal ileal resections, the site of reabsorption of the bile acids and, for vitamin B12 absorption is lost. Parenteral supplementation of vitamin B12 is necessary in cases with ileal resections over 60 cm. In cases with ileal resections larger that 100 cm, the enterohepatic circuit is significantly affected and the reduction of bile acid absorption and loss of bile acids exceed the synthetic capacity of the liver, determining a decreased bile acid pool, which significantly impacts lipid digestion and determines steatorrhea and fat-soluble vitamins deficiency [17].

For jejunoileostomy anastomosis, we can anticipate variable requirements for parenteral nutrition and fluid and electrolyte supplementation. Vitamin B12 and fat-soluble vitamin supplementation are needed.

3.2.3 The Role of the Colon (Jejunocolic or Jejunoileocolic Anastomosis)

The presence of the ileocecal valve can contribute to the slowing of the intestinal transit time in SBS patients. The ileocecal valve has a definite role in preventing the backward movement of colonic content by constituting a physical barrier for the large colonic bacterial population, obstructing colonic flora to reach the small bowel. The colon delays gastric emptying and increases intestinal transit time by secreting specific hormones, contributing to the "ileal brake" and enhancing absorption of nutrients. In the presence of the colon, larger ileal resections are associated with worse outcome, and diarrhea is more likely to occur in patients with ileal resections as compared to jejunal resections, especially if part of the colon is resected along with the ileum. This is due to the enhanced water absorbing capacity of the ileum. Remnant ileum and intact colon can compensate for the absence of the jejunum.

In general, lifelong PN is required in patients with a jejunocolic anastomosis and less than 50 cm of jejunum attached to colon. The presence of at least half of the colon is considered to be equivalent to about 50 cm of small bowel [18].

It has been stated that the intestinal failure is more likely reversible in the following clinical scenarios [19]:

1. When there are more than 115 centimeters of remaining jejunum with an end jejunostomy.
2. When there are more than 60 centimeters of small bowel with a jejunocolonic anastomosis.
3. When there are more than 35 centimeters of small bowel along with a jejunoileal anastomosis and an intact ileocecal valve and colon.

For jejunoileocolic anastomosis with intact ileocecal valve, we can anticipate that usually only short-term parenteral nutrition and fluid/electrolyte supplementation are needed; most patients can be weaned from parenteral nutrition.

The main function of the colon is the absorption of water and electrolytes. Normally, when the chyme reaches the colon, almost all nutrients have been absorbed, and only electrolytes and indigestible dietary fiber are left. It is the part of the digestive tract that has physiologically the slowest transit time. It has the tightest intercellular junctions so that in normal conditions, from a mean of 1–1.5 L of fluids that are passing daily through the ileocecal valve, only around 150 mL is excreted in the feces. It has been shown that the capacity of the colon to absorb water can increase to 6 L/day [8]. But, if distal ileum is resected, the unabsorbed bile acids stimulate colonic motility and enhance water secretion, with consequent increase fluid losses.

Another important role of the colon is as supplemental energy source, salvaging calories by the process of anaerobic bacterial fermentation of malabsorbed carbohydrates to short-chain fatty acids (SCFAs) and by improved absorption of medium-chain triglycerides. SCFAs (butyrate, propionate, acetate) can be used both systemically, after absorption and can also be utilized at colonic level by the colonocytes as their main energy source. The amount of energy that can be salvaged in this way can reach 1000 kcal per day [12, 13, 20], underscoring the importance of a remnant colon in SBS patients. It has been shown that starch is a very important dietary carbohydrate for SBS patients and the intake of both starch and soluble fiber (specifically pectin) increases production of SCFA [20]. In patients with preserved colon, the changes in microbiota with overgrowth of bacteria at the site of anastomosis (jejunocolic or ileocolic) may further contribute to energy salvage by the supplemental fermentation of starch to SCFA [20].

In SBS, changes in microflora occur with reduced microbial diversity in all types of SBS patients when compared with healthy controls [21]. Reduction in Bacteroidetes and increase in Protobacteria were reported. An abundance of

Lactobacillaceae and Enterobacteriaceae at the order level and Veillonellaceae and Enterobacteriaceae at the family level was observed [21]. The microbiome of SBS patients with a colon in continuity is enriched with Bacteroidetes and Actinobacteria, and the microbiome of SBS patients with ileostomy or jejunostomy is enriched with Proteobacteria. A shorter bowel was associated with more proteobacteria and a longer remnant bowel with more Firmicutes. In PN-dependent SBS, there are more Bacteroidetes, and in PN-independent cohort, an increased number of Firmicutes was observed (Clostridium family that regulates production of SCFA, specifically of butyrate).

The complex role and interactions generated by the modified microbiota of SBS patients are still to be defined. It has been shown that fecal transfer from a patient with SBS to germ-free rats was associated with an increase in crypt depth and that plasma levels of GLP-1 (glucagon-like peptide 1) and ghrelin, hormones that are involved in intestinal adaptive mechanisms, are increased by SBS lactobacillus species [22].

While intestinal flora can have benefic effects, the excessive multiplication of bacteria can also bring harm. It can determine the deconjugation of biliary acids contributing to lipid malabsorption, can determine vitamin B12 deficit by utilizing it for bacterial growth, impending its absorption, and can have an inflammatory effect on the epithelium. Overgrowth of bacteria in the small bowel (small intestinal bacterial overgrowth [SIBO]) is defined by the high levels of CFU (colony-forming units): over 10^5 CFU/ml or over 10^3CFU/ml of typical colonic bacterial species [23]. SIBO can determine various clinical symptoms: abdominal pain, bloating, and diarrhea. If not diagnosed promptly, SIBO can induce reversible loss of intestinal villi, with decreased surface of absorption and accelerated intestinal motility, thus aggravating malabsorption [24]. In SBS patients, due to malabsorption, an increased quantity of unabsorbed carbohydrates reaches the colon and serves as a substrate for the fermentation by the increased gut lactobacilli population. In this way, the high levels of D-lactate can be produced, up to a ten-fold increase compared with non-SBS patients. As a consequence of lactate absorption, metabolic D-acidosis can occur, with an elevated ratio of D-lactate (exogenous) and L-lactate (endogenous); it can clinically manifest usually by excessive gas (bloating, flatulence); but, in severe cases, it can manifest as D-lactic encephalopathy (confusion, slurred speech, headache, ataxia, convulsions, and even coma).

In conclusion, various factors are associated with the degree of intestinal failure: the length of the remnant small bowel; the presence and length of the remnant colon; the presence of the ileocecal valve; the presence or absence of disease in the remnant bowel; and the time elapsed since the surgery, which determines the occurrence and grade of intestinal adaptation.

Due to variable absorptive capacity of the remnant bowel, individualized nutritional plans are needed in order to reach the best patient outcomes.

References

1. Nightingale J, Spiller R. Normal intestinal anatomy and physiology. In: Nightingale J, editor. Intestinal Failure. London: Greenwich Medical Media Limited; 2001. p. 15–36.
2. Underhill BM. Intestinal length in man. Br Med J. 1955;2(4950):1243–6. https://doi.org/10.1136/bmj.2.4950.1243. PMID: 13269841; PMCID: PMC1981305
3. Nightingale JM, Bartram CI, Lennard-Jones JE. Length of residual small bowel after partial resection: correlation between radiographic and surgical measurements. Gastrointest Radiol. 1991;16(4):305–6. https://doi.org/10.1007/BF01887374. PMID: 1936771
4. Cheng W, Zhang S, Wang J, Zhou C, Li Y, Li J. Three-dimensional CT enterography versus barium follow-through examination in measurement of remnant small intestinal length in short bowel syndrome patients. Abdom Radiol (NY). 2018;43(11):2955–62. https://doi.org/10.1007/s00261-018-1597-x. PMID: 29700592
5. Tappenden KA. Pathophysiology of short bowel syndrome: considerations of resected and residual anatomy. JPEN J Parenter Enteral Nutr. 2014;38(1 Suppl):14S–22S. https://doi.org/10.1177/0148607113520005. Epub 2014 Feb 5
6. Jeejeebhoy KN. Short bowel syndrome: a nutritional and medical approach. CMAJ. 2002;166(10):1297–302. PMID: 12041848; PMCID: PMC111082
7. Feldman EJ, Dowling RH, McNaughton J, Peters TJ. Effects of oral versus intravenous nutrition on intestinal adaptation after small bowel resection in the dog. Gastroenterology. 1976;70:712–9.
8. Menge H, Grafe M, Lorenz-Meyer H, Riecken EO. The influence of food intake on the development of structural and functional adaptation following ileal resection in the rat. Gut. 1975;16:468–72.
9. Le Beyec J, Billiauws L, Bado A, Joly F, Le Gall M. Short bowel syndrome: a paradigm for intestinal adaptation to nutrition? Annu Rev Nutr. 2020;40:299–321. https://doi.org/10.1146/annurev-nutr-011720-122203. Epub 2020 Jul 6
10. Seidl H, Gundling F, Pfeiffer A, Pehl C, Schepp W, Schmidt T. Comparison of small-bowel motility of the human jejunum and ileum. Neurogastroenterol Motil. 2012;24:e373–80.
11. Nightingale JM, Kamm MA, van der Sijp JR, et al. Disturbed gastric emp tying in the short bowel syndrome: evidence for a 'colonic brake'. Gut. 1993;34:1171–6.
12. Nightingale JMD. How to manage a high-output stoma. Frontline Gastroenterol. 2021;13(2):140–51. https://doi.org/10.1136/flgastro-2018-101108. PMID: 35300464; PMCID: PMC8862462
13. Sanaksenaho G, Mutanen A, Godbole N, Kyrönlahti A, Koivusalo A, Lohi J, Pihlajoki M, Heikinheimo M, Pakarinen MP. Parenteral nutrition-dependent children with short-bowel syndrome lack duodenal-adaptive hyperplasia but show molecular signs of altered mucosal function. JPEN J Parenter Enteral Nutr. 2020;44(7):1291–300. https://doi.org/10.1002/jpen.1763. Epub 2020 Jan 27. PMID: 31985858
14. Doldi SB. Intestinal adaptation following jejuno-ileal bypass. Clin Nutr. 1991;10(3):138–45. https://doi.org/10.1016/02615614(91)90049-i.
15. Joly F, Mayeur C, Messing B, et al. Morphological adaptation with preserved proliferation/transporter content in the colon of patients with short bowel syndrome. Am J Physiol Gastrointest Liver Physiol. 2009;297(1):G116–23. https://doi.org/10.1152/ajpgi.90657.2008.
16. Tappenden KA. Anatomical and physiological considerations in short bowel syndrome: emphasis on intestinal adaptation and the role of enterohormones. Nutr Clin Pract. 2023;38:S27–34. https://doi.org/10.1002/ncp.10991.
17. Matarese LE. Nutrition and fluid optimization for patients with short bowel syndrome. JPEN J Parenter Enteral Nutr. 2013;37(2):161–70. https://doi.org/10.1177/0148607112469818. Epub 2012 Dec 21
18. Pironi L, Steiger E, Joly F, et al. Characteristics of adult patients with chronic intestinal failure due to short bowel syndrome: an international multicenter survey. Clin Nutr ESPEN. 2021;45:433–41. https://doi.org/10.1016/j.clnesp.2021.07.004.

19. Amiot A, Messing B, Corcos O, Panis Y, Joly F. Determinants of home parenteral nutrition dependence and survival of 268 patients with non-malignant short bowel syndrome. Clin Nutr. 2013;32(3):368–74. https://doi.org/10.1016/j.clnu.2012.08.007. Epub 2012 Aug 23
20. Atia A, Girard-Pipau F, Hébuterne X, Spies WG, Guardiola A, Ahn CW, Fryer J, Xue F, Rammohan M, Sumague M, Englyst K, Buchman AL. Macronutrient absorption characteristics in humans with short bowel syndrome and jejunocolonic anastomosis: starch is the most important carbohydrate substrate, although pectin supplementation may modestly enhance short chain fatty acid production and fluid absorption. JPEN J Parenter Enteral Nutr. 2011;35(2):229–40. https://doi.org/10.1177/0148607110378410.
21. Boutte HJ Jr, Chen J, Wylie TN, Wylie KM, Xie Y, Geisman M, Prabu A, Gazit V, Tarr PI, Levin MS, Warner BW, Davidson NO, Rubin DC. Fecal microbiome and bile acid metabolome in adult short bowel syndrome. Am J Physiol Gastrointest Liver Physiol. 2022;322(1):G154–68. https://doi.org/10.1152/ajpgi.00091.2021. Epub 2021 Nov 24. PMID: 34816756; PMCID: PMC8793869
22. Gillard L, Mayeur C, Robert V, Pingenot I, Le Beyec J, Bado A, Lepage P, Thomas M, Joly F. Microbiota is involved in post-resection adaptation in humans with short bowel syndrome. Front Physiol. 2017;8:224. https://doi.org/10.3389/fphys.2017.00224. PMID: 28469580; PMCID: PMC5395573
23. Carter J, Bettag J, Morfin S, Manithody C, Nagarapu A, Jain A, Nazzal H, Prem S, Unes M, McHale M, Lin CJ, Hutchinson C, Trello G, Jain A, Portz E, Verma A, Swiderska-Syn M, Goldenberg D, Kurashima K. Gut microbiota modulation of short bowel syndrome and the gut-brain Axis. Nutrients. 2023;15(11):2581. https://doi.org/10.3390/nu15112581. PMID: 37299543; PMCID: PMC10255811
24. Hirsch TI, Wang SZ, Fligor SC, Quigley M, Gura KM, Puder M, Tsikis ST. Fat malabsorption in short bowel syndrome: a review of pathophysiology and management. Nutr Clin Pract. 2024;39(Suppl 1):S17–28. https://doi.org/10.1002/ncp.11119. PMID: 38429962; PMCID: PMC10914324

Humanistic Burden of Short Bowel Syndrome

4

Anca Trifan, Ana-Maria Singeap, Ermina Stratina, and Carol Stanciu

4.1 Introduction

Short bowel syndrome (SBS) is a rare and complex condition characterized by the inability of the remaining intestine to absorb sufficient nutrients, fluids, and electrolytes due to extensive loss or functional impairment of the small intestine. While advances in clinical management have improved survival and physiological outcomes, SBS imposes profound challenges that extend far beyond medical complications. It is not merely a medical condition but a life-altering challenge that permeates the physical, emotional, social, and financial aspects of daily living, including the substantial resources required for ongoing care [1]. Addressing the humanistic burden of SBS is paramount, as it highlights the need for holistic approaches that go beyond clinical treatment to consider the lived experiences of patients, fostering better long-term outcomes and improved well-being.

4.2 Physical and Health-Related Burden

4.2.1 Chronic Symptoms and Complications

SBS is associated with a range of chronic symptoms and complications that significantly impact patients' physical health and daily functioning. These challenges stem from the impaired ability of the shortened intestine to absorb essential nutrients, fluids, and electrolytes, leading to cascading effects on various physiological

A. Trifan · A.-M. Singeap (✉) · E. Stratina · C. Stanciu
Gastroenterology Department, Grigore T. Popa University of Medicine and Pharmacy, Iaşi, Romania

Institute of Gastroenterology and Hepatology, St. Spiridon Emergency Hospital, Iaşi, Romania

A. Trifan et al. (eds.), *Short Bowel Syndrome in Adults*, https://doi.org/10.1007/978-3-031-95848-9_4

systems. Frequent and often severe diarrhea is a defining symptom of SBS, resulting from the reduced intestinal surface area and altered gut motility. This symptom exacerbates dehydration and electrolyte imbalances, posing a constant threat of kidney dysfunction and requiring vigilant fluid management to prevent acute complications. The extent of malabsorption and the specific nutrient deficiencies experienced depend on factors such as the remaining length and structure of the bowel [2]. Other contributing factors, including the presence of underlying conditions like active Crohn's disease, can further hinder the ability of the remaining bowel to adapt and compensate [3].

The hallmark of SBS is malabsorption, which results in deficits in macronutrients (proteins, fats, and carbohydrates) and micronutrients (vitamins and minerals). Deficiencies in fat-soluble vitamins (A, D, E, and K), vitamin B12, and trace elements like zinc, selenium, and magnesium are common, contributing to systemic complications such as anemia, weakened immunity, and bone demineralization. In addition to impairing the absorption of essential nutrients, SBS can also hinder the absorption of critical medications [4]. For individuals with chronic conditions such as diabetes, cardiovascular disease, or infections, this presents a substantial challenge, as the effectiveness of prescribed treatments may be compromised. In turn, this can lead to treatment failures, the need for dose adjustments, and more frequent monitoring, further complicating the clinical management of SBS patients.

Malnutrition not only affects overall health but also increases patients' vulnerability to various diseases. Patients with malnutrition often face a higher risk of experiencing adverse outcomes from surgery or illness. Their ability to recover from procedures is diminished, and the healing process is delayed due to insufficient nutrient stores [5].

A significant proportion of individuals with SBS rely on parenteral nutrition (PN) to meet their nutritional needs. While PN is lifesaving, it comes with long-term risks, including catheter-related infections, thrombosis, bone disease, and liver dysfunction [6]. Depending on PN also imposes logistical challenges and significantly disrupts patients' autonomy and daily routines. Parenteral support is typically administered overnight, with a frequency depending on individual needs. This nocturnal infusion schedule helps improve nitrogen balance and encourages oral alimentation during the day. However, it may also interfere with sleep patterns or may experience discomfort related to the infusion process. For many patients, particularly those with extremely short intestinal remnants, long-term PN becomes a necessary part of their daily life. However, dependence on PN or intravenous support comes with significant risks, and complications are responsible for about 15–20% of all deaths in patients on long-term PN [7]. The challenges associated with long-term PN can lead to life-threatening conditions, dramatically affecting patients' overall prognosis and quality of life (QoL). The most common PN complications are catheter-related infections, which contribute to a huge portion of PN-related deaths. Septicemia is particularly concerning, accounting for nearly three-quarters of hospitalizations among PN patients [8]. Other complications include venous thrombosis, catheter occlusions, and issues related to catheter maintenance, such as fracture, breakage, or placement difficulties, all of which can disrupt the delivery of adequate PN support [9]. Liver complications are common in patients receiving long-term PN and can contribute to PN-related mortality. Around 15% of PN-dependent patients develop end-stage liver disease, which has a poor prognosis [10]. Studies have shown that the longer the dependence on PN, the higher the risk of developing severe liver conditions such as fibrosis, cirrhosis, and liver failure [11].

Patients who rely on PN for over 5 years are particularly susceptible to significant liver damage [12].

Fatigue is one of the most common and debilitating symptoms experienced by patients with SBS, often significantly affecting their daily functioning and overall QoL [13]. This fatigue is multifactorial, arising from the combination of malnutrition, chronic dehydration, anemia, and the constant physical strain of managing gastrointestinal and metabolic imbalances. The persistent energy depletion due to inadequate nutrient absorption leaves patients feeling exhausted, which can limit their ability to participate in normal activities, such as work, social interactions, or even basic self-care tasks. The resulting feeling of sadness and frustration can influence patients' adherence and motivation to follow the therapeutic plan.

4.2.2 Impact on Quality of Life

The impact of SBS extends well beyond physical health, profoundly affecting the QoL of individuals living with this condition. Due to the complexity and chronic nature of the disease, patients face substantial challenges in their daily lives, encountering limitations in various domains such as physical activity, pain management, and access to healthcare. These factors often combine to create a multifaceted burden, hindering both personal well-being and social participation.

The complexity of QoL impairment is highlighted by the wide range of assessment tools used across studies. General questionnaires, such as the SF-36, SF-12, and EQ-5D-5L, have been employed alongside disease-specific instruments designed to capture the full spectrum of QoL dimensions in SBS patients [1, 14, 15]. These tailored tools address the unique challenges faced by SBS patients, including nutritional deficiencies, dependence on PN, gastrointestinal symptoms, and the emotional and social impacts of living with the condition. The SBS-QoL, for example, focuses on these specific aspects, evaluating physical, emotional, and social well-being in the context of SBS [16]. Similarly, the home parenteral nutrition (HPN)-QoL scale is designed to assess the impact of long-term HPN on patients, considering the physical, psychological, and social burdens of managing this treatment daily [15].

Patients with SBS and chronic intestinal failure often report significantly lower QoL scores compared to the general population and individuals living with other chronic conditions [1]. This diminished QoL reflects the unique and ongoing challenges they face, such as persistent physical symptoms, dependence on medical interventions like PN, and the emotional and psychological toll of managing a life-altering condition. One of the most noticeable effects of SBS on QoL is the restriction on physical activity. Many individuals with SBS experience fatigue, muscle weakness, and reduced endurance, which can limit their ability to engage in even simple physical tasks. This includes difficulty participating in work, recreational activities, or daily routines such as shopping or walking. Physical limitations are often a result of the underlying malnutrition, chronic dehydration, and systemic effects of the condition. The inability to maintain a normal level of physical activity not only affects physical fitness but also impacts mental health, leading to feelings of frustration, isolation, and a diminished sense of independence [17]. The persistent discomfort associated with abdominal pain or frequent bloating can lead to poor sleep, reduced appetite, and a diminished quality of life. Additionally, for many patients, the need for continuous intravenous nutrition or the presence of central venous catheters can contribute to physical discomfort or localized pain. The combination of gastrointestinal and procedural pain can create a relentless cycle of physical and emotional strain, further impacting a patient's ability to function normally on a day-to-day basis.

Several studies have highlighted the significant role of treatment modalities in influencing QoL of patients with SBS. A study comparing four treatment approaches—no treatment, surgical intervention, bowel rehabilitation, and nutritional therapy—found that individuals who received no treatment or surgery reported lower QoL scores. In contrast, those who underwent surgery demonstrated improved QoL outcomes [1]. This emphasizes the impact that different treatment options can have on patients' well-being.

Further research on PN and HPN revealed a consistently negative impact on QoL. One study with patients receiving HPN for an average of 6 years found that the treatment led to a significant decline in QoL, even surpassing the adverse effects of having a stoma [18]. Another investigation showed that the higher volumes of PN negatively correlated with QoL, with an increase of just 1 l/day causing a marked deterioration in patient outcomes [19].

Similarly, an increase in the number of days on PN led to a decline in patients' health-related QoL, as measured by the time trade-off (TTO) method, which evaluates individuals' willingness to trade a portion of their remaining lifespan for improved health or a higher QoL [20]. On a more positive note, the use of teduglutide (Ted), a GLP-2 analog, was shown to reduce dependence on PN. In one study, patients treated with Ted for 24 weeks experienced a 32% reduction in weekly PN volume, and 54% were able to reduce their PN days, leading to potential QoL improvements. However, while the overall SBS-QoL score improved, statistical significance was not achieved when compared to the placebo group [13]. Another study revealed that after 6 months of treatment, patients treated with Ted showed significant improvements in SBS-QoL, though no significant changes were found in other scales, such as the SF-12 [16]. SBS patients with stoma were found to have slightly lower QoL scores compared to those without one [21]. This difference may be attributed to the additional physical and psychological burdens, such as challenges in managing stoma output and maintaining skin integrity and the risk of complications. Furthermore, social and emotional challenges contribute to a more pronounced negative impact on their overall QoL.

Several studies have explored the impact of age on the QoL in patients with SBS. While one study concluded that age had a minimal effect on QoL [17], most of the research indicated that increasing age tends to negatively influence QoL outcomes in SBS patients. One study stratifying patients into three age-groups (15–34, 35–59, and ≥60 years) found a significant decline in QoL with advancing age ($P < 0.05$) [14]. Another study, with a median patient age of 56 years, reported a negative correlation between age and overall QoL scores, though the results were not statistically significant ($P > 0.05$) [19]. Interestingly, a study focusing on children with SBS revealed that while age did not impact QoL, children aged 11 years and older had significantly lower QoL than their peers in the general population ($P < 0.05$) [22].

In terms of caregivers, one study found that parents of children under 5 years old experienced a lower QoL, while no significant differences in QoL were observed between families with children under or above the age of five ($P > 0.05$) [23]. These findings suggest that age can play a role in shaping the QoL outcomes for both patients and their caregivers, though the degree of impact may vary. Additionally, a study focusing on caregivers revealed that following an autologous gastrointestinal reconstruction procedure in children, parents experienced a significant improvement in QoL, highlighting the broader impact of SBS treatment on family dynamics as well [24].

4.3 Emotional and Psychological Impact

4.3.1 Mental Health Challenges

Living with SBS presents significant emotional and psychological challenges, stemming from the chronic nature of the condition and its profound impact on daily life. The physical burden of SBS often coexists with mental health struggles. Many patients experience heightened levels of anxiety and depression, which can be attributed to the uncertainty surrounding their health and the relentless demands of managing a complex medical condition.

Anxiety may arise from fears of complications such as infections related to PN or malnutrition.

Depression is frequently reported due to the chronic fatigue, social isolation, and limitations imposed by the disease [17]. For many, the diagnosis of SBS marks a significant turning point in their lives. The loss of autonomy, dependence on medical devices such as central venous catheters for PN, and frequent hospital visits can lead to feelings of helplessness and frustration. The psychological toll of living with a life-altering condition is compounded by the need to constantly monitor food intake, fluid balance, and overall health. The unpredictability of SBS can be emotionally taxing. Patients often live with fear of serious complications, such as catheter-related bloodstream infections, severe dehydration, or further intestinal deterioration. This constant vigilance can contribute to chronic stress and emotional exhaustion.

4.3.2 Coping Mechanisms and Resilience

Coping with SBS requires a multifaceted approach that integrates dietary adaptation, psychological support, community engagement, and multidisciplinary care. Learning to navigate dietary restrictions is a significant adjustment, as individuals must develop personalized routines to optimize nutrition while minimizing gastrointestinal symptoms. For those reliant PN, adapting to the regimen—including managing commitment and potential risks—is essential for maintaining a sense of control and normalcy. Psychological support plays a crucial role in addressing the emotional and mental health challenges associated with SBS.

Access to individual or group counseling provides a safe space to express fears, frustrations, and hopes, while mental health professionals offer strategies to manage stress, cope with uncertainty, and foster resilience [25]. Engaging with peers who share similar experiences can also be empowering, as support groups and online communities facilitate the exchange of advice, coping strategies, and encouragement, fostering a sense of belonging. Additionally, a multidisciplinary approach involving healthcare providers, nutritionists, mental health professionals, and social workers enhances coping strategies by ensuring comprehensive care. This team-based model addresses both the physical and psychological burdens of SBS, ultimately improving overall well-being and QoL.

4.4 Social and Relational Burden

Living with SBS not only affects the individual but also places significant strain on family members and caregivers, influencing relationships, social interactions, and overall QoL. The complexity of managing the condition, including dietary restrictions, medical treatments, and emotional challenges, contributes to a substantial social and relational burden.

4.4.1 Impact on Family and Caregivers

Caregivers, often family members, play a crucial role in supporting individuals with SBS, but this responsibility can lead to caregiver fatigue and emotional strain [15]. The constant need for assistance with meal planning, medical treatments such as PN, and hospital visits can be physically and mentally exhausting. Many caregivers experience heightened stress, anxiety, and even burnout due to the chronic nature of SBS and the unpredictability of symptoms.

Additionally, family dynamics often shift, with roles and responsibilities being redistributed to accommodate the needs of the affected individual. Spouses, parents, or children may take on caregiving roles, which can alter relationships and create emotional tensions. These changes can affect family cohesion, financial stability, and overall household well-being, making emotional support and caregiver resources essential for maintaining balance.

4.4.2 Social Isolation

Individuals with SBS frequently experience social isolation due to limitations on travel, work, and social interactions. The need for strict dietary control, reliance on medical equipment, and the unpredictability of symptoms such as diarrhea or fatigue can make it challenging to participate in everyday activities. Many individuals find it difficult to maintain a regular work schedule, attend social gatherings, or engage in recreational activities, leading to feelings of loneliness and detachment from social circles. Furthermore, stigma or embarrassment related to symptoms, body image concerns, and the use of external medical appliances can contribute to withdrawal from public settings. Individuals who require visible medical devices, such as central venous catheters for PN or ostomy bags, may feel self-conscious, impacting their self-esteem and willingness to engage in social interactions [26]. The discomfort or inconvenience associated with these appliances can further limit mobility and participation in daily activities.

Fear of accidents, the need for frequent bathroom access, or the physical restrictions imposed by medical equipment may create additional barriers to an active social life. Over time, these challenges can negatively impact mental health, increasing the risk of anxiety and depression. Support systems, both within the family and in patient advocacy groups, are crucial in mitigating these effects by fostering understanding, reducing stigma, and encouraging meaningful social connections.

4.5 Economic and Financial Burden

Short bowel syndrome imposes a substantial economic and financial burden on individuals, families, and healthcare systems. The high costs associated with ongoing medical care, specialized nutrition, and frequent hospitalizations contribute to significant financial strain.

Beyond direct medical expenses, the impact of SBS extends to lost productivity, employment challenges, and broader implications for public and private healthcare systems.

4.5.1 Direct Costs

Managing SBS requires lifelong medical interventions, leading to significant direct healthcare expenses. One of the most substantial costs is PN, which is essential for many individuals with SBS to maintain adequate hydration and nutrition. The expense of PN includes not only the specialized nutrient solutions but also the equipment, supplies, and home healthcare services required for safe administration. Additionally, patients often require multiple medications, including antimotility agents, antibiotics, and vitamin or mineral supplements, further increasing healthcare expenditures. Frequent hospitalizations due to complications such as infections, catheter-related bloodstream infections, dehydration, and metabolic imbalances add to the financial burden. Regular medical appointments with gastroenterologists, dietitians, and other specialists are also necessary to monitor the patient's condition and adjust treatment plans, leading to ongoing out-of-pocket expenses for consultations, diagnostic tests, and interventions. A study assessing the cost of comprehensive care for pediatric SBS patients over 5 years found that the mean total cost per child was approximately US$1,619,851, with the first-year accounting for US$505,250 [27]. Inpatient hospitalization was the primary expense, constituting 82% of the total cost in the first year. Notably, home care services' costs increased annually, reaching US$184,520 in the fifth year, primarily due to complications associated with PN [27]. For adults with SBS, annual costs per patient range between US$100,000 and US$150,000 [28]. While HPN significantly reduces in-hospital costs, the overall annual expenses associated with a prolonged HPN regimen remain high. Interestingly, after 2 years, the total costs of a successful intestinal transplant can be lower than the ongoing costs of extended HPN treatment [29].

Teduglutide, a novel therapy promoting intestinal adaptation in SBS patients, is associated with high annual costs exceeding US$400,000 [30]. A cost-effectiveness study conducted using Markov modeling showed that teduglutide does not meet the conventional cost-effectiveness criteria as a treatment for reducing PN use in adult patients with SBS when compared to standard intestinal rehabilitation. However, certain subgroups that experience the greatest benefit from the treatment may find it cost-effective, while complete avoidance of teduglutide could result in financial losses. Teduglutide becomes economically viable only if its price is significantly lowered [31]. Similarly, a cost-effectiveness analysis in the USA found that teduglutide's incremental cost-effectiveness ratio (ICER) was US$285,334 per quality-adjusted life year (QALY) gained, indicating that while the treatment is effective, it is not cost-effective based on traditional threshold [32]. A European study determined that teduglutide for treating patients with SBS-IF aligns with the established cost-effectiveness standards from a societal perspective. However, the varying levels of efficacy observed with teduglutide introduce some uncertainty into the overall economic analysis [33]. In pediatric patients, teduglutide treatment was associated with a significant reduction in annual HPN costs.

However, when the cost of teduglutide was included, the total annual costs remained high, underscoring the need for cost-saving strategies [34].

4.5.2 Indirect Costs

Beyond the direct medical expenses, SBS significantly impacts employment and financial stability. Many individuals with SBS face challenges in maintaining full-time employment due to the physical limitations imposed by their condition, including fatigue, frequent bathroom needs, and the time-consuming nature of medical treatments [26]. Some are forced to reduce their working hours, switch to less demanding jobs, or leave the workforce entirely, resulting in lost income and long-term financial insecurity. Caregivers, often family members, may also experience employment disruptions as they take on responsibilities for managing medical care, attending appointments, and providing emotional and physical support. This loss of productivity, combined with the ongoing costs of care, can place a severe financial strain on families, potentially leading to debt or reliance on financial assistance programs. The emotional toll of financial stress can further exacerbate the psychological burden already experienced by both patients and caregivers.

4.5.3 Healthcare System Implications

The economic impact of SBS extends beyond individual patients and families to healthcare systems. The condition places a significant burden on both public and private healthcare systems due to the high costs of long-term medical management. Government-funded healthcare programs and insurance providers face substantial expenditures related to PN, hospitalizations, specialist care, and complications arising from the disease. Additionally, healthcare resources must be allocated for multidisciplinary care teams, home healthcare services, and research into more effective treatments. The financial strain on healthcare systems underscores the need for cost-effective management strategies, including preventive measures to reduce complications, advancements in intestinal rehabilitation therapies, and potential innovations such as intestinal transplantation for select patients [35]. Addressing these economic challenges requires coordinated efforts among policymakers, healthcare providers, and patient advocacy groups to improve access to care while minimizing financial hardship. By understanding the full economic and financial burden of SBS, healthcare systems can work toward solutions that enhance patient care, reduce costs, and support both individuals and their families in managing the challenges of this complex condition.

Despite the numerous challenges and disadvantages associated with SBS, surgeons (or, more broadly, the physicians responsible for decision-making) should not automatically dismiss small bowel resection in life-threatening, critical situations or even in cases where surgery represents the last resort for, if not curing, at least improving the condition of a critically ill patient. In such cases, surgery remains a necessary intervention to preserve life, even if it comes at the cost of managing the burdens of short bowel syndrome. Ensuring survival, albeit with significant medical and nutritional challenges, is a fundamental priority, and the subsequent management of short bowel syndrome can provide patients with a chance at a functional and sustainable quality of life.

4.6 Patient Advocacy and Support

Patient education plays a crucial role in improving the overall quality of care and outcomes for individuals living with SBS. By equipping patients with knowledge about their diagnosis, treatment options, and the long-term management of their condition, they become active participants in their own care. Empowering patients through education enables them to make informed decisions about their treatment plans, fostering a sense of autonomy and control. This can lead to better adherence to prescribed therapies, such as HPN, and more effective management of symptoms and complications. Educational interventions also help patients understand how lifestyle changes, such as dietary adjustments and the proper use of medical devices, can improve their health outcomes. When patients are educated, they are better able to engage in preventive care strategies, which can reduce hospitalizations, improve self-management, and ultimately enhance their QoL.

Support groups and patient advocacy organizations play an essential role in providing emotional, informational, and practical support to individuals with chronic conditions like SBS. These organizations serve as a valuable resource for patients and their families, offering a network of shared experiences, practical advice, and coping strategies [36]. By connecting with others facing similar challenges, patients can reduce feelings of isolation, increase their emotional resilience, and gain insight into the real-world management of their condition. Clinicians can integrate the patient- and family-centered care (PFCC) approach by focusing on whole-person care, building strong partnerships with patients and families, enhancing communication, and providing clear information. Encouraging patients to take an active role in managing their condition is a key aspect of PFCC and can improve coping with the chronic nature of SBS. Advocacy organizations also work to raise awareness about SBS, educate the public and healthcare professionals, and advocate for policy changes that can improve access to care and reduce the financial burden of long-term treatments [37]. Additionally, many organizations offer a structured platform for patients to voice their concerns, which can influence policy decisions and drive the development of more effective treatments [35].

Support groups are also instrumental in providing guidance on navigating the complexities of insurance coverage and healthcare systems. By facilitating access to essential resources and peer support, these groups can significantly alleviate both the emotional and financial burdens associated with chronic illnesses.

4.7 Future Directions

Despite significant advancements in the medical management of SBS, there are still considerable gaps in our understanding of the humanistic burden of the condition. Research has largely focused on clinical aspects, such as nutritional management and surgical interventions. However, there is a need for comprehensive studies that explore the psychological, emotional, and social impacts on patients with SBS and their families.

Longitudinal studies assessing the effects of SBS on mental health, quality of life (QoL), social relationships, and overall well-being could provide invaluable insights into the broader implications of living with this condition. Additionally, research examining the role of healthcare systems in addressing these nonclinical factors is crucial in developing more holistic care models that encompass the full spectrum of challenges faced by SBS patients. Medical advancements continue to offer hope for improving the lives of SBS patients, particularly through novel therapies and technological innovations. The development of improved intestinal rehabilitation techniques, new medications, and advanced nutritional support systems can help reduce the physical burden of SBS. However, equally important is the focus on improving QoL through supportive care strategies, such as better pain management, mental health support, and patient education programs [38]. Empowering patients to self-manage their condition with the help of digital health tools and telemedicine platforms could enhance both clinical and emotional well-being. Furthermore, the integration of complementary therapies, like psychological counseling and social support networks, can be key components in improving QoL, offering SBS patients a more holistic approach to managing their condition.

4.7.1 Importance of Interdisciplinary Approach

Addressing the complex challenges of SBS requires a coordinated, interdisciplinary approach.

Collaboration among healthcare professionals, including gastroenterologists, surgeons, dietitians, psychologists, social workers, and nurses, is essential in delivering comprehensive care. Such teams can ensure that all aspects of a patient's health—physical, emotional, and psychological—are considered in the management plan. Moreover, partnerships between healthcare providers and patient advocacy groups are critical in addressing the broader social and economic challenges of SBS, such as financial burdens, healthcare access, and patient education. These interdisciplinary efforts will be vital in ensuring that SBS patients receive the most effective and compassionate care possible, leading to improved long-term outcomes.

4.7.2 Call to Action for Healthcare Professionals and Policymakers

Given the profound humanistic burden of SBS, it is imperative that healthcare professionals, researchers, and policymakers work together to address not only the clinical but also the nonclinical aspects of the condition. Healthcare providers must adopt a more holistic approach to care that incorporates the psychological, emotional, and social needs of SBS patients.

Researchers should focus on bridging the gaps in understanding the humanistic impact of the disease, while policymakers should advocate for more accessible resources, including financial support and mental health services. Collaborative efforts are essential to improving the lives of SBS patients, ensuring they receive comprehensive care that truly addresses the full range of challenges they face.

4.8 Conclusion

Patients with SBS face numerous humanistic challenges that extend beyond the clinical management of the condition. The daily struggles with malabsorption, dependence on PN, and the physical limitations imposed by the disease are compounded by psychological and emotional difficulties, such as anxiety, depression, and social isolation. The financial strain of long-term therapies and the ongoing burden on families further exacerbate the impact of SBS.

These nonclinical aspects are often under-recognized but play a critical role in the overall experience of patients, making them essential considerations in the development of effective care strategies.

References

1. Chen Y, et al. A systematic review of quality of life in patients with short bowel syndrome and their caregivers. Patient Prefer Adherence. 2024;18:1217–30.
2. Tappenden KA. Anatomical and physiological considerations in short bowel syndrome: emphasis on intestinal adaptation and the role of enterohormones. Nutr Clin Pract. 2023;38(Suppl 1):S27–34. https://doi.org/10.1002/ncp.10991.
3. Thompson JS, Iyer KR, DiBaise JK, Young RL, Brown CR, Langnas AN. Short bowel syndrome and Crohn's disease. J Gastrointest Surg. 2003;7(8):1069–72. https://doi.org/10.1016/j.gassur.2003.08.007.
4. Azuz S, Poulsen JL, Vinter-Jensen L, Olesen AE. Drug absorption from oral formulations in patients with short bowel syndrome: a comprehensive update of the literature. Expert Opin Drug Metab Toxicol. 2023;19(9):577–600. https://doi.org/10.1080/17425255.2023.2256216. Epub 2023 Sep 8
5. Stratton RJ, Hackston A, Longmore D, Dixon R, Price S, Stroud M, King C, Elia M. Malnutrition in hospital outpatients and inpatients: prevalence, concurrent validity and ease of use of the 'malnutrition universal screening tool' ('MUST') for adults. Br J Nutr. 2004;92(5):799–808. https://doi.org/10.1079/bjn20041258.
6. Pironi L, Boeykens K, Bozzetti F, Joly F, Klek S, Lal S, Lichota M, Mühlebach S, Van Gossum A, Wanten G, Wheatley C, Bischoff SC. ESPEN guideline on home parenteral nutrition. Clin Nutr. 2020;39(6):1645–66. https://doi.org/10.1016/j.clnu.2020.03.005. Epub 2020 Apr 18
7. Dibb M, Soop M, Teubner A, Shaffer J, Abraham A, Carlson G, Lal S. Survival and nutritional dependence on home parenteral nutrition: three decades of experience from a single referral centre. Clin Nutr. 2017;36(2):570–6. https://doi.org/10.1016/j.clnu.2016.01.028. Epub 2016 Feb 22
8. O'Keefe SJ, Burnes JU, Thompson RL. Recurrent sepsis in home parenteral nutrition patients: an analysis of risk factors. JPEN J Parenter Enteral Nutr. 1994;18(3):256–63. https://doi.org/10.1177/0148607194018003256.
9. Zaccone V, Santoro L, Guerrieri E, Diblasi I, Roncarati I, Viticchi G, Vecchiarelli P, Santoliquido A, Fiore F, Molfino A, Landi F, Moroncini G, Gasbarrini A, Muscaritoli M, Falsetti L. Prevention and treatment of catheter-related venous thrombosis in long-term parenteral nutrition: a SINuC position statement. Front Nutr. 2023;10:1106327. https://doi.org/10.3389/fnut.2023.1106327. PMID: 36814508; PMCID: PMC9940014
10. Chan S, McCowen KC, Bistrian BR, Thibault A, Keane-Ellison M, Forse RA, Babineau T, Burke P. Incidence, prognosis, and etiology of end-stage liver disease in patients receiving home total parenteral nutrition. Surgery. 1999;126(1):28–34. https://doi.org/10.1067/msy.1999.98925.

11. Mitra A, Ahn J. Liver disease in patients on total parenteral nutrition. Clin Liver Dis. 2017;21(4):687–95. https://doi.org/10.1016/j.cld.2017.06.008. Epub 2017 Aug 19
12. Cavicchi M, Beau P, Crenn P, Degott C, Messing B. Prevalence of liver disease and contributing factors in patients receiving home parenteral nutrition for permanent intestinal failure. Ann Intern Med. 2000;132(7):525–32. https://doi.org/10.7326/0003-4819-132-7-200004040-00003.
13. Jeppesen PB, Shahraz S, Hopkins T, Worsfold A, Genestin E. Impact of intestinal failure and parenteral support on adult patients with short-bowel syndrome: a multinational, noninterventional, cross-sectional survey. JPEN J Parenter Enteral Nutr. 2022;46(7):1650–9. https://doi.org/10.1002/jpen.2372. Epub 2022 Apr 13. PMID: 35289416; PMCID: PMC9543571
14. Dai R, Xiaohong G. Study on health-related quality of life in patients with short bowel syndrome and its influencing factors. Chinese J Gene Sur. 2016;106:486–9.
15. Beurskens-Meijerink J, Huisman-de Waal G, Wanten G. Evaluation of quality of life and caregiver burden in home parenteral nutrition patients: a cross sectional study. Clin Nutr ESPEN. 2020;37:50–7. https://doi.org/10.1016/j.clnesp.2020.03.023.
16. Joly F, Quilliot D, Chambrier C, et al. Equative: quality of life in adult patients with short bowel syndrome treated by teduglutide, a French real-world study. Clin Nutr ESPEN. 2021;46:S665. https://doi.org/10.1016/j.clnesp.2021.09.346.
17. Kalaitzakis E, Carlsson E, Josefsson A, Bosaeus I. Quality of life in short-bowel syndrome: impact of fatigue and gastrointestinal symptoms. Scand J Gastroenterol. 2008;43(9):1057–65. https://doi.org/10.1080/00365520802078325.
18. Carlsson E, Bosaeus I, Nordgren S. Quality of life and concerns in patients with short bowel syndrome. Clin Nutr. 2003;22(5):445–52. https://doi.org/10.1016/S0261-5614(03)00042-6.
19. Nordsten CB, Molsted S, Bangsgaard L, et al. High parenteral support volume is associated with reduced quality of life determined by the short-bowel syndrome quality of life scale in nonmalignant intestinal failure patients. J Parenteral Enteral Nutr. 2021;45(5):926–32. https://doi.org/10.1002/jpen.1958.
20. Lachaine J, Gouault Laliberté A, Miron A, Xenopoulos A. Time trade off study for parenteral support in short bowel syndrome in Canada. Value Health. 2016;19(3):A251. https://doi.org/10.1016/j.jval.2016.03.99928.
21. Dabirian A, Yaghmaei F, Rassouli M, Tafreshi MZ. Quality of life in ostomy patients: a qualitative study. Patient Prefer Adherence. 2010;5:1–5. https://doi.org/10.2147/PPA.S14508.
22. Olieman JF, Penning C, Poley MJ, Utens EMWJ, WCJ H, Tibboel D. Impact of infantile short bowel syndrome on long-term health-related quality of life: a cross-sectional study. J Pediatr Surg. 2012;47(7):1309–16. https://doi.org/10.1016/j.jpedsurg.2012.01.005.
23. Pederiva F, Khalil B, Morabito A, Wood S. Impact of short bowel syndrome on quality of life and family: the patient's perspective. Eur J Pediatr Surg. 2019;29(02):196–202. https://doi.org/10.1055/s-0037-162173714.
24. Edge H, Hurrell R, Bianchi A, Carlson G, Zaidi T, Gozzini S, Khalil BA, Morabito A. Caregiver evaluation and satisfaction with autologous bowel reconstruction in children with short bowel syndrome. J Pediatr Gastroenterol Nutr. 2012;54(4):510–5. https://doi.org/10.1097/MPG.0b013e3182369dc8.
25. Belcher E, Mercer D, Raphael BP, Salinas GD, Stacy S, Tappenden KA. Management of short-bowel syndrome: a survey of unmet educational needs among healthcare providers. JPEN J Parenter Enteral Nutr. 2022;46(8):1839–46. https://doi.org/10.1002/jpen.2388. Epub 2022 May 24. PMID: 35511707; PMCID: PMC9790246
26. Silva R, et al. Clinical, economic, and humanistic impact of short-bowel syndrome/chronic intestinal failure in Portugal (PARENTERAL study). GE Port J Gastroenterol. 2022;30(4):293–304.
27. Spencer AU, et al. Pediatric short-bowel syndrome: the cost of comprehensive care. Am J Clin Nutr. 2008;88(6):1552–9.
28. Schalamon J, et al. Mortality and economics in short bowel syndrome. Best Pract Res Clin Gastroenterol. 2003;17(6):931–42.

29. Canovai E, Ceulemans LJ, Peers G, De Pourcq L, Pijpops M, Hoffman I, De Hertogh G, Hiele M, Jochmans I, Monbaliu D, Vanuytsel T, Pirenne J. Cost-effectiveness of intestinal transplantation compared to parenteral nutrition in adults. Transplantation. 2021;105(4):897–904. https://doi.org/10.1097/TP.0000000000003328.
30. Pironi L, Allard JP, Joly F, Geransar P, Genestin E, Pape UF. Use of teduglutide in adults with short bowel syndrome-associated intestinal failure. Nutr Clin Pract. 2024;39(1):141–53. https://doi.org/10.1002/ncp.11015. Epub 2023 Jun 9
31. Raghu VK, Binion DG, Smith KJ. Cost-effectiveness of teduglutide in adult patients with short bowel syndrome: Markov modeling using traditional cost-effectiveness criteria. Am J Clin Nutr. 2020;111(1):141–8. https://doi.org/10.1093/ajcn/nqz269. PMID: 31665212; PMCID: PMC7307185
32. Gattini D, et al. Cost-utility analysis of teduglutide compared to standard care in weaning parenteral nutrition support in children with short bowel syndrome. Clin Nutr. 2023;42(12):2363–71.
33. Walter E, et al. Cost-effectiveness of teduglutide in adult patients with short bowel syndrome—a European socioeconomic perspective. Am J Clin Nutr. 2024;119(5):1187–99.
34. Cucinotta U, et al. The impact of teduglutide on real-life health care costs in children with short bowel syndrome. J Pediatr. 2024;272:113882.
35. Winkler M, Tappenden K. Epidemiology, survival, costs, and quality of life in adults with short bowel syndrome. Nutr Clin Pract. 2023;38(Suppl 1):S17–26. https://doi.org/10.1002/ncp.10964.
36. Zigdon A, Eckhaus E, Rosenfeld M, Zigdon O. Chronically ill patients' perspectives on support services and activities of patient organizations. Isr J Health Policy Res. 2024;13(1):47. https://doi.org/10.1186/s13584-024-00635-7. PMID: 39285503; PMCID: PMC11403880
37. Kumpf VJ, Neumann ML, Kakani SR. Advocating for a patient- and family centered care approach to management of short bowel syndrome. Nutr Clin Pract. 2023;38(Suppl 1):S35–45. https://doi.org/10.1002/ncp.10966.
38. Sowerbutts AM, Panter C, Dickie G, Bennett B, Ablett J, Burden S, Lal S. Short bowel syndrome and the impact on patients and their families: a qualitative study. J Hum Nutr Diet. 2020;33(6):767–74. https://doi.org/10.1111/jhn.12803. Epub 2020 Aug 10

Intestinal Adaptation: Mechanisms and Therapy Goals

5

Cristina Muzica, Horia Minea, and Irina Girleanu

5.1 Introduction

Intestinal adaptation represents a progressive and extensive rehabilitation process following significant resection, wherein the surviving intestine develops structural and functional modifications in order to enhance absorptive capacity and restore enteral autonomy [1].

The degree of resection and the preserved gut structure are determinants for the potential adaptation and the necessity for continuous parenteral nutrition (PN) [2].

There is inadequate evidence regarding the onset of intestinal adaptation in adult humans. The majority of adults exhibit the beginning of the restructuring process within 48 hours postsurgery and continue during the initial 24 months [3].

The process of the residual intestine is divided into three stages. The first step, known as the hypersecretion, or acute phase, goes immediately postsurgery and could potentially last from 1 month to a maximum of 6 months. Decreased fluid losses and enhanced absorption of macronutrients and micronutrients characterize the second stage. This is accomplished through the secretion of hormones and growth factors from the gut, facilitating structural and functional adaptations. The remaining portions are structured to increase the operational efficiency. The final part of the process, known as the maintenance phase, occurs roughly 2 years postresection, during which the residual part of the intestine achieves its maximal capability, resulting in stabilized nutrient absorption and a decreased need for parenteral nourishment [4].

C. Muzica (✉) · H. Minea · I. Girleanu
Gastroenterology Department, Grigore T. Popa University of Medicine and Pharmacy, Iaşi, Romania

Institute of Gastroenterology and Hepatology, St. Spiridon Emergency Hospital, Iaşi, Romania

A. Trifan et al. (eds.), *Short Bowel Syndrome in Adults*,
https://doi.org/10.1007/978-3-031-95848-9_5

The process of physiological restructuring in short bowel syndrome (SBS) is different from the stages of intestinal failure (IF), where patients are classified based on the duration of their dependence on parenteral nutrition (PN) or intravenous (IV) fluids. The acute postoperative phase of Type I IF is self-limiting, allowing the patient to discontinue PN/IV fluids shortly thereafter. The intermediate duration of Type II IF is the period when the patient could need hydration and parenteral nutrition for 28 days. In individuals categorized as Type III IF, intravenous administration persists over an extended duration [5].

5.2 Optimizing Intestinal Function: Key Rehabilitation Goals

The primary objective is to enhance and optimize intestinal adaptability, enabling these patients to achieve enteral independence. The immediate targets are to focus on decreasing SBS symptoms, providing energy, nutrition, and hydration needs via parenteral assistance [6].

Patients could possess varying degrees of enteral independence, including designated days off per week, which is crucial for certain individuals as it facilitates their entire independence from parenteral assistance. By reducing a patient's necessity for parenteral nutrition and intravenous fluids, it is anticipated to diminish long-term issues associated with intravenous feeding, and central line-related bloodstream infections, improve the quality of life, and reduce long-term healthcare cost and utilization [7].

In the majority of cases, the process of recovery usually reaches a plateau level after one and a half years, called spontaneous adaptation. In this amount of time, intestinal rehabilitation could be modulated according to the primary objectives. Hence, two possible situations are distinguished. The first, called accelerated adaptation, is when the therapies are used to achieve the plateau phase in a shorter amount of time. It is often used for patients who find it difficult to maintain parenteral nutrition or for those who do not want to use intravenous supplements. The second possibility is enhanced adaptation, when there is a requested need for a superior recovery in order to stimulate the remaining functional absorptive capacity [8].

5.3 Structural and Functional Changes in Short Bowel Syndrome

5.3.1 Adaptation Patterns According to the Remaining Intestinal Segments

The autonomy of the patient after surgical intervention depends on the variety of structural and functional adaptations of the organism as well as the external factors, such as nutrient components of the diet, which influence gastrointestinal secretions and hormones. Moreover, the entire process is dependent on the remaining intestinal segment, given their different functions and absorption capacity [4].

For example, the jejunum presents a reduced adaptive capacity in comparison to the ileum, with the functional changes being the main factors involved in the rehabilitation process than structural changes. Therefore, patients with anastomosis between the jejunum and the colon prove an increased ability to restore autonomy in comparison to those with a stoma related to the jejunum [9].

In contrast, the ileum poses an increased adaptation capacity after surgical intervention on the small bowel, having markedly increased growth of the villus as well as length, diameter, and functional mechanism [10].

Nonetheless, there is evidence indicating functional enhancement of absorption via the overexpression of transporters and brush border enzymes. These adaptive modifications result in a progressive enhancement in macronutrient absorption throughout the initial 1–3 years following jejunal resection [11].

A significant aspect that is involved in an efficient structural adaptation is represented by the presence of continuity between the small intestine and colon in order to increase the reabsorption of fluids and electrolytes.

5.3.2 Structural Adaptation Mechanism

A continuous process of renewal of the remaining epithelial layer involves the axis crypt–villus, which implies the migration and differentiation of immature cells, turning into specialized cells to restabilize the normal function of the intestine [12].

The new layer would follow the life cycle of cell proliferation and then apoptosis. Moreover, it was noticed that the process of apoptosis is not specific and determinant for the restructuring process [13].

However, the rate of cell elimination could be slightly increased due to the permanent formation of new enterocytes. Instead, studies on animal models concluded a significant increase in crypt cell proliferation for improving the absorption function. Moreover, accelerated cellular metabolism leads to an increasing depth of the intestinal crypt and elongation of the villus [14].

Another important structural aspect is represented by the formation of new blood vessels, which implies an increased blood flow, allowing better oxygenation of the surface.

Therefore, the entire process involves not only the growth of the mucosal layer and an increase in its absorptive capacity but also the increase in muscular thickness [15].

Regarding human adaptive capacity, there are a reduced number of studies focused on the microscopic evaluation after the intervention. The main research is mostly conducted on pediatric cohorts [16].

In the adult population, the findings rely on the small number of patients observed in the evolution of the remaining small bowel after the surgical cut or jejunoileal bypass. Another disadvantage refers to the single histological analysis performed and not in the dynamic evolution [7].

The main results are from the prospective studies conducted by Doldi et al., whose conclusions suggest that the hyperplasia of enterocytes and almost 75% increase in the height of the villus are responsible for the efficiency of adaptation 24 months after resection [17]. Another study by Joly et al. examined patients with jejunocolonic anastomosis, reporting a 35% increase in crypt depth and a 22% rise in cell count per crypt in the colon. Unfortunately, no histological data from the small intestine were evaluated.

Other studies have reported no significant differences in epithelial proliferation, crypt depth, or villus height when comparing patients with SBS to healthy controls. Therefore, the main conclusions of the studies stress that the principal mechanism relies on functional modification rather than anatomical restructuring, with additional prospective studies required for a definitive conclusion [18].

5.3.3 Functional Changes in Short Bowel

Functional modification represents the main characteristic essential for the remaining bowel to maintain internal homeostasis. Therefore, increasing the activity of intestinal enzymes and overexpression of transmembrane transporters, as well as the motility and the microbiota of the gut, drastically influences the nutritional status of the patients [19].

Following the reduction of the surface, key transporters present increased activity in order to accelerate the absorption of necessary factors for survival, such as ions, carbohydrates, or water. Among cotransporters, there are distinguished Na^+/H^+ exchangers and Na^+/K^+ ATPases. Interestingly, their upregulation is not the result of hyperplasia of the remaining enterocytes; however, it is the consequence of the increased activity of the resting cells [20].

The main results of the research on intestinal human adaptation present different conclusions. For example, a study conducted by Ziegler objected to an increased expression of a specific transporter, peptide transporter 1 (PepT1), essential for the accumulation of dipeptide and tripeptide.

Moreover, its increased function is distinguished in the colon of patients with SBS, not in the remaining small intestine, as expected. However, the results of further prospective studies state different conclusions, having as the main finding the lack of differential protein expression of PepT1 mRNA between healthy patients and those diagnosed with SBS [21].

A significant difference between the conclusions could be influenced by the time after the surgical intervention when the evaluation was performed. Therefore, in the first analysis, the study was conducted on patients who were under parenteral supplements for almost 3 years, while in the second one, the conclusions were stated for patients with SBS over 10 years after surgery. Hence, the comparison concludes that the expression of PepT1 presents increased levels in the early phase of intestinal adaptation among SBS [22].

The reduction of small bowel movements represents an essential mechanism of adaptation that enables better absorption of nutrients due to prolonged contact between the intestinal epithelium and the dietary content. The results on animal models highlight the increased absorption capacity of the intestine due to the prolonged transit time that has increased 3 months after the intervention, without any difference regarding the percentage of the remaining bowel [23].

Moreover, the adaptive mechanism significantly influences avoiding accelerated diarrhea during the primary adaptive phase due to the increased absorption of fluid. The entire process is generally mediated by an intestinal hormone generated by the distal part of the intestine, namely peptide YY (PYY), which reduces gastric evacuation and the peristalsis of the remaining intestine and colon. The theory is supported by the studies that included patients with surgical intervention on ileum and colon continuity; there are markedly elevated levels of PYY in the plasma compared with controls [24].

In patients with a reduced surface area of the small intestine, there are proven modifications of the composition of the microbiota, the immune adaptive system, and an increased permeability of the intestinal barrier. Even though these changes are less understood, this adaptive modification might be influenced by the regulation of the inflammatory response, changes in the metabolism of bile acids, and increased production of short-chain fatty acids [25].

5.4 Conclusions

Intestinal adaptation is a progressive and complex process following extensive resection which enables the remaining bowel to enhance nutrient absorption and reduce dependence on parenteral nutrition. The efficacy of intestinal adaptation depends on the length and type of preserved segments and the continuity with the colon, and is modulated by nutritional and hormonal factors. The functional adaptations occurring during structural changes are represented by upregulation of transporters, modulation of motility and microbiota shifts. Current therapy strategies aim to alleviate symptoms, meet nutritional needs and accelerate or enhance adaptation to achieve enteral autonomy.

References

1. Tappenden KA. Intestinal adaptation following resection. JPEN J Parenter Enteral Nutr. 2014;38:23S.
2. Guo M, Li Y, Wang Z, Wu B, Wang J, Li J. Morphologicaladaptationinadultshortbowelsyndrome undergoing intestinal rehabilitation. J Investig Surg. 2013;26(1):1–5.
3. Buchman AL, Scolapio J, Fryer J. AGA technical review on short bowel syndrome and intestinal transplantation. Gastroenterology. 2003;124:1111–34.
4. Pape UF, Maasberg S, Pascher A. Pharmacological strategies to enhance adaptation in intestinal failure. Curr Opin Organ Transplant. 2016;21(2):147–52. https://doi.org/10.1097/MOT.0000000000000296. PMID: 26881493
5. Cuerda C, Pironi L, Arends J, et al. ESPEN practical guideline: clinical nutrition in chronic intestinal failure. Clin Nutr. 2021;40(9):5196–220. https://doi.org/10.1016/j.clnu.2021.07.002.

6. Tappenden KA. Anatomical and physiological considerations in short bowel syndrome: emphasis on intestinal adaptation and the role of enterohormones. Nutr Clin Pract. 2023;38(Suppl 1):S27–34. https://doi.org/10.1002/ncp.10991.
7. Rubin DC, Levin MS. Mechanisms of intestinal adaptation. Best Pract Res Clin Gastroenterol. 2016;30(2):237–48. https://doi.org/10.1016/j.bpg.2016.03.007. Epub 2016 Mar 16. PMID: 27086888; PMCID: PMC4874810
8. Rintala RJ, Pakarinen M, Wester T, editors. Current concepts of intestinal failure. Switzerland: Springer International Publishing; 2016. https://doi.org/10.1007/978-3-319-42551-1.
9. Buchman AL, Scolapio J, Fryer J. AGA technical review on short bowel syndrome and intestinal transplantation. Gastroenterology. 2003;124(4):1111–34. https://doi.org/10.1016/s0016-5085(03)70064-x.
10. Qandeel HG, Alonso F, Hernandez DJ, Madhavan S, Duenes JA, Zheng Y, Sarr MG. Peptide absorption after massive proximal small bowel resection: mechanisms of ileal adaptation. J Gastrointest Surg. 2011;15(9):1537–47. https://doi.org/10.1007/s11605-011-1581-z. Epub 2011 Jun 7. PMID: 21647767; PMCID: PMC3160514
11. Jeong SH, Lee HJ, Bae HJ, Kim Y, Yoo MW, Yoon YK, Yang HK. Factors affecting postoperative dietary adaptation in short bowel syndrome. Hepato-Gastroenterology. 2009;56(93):1049–52.
12. Umar S. Intestinal stem cells. Curr Gastroenterol Rep. 2010;12:340–8.
13. Hall PA, Coates PJ, Ansari B, Hopwood D. Regulation of cell number in the mammalian gastrointestinal tract: the importance of apoptosis. J Cell Sci. 1994;107(pt 12):3569–77.
14. Williamson RC. Intestinal adaptation (first of two parts). Structural, functional and cytokinetic changes. N Engl J Med. 1978;298:1393–402.
15. Martin CA, Perrone EE, Longshore SW, et al. Intestinal resection induces angiogenesis within adapting intestinal villi. J Pediatr Surg. 2009;44:1077–82. discussion 1
16. McDuffie LA, Bucher BT, Erwin CR, Wakeman D, White FV, Warner BW. Intestinal adaptation after small bowel resection in human infants. J Pediatr Surg. 2011;46:1045–51.
17. Doldi SB. Intestinal adaptation following jejuno-ileal bypass. Clin Nutr. 1991;10:138–45.
18. Jarboe MD, Juno RJ, Bernal NP, Knott AW, Zhang Y, Erwin CR, Warner BW. Bax deficiency rescues resection-induced enterocyte apoptosis in mice with perturbed EGF receptor function. Surgery. 2004;136:121–6.
19. Sigalet DL, Martin GR. Mechanisms underlying intestinal adaptation after massive intestinal resection in the rat. J Pediatr Surg. 1998;33:889–92.
20. Musch MW, Bookstein C, Rocha F, et al. Region-specific adaptation of apical Na/H exchangers after extensive proximal small bowel resection. Am J Physiol Gastrointest Liver Physiol. 2002;283:G975–85.
21. Ziegler TR, Fernandez-Estivariz C, Gu LH, et al. Distribution of the H+/ peptide transporter PepT1 in human intestine: up-regulated expression in the colonic mucosa of patients with short-bowel syndrome. Am J Clin Nutr. 2002;75:922–30.
22. Joly F, Mayeur C, Messing B, et al. Morphological adaptation with preserved proliferation/transporter content in the colon of patients with short bowel syndrome. Am J Physiol Gastrointest Liver Physiol. 2009;297:G116–23.
23. Quigley EM, Thompson JS. The motor response to intestinal resection: motor activity in the canine small intestine following distal resection. Gastroenterology. 1993;105:791–8.
24. Nightingale JM, Kamm MA, van der Sijp JR, Ghatei MA, Bloom SR, Lennard-Jones JE. Gastrointestinal hormones in short bowel syndrome: peptide YY may be the "colonic brake" to gastric emptying. Gut. 1996;39:267–72.
25. Macfarlane S, Macfarlane GT. Regulation of short-chain fatty acid production. Proc Nutr Soc. 2003;62:67–72.

Free Water, Electrolytes, and Acid–Base Balance Disturbances in Short Bowel Syndrome

6

Liliana Mirea, Ana Maria Dumitriu, and Ioana Marina Grintescu

6.1 Physiology of Fluid and Electrolyte Absorption

6.1.1 Water and Electrolyte Absorption in the Gastrointestinal Tract

The gastrointestinal tract (GI tract) processes between 8000 and 9000 ml of fluid daily, including both the ingested food and drink, as well as the gastrointestinal secretions. Water absorption in the GI tract occurs primarily by osmosis—movement from areas of lower solute concentration to areas of higher solute concentration. The *small intestine* absorbs around *85–90% of this water*, particularly the jejunum, with the *colon* responsible for absorbing most of the remainder [1, 2]. Solutes carriage across the GI tract relies on various specialized transport proteins located in the brush border membranes of both the small and large intestines. The main types are sodium pump (Na^+/K^+-ATPase) and the proton pump (H^+/K^+-ATPase), selective channels for sodium ($Na^{+)}$ and chloride (Cl^-), as well as different carrier proteins. The last category includes three primary types. *Uniport carriers* move a single ion or molecule, such as the glucose transporter type 2 (GLUT2), which carries glucose independently. *Symport carriers* transport multiple molecules simultaneously, using the gradient of one (e.g., sodium) to carry another, as seen with the sodium–glucose cotransporter SGLT1.

L. Mirea · A. M. Dumitriu (✉) · I. M. Grintescu
Faculty of Medicine, Carol Davila University of Medicine and Pharmacy, Bucharest, Romania

Anesthesiology and Intensive Care Clinic, Clinical Emergency Hospital, Bucharest, Romania
e-mail: ioana.grintescu@rospen.ro

A. Trifan et al. (eds.), *Short Bowel Syndrome in Adults*,
https://doi.org/10.1007/978-3-031-95848-9_6

Antiport carriers exchange molecules across the membrane, such as chloride/bicarbonate and sodium/hydrogen exchangers, which help regulate pH and ion balance [3]. Together, these pumps, channels, and carrier proteins work dynamically to maintain the gut's electrolyte balance, supporting both nutrient absorption and overall fluid homeostasis.

6.1.2 Role of the Small and Large Intestine in Electrolyte Homeostasis

The small and large intestines both play essential roles in maintaining electrolyte homeostasis, managing the absorption and regulation of key ions such as sodium (Na^+), chloride (Cl^-), and potassium (K^+). Na^+ and Cl^- are absorbed by the intestinal mucosa through distinct, region-specific mechanisms. In the *proximal small intestine*, sodium is absorbed through nutrient-dependent cotransport mechanisms, particularly in the upper regions (duodenum and jejunum). This process involves sodium–glucose and sodium–amino acid cotransporters that facilitate significant sodium absorption. In the jejunum, sodium is also absorbed via Na^+/H^+ exchangers on the luminal membrane. In this region, Na^+ absorption is not linked to Cl^- exchange, resulting in bicarbonate (HCO_3^-) absorption as protons are extruded, leading to CO_2 formation and increased cellular bicarbonate. In the *distal small intestine and proximal colon*, Na^+ and Cl^- are absorbed together through two exchangers: Na^+/H^+ and Cl^-/HCO_3^-.

These exchangers balance pH by forming HCO_3^- and protons. In the *distal colon*, active Na^+ absorption occurs against strong electrochemical gradients through an electrogenic, amiloride-sensitive Na^+ channel. This area has low paracellular permeability, limiting ion back diffusion and allowing large potential differences that aid Cl^- absorption. Unlike passive K^+ transport in the small intestine, K^+ is actively absorbed in the rectosigmoid colon, likely via a K^+/H^+ exchanger and a recently identified H^+/K^+-ATPase [4–6].

Active water and electrolyte secretion in the intestine supports digestion and nutrient absorption. *Cl^- secretion* is well studied and involves four membrane proteins: a Cl^- selective channel, an $Na^+/K^+/2Cl^-$ cotransporter, K^+ channels, and the Na^+/K^+-ATPase pump. Cl^- enters cells and exits into the lumen, driving Na^+ secretion passively via transepithelial potential. *HCO_3^- secretion* aids digestion, involving different transporters and varying mechanisms along the intestine. In the colon, *K^+ active secretion* occurs through K^+ conductance in the apical membrane, regulated by cyclic adenosine monophosphate (cAMP) and calcium ion (Ca^{2+}) [7].

Intestinal secretion is regulated by a complex array of stimuli, including mechanical and chemical signals within the gut, systemic metabolic changes (e.g., dehydration and acid–base imbalances), and even neural signals from higher brain centers. These stimuli interact with receptors on gut cells, involving neural, hormonal, and autocrine modulators that manage both baseline and stimulated secretion levels.

Various peptides, bioactive amines, and other substances produced in different layers of the gut can influence the transport of fluids and electrolytes within the intestines, and they are categorized as either secretagogues or proabsorptive agents. Secretagogues, such as vasoactive intestinal peptide (VIP), serotonin, gastrin, histamine, prostaglandins, and guanylin, promote fluid secretion into the intestinal lumen. Conversely, proabsorptive agents, including somatostatin, corticosteroids, mineralocorticoids, norepinephrine, and neuropeptide Y, enhance fluid and electrolyte absorption by reducing secretion or increasing transport across intestinal cells [4].

Responses to these agents vary in duration based on receptor type and ligand interaction. Short-lived responses, like those triggered by calcium-dependent secretagogues and prostaglandins, handle immediate changes in the gut environment, while steroid-mediated responses have longer-lasting effects. For example, in the distal colon, steroids regulate transport proteins over the long term, aiding in fluid and electrolyte balance under conditions such as dehydration or low sodium intake [8, 9].

6.1.3 How SBS Disrupts These Processes Due to Reduced Absorptive Surface Area

The primary cause of malabsorption in short bowel syndrome (SBS) is the loss of the small intestine's absorptive surface area due to surgical resection or loss of function. The extent of malabsorption is inversely related to the length of the remaining small bowel and is worsened when the colon is partially or completely removed. Patients who have undergone extensive intestinal resection are particularly vulnerable to dehydration and electrolyte imbalances, especially in cases involving an end jejunostomy or proximal ileostomy. The loss of intestinal surface area leads to increased fluid losses, and patients often experience deficiencies in electrolytes like sodium, potassium, and magnesium. The loss of specific anatomical sites leads to deficiencies in key nutrients. For example, the absence of the terminal ileum impairs the absorption of vitamin B12, fat-soluble vitamins, and bile acids. When the distal ileum and ileocecal valve are lost, there is a disruption of inhibitory hormonal signals that control intestinal motility, leading to accelerated transit, increased gastric secretion, and conditions like dumping syndrome [10, 11]. Additionally, rapid transit, reduced mucosal contact, and small intestinal bacterial overgrowth (SIBO), which is common after loss of the ileocecal valve, further exacerbate malabsorption by consuming nutrients (e.g., vitamin B12) and interfering with bile acid absorption, which can cause fat malabsorption [12].

The clinical presentation and complications of SBS vary based on the presence or absence of the colon. Surgical removal of the colon drastically impairs the body's ability to absorb sodium and water, significantly increasing the risk of dehydration and kidney dysfunction. Additionally, without the colon, the body loses the ability to recover energy from unabsorbed carbohydrates, which would normally be fermented by gut bacteria into short-chain fatty acids (SCFAs) and absorbed. Conversely, retaining the colon can increase the likelihood of enteric hyperoxaluria, a condition that promotes kidney stone formation and contributes to lactic acidosis [13].

Table 6.1 Types of SBS: anatomical features and clinical implications [14, 15]

Type of SBS	Minimal small intestine length needed for nutritional autonomy	Description	Clinical features
Type I End jejunostomy	≥115 cm	Complete removal of the ileum and colon, leaving only a portion of the jejunum	High risk of dehydration, electrolyte imbalances (e.g., low magnesium), hypotension, and kidney failure
Type II Jejunocolonic anastomosis	≥60 cm	Removal of the ileum with preservation of the colon	Malnutrition, diarrhea, steatorrhea (fatty stools), and vitamin/mineral deficiencies
Type III Jejunoileal anastomosis	≥35 cm	Mainly resection of the jejunum while leaving at least 10 cm of the terminal ileum and the entire colon intact	Generally, does not require extensive nutritional support

Table 6.1 presents an overview of the different types of SBS, highlighting the anatomical changes, retained sections of the digestive tract, and common clinical features associated with each type.

In addition to the anatomical classification of SBS, intestinal failure (IF) is also categorized into three phases—acute, prolonged acute, and chronic—based on expected duration, metabolic stability, and outcomes [16].

Following extensive small bowel resection, the body enters an adaptation phase that typically lasts between 1 and 2 years. During this period, the remaining intestine undergoes structural and functional modifications to enhance its ability to absorb nutrients. One notable change is an approximate 30% increase in villus height due to mucosal expansion, which enlarges the surface area available for digestion and absorption. Additionally, intestinal motility tends to slow, allowing for prolonged contact time between nutrients and the absorptive mucosa, thereby improving nutrient uptake.

The exact biological mechanisms driving these adaptations are not yet fully understood. However, several factors within the intestinal lumen are believed to play a role, including the presence of nutrients, pancreatic and bile secretions, and key hormones. Hormones such as gastrin, ghrelin, peptide YY (PYY), glucagon-like peptide-1 (GLP-1), and glucagon-like peptide-2 (GLP-2) contribute to mucosal growth and functional improvement of the remaining intestine. These factors work together to boost the digestive and absorptive capacity of the remaining intestine, helping to mitigate the effects of the lost gut surface [15, 17].

6.2 Water and Electrolyte Disturbances in SBS

6.2.1 Fluid and Electrolyte Imbalances in SBS: Mechanisms and Treatment

The loss of intestinal surface area, especially in patients with a *proximal jejunostomy*, means that these individuals cannot reabsorb the normal volumes of water and electrolytes. This results in *excessive stool output* and complications such as *hypovolemia, hyponatremia, and hypokalemia.* For instance, in a study involving jejunostomy patients with a mean jejunal length of *50 cm*, bowel output ranged from *3.2 to 8.3 liters per day, with negative Na^+* and *water balance*, and *negative K^+* in some patients [18]. In contrast, patients with longer jejunal lengths (mean 120 cm) maintained positive sodium and water balance, highlighting the importance of *jejunal length* in managing water and electrolyte absorption. Generally, at least *100 cm of intact jejunum* is needed for the maintenance of a positive fluid and electrolyte balance.

Patients with a jejunostomy typically lose up to 100 mEq of Na^+ and up to 20 mEq of K^+ per liter of stomal output. The high volume is primarily due to the loss of normal digestive secretions (around *4 liters/day*) that would typically be absorbed in the small intestine [19]. This substantial loss leads to decreased urinary sodium excretion and increased plasma aldosterone levels [20]. Some patients require long-term *parenteral supplementation* for fluids and electrolytes, while others can manage through the consumption of a *glucose-saline oral rehydration solution (ORS)* throughout the day. This solution takes advantage of the coupled active transport of sodium with glucose and amino acids in the jejunum, enhancing *Na^+ and water absorption* [21]. The tight junctions in the jejunum are more permeable compared to the ileum and colon, thus requiring a *high NaCl concentration* (>90 mmol/L) in the ORS to optimize absorption [22].

The colon, however, absorbs up to *3 to 4 liters* of isotonic salt solution per day and plays a *key role* in *sodium and water absorption*. In patients with SBS who have a preserved colon, the large absorptive capacity of the colon significantly reduces the likelihood of negative water and sodium balance. These patients experience *lower stomal output* and are generally able to avoid sodium or water supplements unless there is a sodium deficiency. In such cases, a *glucose-saline drink* can be used throughout the day, similar to jejunostomy patients. A comparison of patients with similar jejunal lengths—one group with a *jejunostomy* and the other with a jejunum anastomosed to the colon—showed that the latter group required fewer oral or intravenous (IV) supplements, reinforcing the colon's role in maintaining fluid and electrolyte balance. Additionally, while the colon does secrete potassium, hypokalemia is rare in these patients. The colon's chloride absorption and bicarbonate secretion mechanism can sometimes lead to *bicarbonate loss* in the stools, potentially resulting in *metabolic acidosis* [21].

After significant intestinal resection, the loss of inhibitory hormones such as gastric inhibitory polypeptide (GIP) and VIP—which are normally secreted in the jejunum—leads to elevated gastrin levels and gastric hypersecretion [23]. Factors such as *rapid gastric emptying, increased gastric acid secretion, and accelerated small bowel transit* further contribute to fluid loss. *Transient gastric hypersecretion* is commonly observed in patients with SBS, especially after jejunal resection. This hypersecretion can manifest as early as 24 h postsurgery and is generally more pronounced following jejunal resection compared to ileal resection. While it often resolves within 6 months, basal acid secretion may remain elevated for several months [24]. This excess gastric acid lowers the pH of duodenal contents, which can deactivate pancreatic lipase and *deconjugate bile salts* [25]. These changes disrupt *fat digestion*, worsening fat malabsorption and contributing to an overall increase in malabsorption symptoms. Moreover, patients with substantial bowel resections often experience hypergastrinemia in the early postoperative period further altering digestion and absorption. This process exacerbates dehydration and electrolyte disturbances.

6.2.1.1 Management of Fluid Imbalance

Effective fluid management in SBS requires a tailored approach that accounts for both maintenance needs (20–30 mL/kg/day) and replacement of GI tract fluid losses. Fluid prescriptions must also consider contributions from IV medications, parenteral nutrition (PN), and any oral intake. For patients with high jejunostomy output, replacement fluids may be dosed proportionally (e.g., 0.5–1 mL per 1 mL of jejunostomy loss) to maintain balance.

Chronic IV fluid-dependent patients may receive crystalloids daily, either as needed during the day or intermittently throughout the week, depending on their hydration status. In the home setting, IV fluids should be customized to meet electrolyte needs if PN does not already do so.

ORS plays a crucial role, particularly for patients without a colon, as they facilitate sodium and water absorption via sodium–glucose cotransport. The World Health Organization (WHO) provides standardized ORS formulations that have significantly reduced morbidity and mortality from diarrheal diseases worldwide. However, commercial beverages such as juices, sodas, and sports drinks are unsuitable due to their high osmolarity and low sodium content, while hypotonic fluids like water, tea, and diet sodas should be restricted in patients with high-output stomas.

Despite their benefits, ORS can be unpalatable, making adherence challenging. Patients should be encouraged to sip ORS throughout the day, refrigerate it, or use flavor enhancers, ice cubes, or popsicles to improve palatability. The goal is to consume enough ORS to exceed enterostomy losses and maintain a urine output of at least 1 L/day. Starting with lower-sodium ORS and gradually increasing concentration can help patients adjust. Those with type 1 SBS (end jejunostomy) can use liberal salt intake and restrict oral fluids around meals to enhance sodium absorption. Meanwhile, patients with net secretion and high-output jejunostomy should minimize hypotonic and hypertonic fluids to reduce stoma output and prevent dehydration.

Various pharmacologic agents are used to minimize fluid and electrolyte losses in patients with SBS or high-output stomas. These medications aid in reducing gastric hypersecretion, slowing intestinal transit, enhancing nutrient absorption, and optimizing hydration. Table 6.2 provides a summary of key drug classes, their mechanisms of action, clinical applications, and important considerations.

Table 6.2 Pharmacologic management of gastrointestinal fluid loss in SBS [16, 24, 26]

Drug class	Examples	Mechanism of action	Clinical use	Key considerations and frequently used dosage
Acid-suppressing agents	Proton pump inhibitors (PPIs)—Omeprazole, pantoprazole; H_2-receptor antagonists (H_2RAs)—Ranitidine, famotidine	Reduce gastric acid secretion to prevent excessive fluid loss and improve nutrient absorption	Used in early postresection phase to manage gastric hypersecretion	PPIs preferred for long-term use; IV administration may be required initially Omeprazole: 40 mg twice daily (esomeprazole, lansoprazole, rabeprazole, and pantoprazole as alternatives) Ranitidine: 300 mg twice daily (cimetidine, famotidine, and nizatidine as alternatives)
Antimotility agents	Loperamide, diphenoxylate–atropine, codeine phosphate, tincture of opium	Slow intestinal transit, increase water and sodium absorption, and reduce diarrhea	Taken before meals to decrease fluid losses and improve absorption	Loperamide is preferred due to minimal CNS effects; codeine can cause sedation Loperamide: 4–6 mg, four times daily Codeine phosphate: 15–60 mg, 2–4 times daily Tincture of opium: 0.6 mL (2.5 mg), 2–4 times daily

(continued)

Table 6.2 (continued)

Drug class	Examples	Mechanism of action	Clinical use	Key considerations and frequently used dosage
Bile acid sequestrants	Cholestyramine, colestipol	Bind bile acids to reduce their colonic toxicity and improve stool consistency	Used in patients with colon in continuity who experience bile salt diarrhea	Should be taken 2 h before or after other medications to prevent interactions Cholestyramine: 4 g once or twice daily
Somatostatin analogs	Octreotide, lanreotide	Inhibit gastrointestinal and pancreatic secretions, slow transit, and enhance sodium and water absorption	Used in patients with high-output stomas or fistulas to reduce enteric losses	May impair intestinal adaptation, increase risk of gallstones, and should be used selectively Octreotide: 50–100 μg SC, 2–3 times daily
α2-adrenergic agonists	Clonidine	Enhances Cl^- absorption, reduces intestinal secretion, and decreases diarrhea	Can be used in SBS to reduce stool output	Transdermal administration can help bypass absorption issues Clonidine: 0.3 mg transcutaneous patch once weekly

6.2.2 Sodium Losses and Management in Short Bowel Syndrome

Sodium losses can be significant in patients with SBS, particularly immediately following a major bowel resection. Although some sodium loss may improve as the bowel adapts, persistent deficits can occur depending on the extent and location of the resected bowel, as well as the health of the remaining bowel [27].

In SBS, hyponatremia usually arises from significant fluid loss and is classified as "hypovolemic hyponatremia." However, borderline dehydration or sodium depletion may also occur. Sodium losses are particularly severe in patients with an end jejunostomy, as the absence of the ileum and colon exacerbates the loss [28, 29].

The remaining length of the jejunum directly influences sodium losses. When less than 100 cm of the jejunum is intact, a *net secretory* response to sodium intake is observed. The permeability of the jejunum's mucosal junctions is higher than that of the ileum and colon, leading to increased secretion of sodium and fluids rather than their absorption. Additionally, the jejunum is less effective at reabsorbing fluid and electrolytes when exposed to osmotic loads, such as during food intake [18].

If significant portions of the ileum are removed, the transit time in the jejunum increases, exacerbating fluid and sodium losses [28]. Even patients with an end ileostomy, who have not undergone further resections, may still experience substantial sodium depletion. This underscores the critical role the colon plays in maintaining fluid and electrolyte balance in SBS patients [30].

6.2.2.1 Management of Sodium Loss

The use of ORS in SBS patients is aimed at optimizing sodium and water absorption. For those with borderline SBS intestinal insufficiency or failure, ORS therapy may help maintain intestinal autonomy, while in cases of intestinal failure (IF), it can reduce the need for parenteral fluids and sodium support [29]. The inclusion of glucose in ORS promotes sodium reabsorption by enhancing the glucose-coupled sodium transport mechanism. Additionally, glucose helps maintain the isotonic nature of the ORS, which aids in reducing sodium and water secretion into the digestive lumen [27]. Also, patients should consume a generous amount of sodium with meals to achieve intraluminal sodium concentrations that promote effective sodium absorption [31].

Patients with high-output ostomies may need to avoid low-sodium, hypotonic, and hypertonic fluids to reduce stoma output, while also requiring long-term intravenous fluids to manage sodium and water losses. In such cases, sodium-rich crystalloids like Lactated Ringer's solution are preferred, as their sodium content closely matches that of small bowel losses. For individuals dependent on parenteral nutrition, sodium supplementation may need to exceed the usual 1–2 mEq/kg/day to properly address ongoing losses [27, 29].

6.2.2.2 Monitoring and Addressing Hyponatremia

It is important to note that low serum sodium levels do not always accurately reflect true sodium stores in patients who are volume overloaded. However, in volume-depleted states, hyponatremia indicates concurrent sodium and fluid deficits, necessitating the targeted replacement of both.

Although clinical balance studies offer valuable insights into individual patients' intestinal fluid and sodium absorption, they are often not feasible in routine clinical practice. As a result, many clinicians rely on less precise methods, such as clinical evaluation, body weight monitoring, and standard blood tests, to assess fluid balance. As an alternative, measuring 24-hour urine volume and sodium excretion can provide useful indicators of fluid and sodium absorption, with sodium levels below 20 mEq/L typically signaling depletion [29].

6.2.3 Potassium Imbalance and Management in Short Bowel Syndrome

Potassium absorption primarily occurs in the jejunum, making its balance particularly susceptible to the effects of significant small bowel resections. When the remaining jejunal length is less than 50 cm, net potassium secretion becomes a critical concern due to limited absorptive capacity [32]. Potassium losses can vary depending on the site of gastrointestinal fluid loss. Small bowel fluids typically contain 5–20 mEq/L of potassium, while colonic output can result in significantly higher potassium losses, with levels reaching up to 60 mEq/L [27].

6.2.3.1 Factors Contributing to Potassium Deficiency

Potassium depletion in SBS arises from various physiological and clinical factors. Metabolic alkalosis can shift potassium into cells, reducing serum levels, while medications like loop diuretics promote renal potassium losses and insulin therapy increases intracellular potassium uptake [33]. Magnesium deficiency further exacerbates potassium wasting by impairing renal retention, making hypokalemia resistant to potassium supplementation alone [34].

Additionally, significant sodium losses in SBS can trigger secondary hyperaldosteronism, increasing potassium excretion through the kidneys [19].

6.2.3.2 Management of Potassium Deficiency

Managing potassium levels in SBS requires a patient-specific approach. In cases of hypokalemia, addressing sodium and water depletion and correcting magnesium deficiency is critical, as potassium supplements are rarely needed [10]. When supplementation is required, oral potassium should be given in divided doses (e.g., 20 mEq every 2 h for a total of 60 mEq/day) to minimize gastrointestinal side effects like osmotic diarrhea. Solid dosage forms, such as film-coated or microencapsulated tablets, are preferred over liquid or powder forms, while wax matrix tablets should be avoided in patients with enterostomies to prevent mucosal irritation or obstruction [35, 36]. Intravenous potassium replacement may be necessary for those who cannot tolerate oral supplementation, typically at a rate of 10 mEq to raise serum potassium by 0.1 mmol/L. IV potassium administration should not exceed 10 mEq/h in unmonitored settings, though rates up to 20 mEq/h may be cautiously used under ECG monitoring [37]. Potassium phosphate may be an alternative for patients with concurrent hypophosphatemia. Regular monitoring is essential, with serum potassium levels reassessed 1–2 h after IV replacement, and dose adjustments required for those with renal impairment to prevent hyperkalemia. Special considerations include pseudohyperkalemia, which may result from hemolyzed blood samples or PN fluid contamination, and renal impairment, where careful monitoring is necessary to avoid excessive potassium accumulation [38].

6.2.4 Magnesium Imbalance and Management in SBS

Magnesium deficiency is a frequent and often underestimated complication in SBS, particularly in patients with a jejunostomy or significant ileal resections. As magnesium is primarily absorbed in the distal small intestine and colon, patients with extensive bowel loss—especially those lacking colonic continuity—are at higher risk for depletion [24, 30].

The condition can manifest as muscle weakness, tremors, ataxia, cardiac arrhythmias, and, in severe cases, seizures [39]. When hypocalcemia is also present, patients may exhibit Chvostek and Trousseau signs due to impaired parathyroid hormone secretion [40].

6.2.4.1 Mechanisms of Magnesium Loss

Magnesium depletion in SBS results from multiple mechanisms, primarily intestinal malabsorption, renal wasting, and medication-induced losses. Magnesium is absorbed in the ileum and colon via passive diffusion, and the loss of these segments increases magnesium losses [41]. Additionally, unabsorbed fatty acids bind to magnesium, forming insoluble complexes that are excreted in stool, a process exacerbated in high-fat diets [42]. Renal magnesium wasting further contributes to deficiency, as chronic sodium and water losses lead to secondary hyperaldosteronism, which promotes increased urinary magnesium excretion [43]. Medication-induced losses also play a role, with long-term use of proton pump inhibitors (PPIs)—commonly prescribed to SBS patients for gastric hypersecretion—being associated with persistent hypomagnesemia, possibly due to impaired intestinal absorption [44]. Assessing magnesium levels can be challenging, as only a small fraction of total body magnesium circulates in serum. Hypoalbuminemia, common in SBS, can lower measured total magnesium levels, sometimes masking true deficits [45]. A serum magnesium level below 0.6 mmol/L is often indicative of magnesium deficiency; however, more precise assessments, such as ionized magnesium levels or 24-h urinary magnesium excretion, may provide better insights into a patient's magnesium status [46].

6.2.4.2 Management of Magnesium Deficiency

Managing magnesium deficiency in SBS requires a comprehensive approach, beginning with the correction of fluid and sodium imbalances, as persistent sodium depletion exacerbates renal magnesium losses [47]. In cases of severe deficiency or poor oral tolerance, intravenous magnesium sulfate is administered at controlled rates ($\leq$1 g/h) to minimize renal excretion, with ongoing postinfusion monitoring to ensure adequate repletion [27]. For long-term maintenance, oral magnesium supplements such as magnesium oxide, citrate, or lactate are commonly used, though their laxative effects may limit tolerability; administering divided doses at night may improve absorption and reduce diarrhea (e.g., 12 mmol magnesium oxide or 10 mmol magnesium aspartate at night) [47]. Magnesium diglycinate, a chelated form, may offer better tolerance with fewer gastrointestinal side effects [48]. Dietary modifications, such as reducing fat intake, can help limit magnesium-binding fatty acid complexes, thereby improving net absorption [42]. Patients with a retained colon generally require lower supplementation doses, emphasizing the colon's role in magnesium conservation. Adjunctive therapies, including 1α-hydroxycholecalciferol in a dose of 1–9 μg/day may enhance magnesium absorption, as well as discontinuing PPIs or switching to alternative acid suppression therapies may be beneficial in refractory cases [29, 49]. In severe or recurrent hypomagnesemia, alternative administration methods such as transdermal magnesium sprays or subcutaneous (SC) injections may be considered, though their efficacy remains uncertain [47].

6.2.5 Calcium Homeostasis and Management in SBS

Calcium plays a strategic role in various physiological processes, but its absorption and balance are significantly disrupted in SBS, especially in patients with fat malabsorption.

6.2.5.1 Mechanisms of Calcium Imbalance

Under normal conditions, dietary calcium binds to oxalate in the GI tract, forming insoluble calcium oxalate, which is excreted in stool. However, in SBS patients with fat malabsorption, calcium preferentially binds to free fatty acids instead of oxalate. This leaves oxalate in its free form, which can be absorbed by the colon. As a result, patients with an intact colon are at increased risk of **enteric hyperoxaluria**, which may lead to the precipitation of oxalate salts and **renal stone formation** [50].

6.2.5.2 Management of Calcium Deficiency

Managing calcium levels in SBS involves dietary intake, supplementation, and careful monitoring. Patients with fat malabsorption and a remnant colon may require calcium supplementation to reduce oxalate absorption, with calcium carbonate or calcium citrate being viable options [29]. Calcium citrate is generally preferred for patients with altered gastric physiology, such as those with gastrectomy, due to its superior absorption in low-acid environments [51]. Since less than 1% of the body's calcium is in the serum and most is protein bound, primarily to albumin, serum calcium levels should be interpreted in context, with correction for hypoalbuminemia using the formula: Corrected Calcium = [0.8 × (Normal Albumin—Patient's Albumin)] + Serum Total Calcium. However, this correction can sometimes overestimate serum calcium, leading to misinterpretations of hypercalcemia or normocalcemia [52]. Optimizing vitamin D (200 IU/day) and magnesium levels is necessary, as hypomagnesemia can reduce parathyroid hormone secretion, leading to urinary calcium loss and impaired calcium absorption [29]. Intravenous calcium, such as calcium gluconate, should be reserved for acute, symptomatic hypocalcemia, while oral calcium supplementation is typically sufficient for long-term management [27]. It is important to note that the solubility of calcium in parenteral nutrition (PN) solutions is restricted due to the potential formation of insoluble salts, such as calcium phosphate, calcium carbonate, and calcium–magnesium salts. To optimize solubility and prevent precipitation, it is recommended to initially administer calcium and phosphate in a ratio of 1:2, adjusting the ratio as necessary.

For example, a typical starting dose may involve adding 15 mEq of calcium and 30 mmol of phosphorus to the PN solution daily [53].

6.2.6 Phosphorus Balance in SBS

Phosphorus is often affected in patients with SBS, particularly those who are hospitalized or malnourished [29]. The causes of hypophosphatemia in these patients can be multifactorial.

Nutritional deficiency, particularly reduced dietary intake, is a common contributor to phosphorus depletion. Additionally, the initiation of dextrose-based nutrition or insulin therapy can drive phosphorus into cells, leading to a reduction in serum levels [54]. This intracellular shifting is particularly concerning in the context of refeeding syndrome, which can be life threatening in malnourished patients undergoing nutritional rehabilitation [55].

Finally, physiological processes such as bone mineralization or tissue healing can increase the body's demand for phosphorus, further contributing to its depletion.

6.2.6.1 Management of Phosphorus Deficiency

In managing phosphorus levels, intravenous phosphorus replacement is generally preferred in hospitalized patients, as oral administration can exacerbate diarrhea, a common issue in SBS.

Sodium phosphate or potassium phosphate are commonly used, with potassium phosphate being particularly beneficial in patients with concurrent hypokalemia. While enteral phosphorus administration is an option, it should be approached cautiously due to the potential for osmotic diarrhea [56]. If enteral supplementation is necessary, it is recommended to administer smaller, divided doses throughout the day to minimize gastrointestinal side effects [57]. Close monitoring of phosphorus levels is imperative, particularly in patients receiving parenteral nutrition or transitioning to oral feeding [58].

Early detection and correction of hypophosphatemia can prevent complications such as muscle weakness, impaired cardiac function, and respiratory distress [59].

6.3 Physiology of Acid–Base Balance in Short Bowel Syndrome

The acid–base balance in patients with SBS is subject to unique challenges due to metabolic stresses and alterations in gastrointestinal physiology. Factors such as dehydration, lactic acidosis, ketoacidosis, renal impairment, and the infusion of acidic parenteral nutrition solutions or saline can disrupt acid–base balance even in otherwise healthy individuals. In the context of SBS, these disturbances are compounded by the reduced absorptive capacity and metabolic stresses associated with shortened or dysfunctional bowel.

6.3.1 Mechanisms of Acid–Base Disturbance in IF/SBS

Acid–base disturbances in patients with SBS arise from multiple factors, including metabolic stressors, alimentary losses, nutritional support, and additional metabolic complications. Net losses of bicarbonate or acid through the GI tract can lead to metabolic acidosis or alkalosis, particularly when compensatory mechanisms fail [60]. Negative water balance, often due to increased stomal output, dehydration, or renal impairment, may exacerbate acid–base disturbances, sometimes resulting in a mixed acid–base disorder [60]. Nutritional support also plays a role, as parenteral nutrition and certain enteral nutrition solutions are often acidic, with elemental or semi-elemental diets contributing to acid loads [21, 61]. Additionally, saline, commonly used for fluid replacement in patients with high intestinal losses, may worsen acidosis rather than restoring balance. Even ORS, while beneficial for hydration, can influence acid–base balance and require careful management [29]. Other contributing factors include D-lactic acidosis, a unique complication in SBS patients with a colon in continuity, and sepsis-related L-lactic acidosis [62]. Phosphate depletion, potassium and magnesium deficiencies, and refeeding syndrome can further worsen acid–base abnormalities [63]. Hepatic dysfunction, particularly thiamine deficiency, can impair lactic acid metabolism and further exacerbate these issues [64, 65].

6.3.2 Detection of Acid–Base Disturbance in SBS

Acid–base disturbances are often underdiagnosed in patients with SBS due to several factors. Routine monitoring of acid–base balance is not consistently integrated into standard care protocols, as key parameters like venous bicarbonate and chloride levels are frequently omitted due to the low detection rate of abnormalities in broader populations. Blood pH alone is an unreliable indicator, as compensatory mechanisms, such as respiratory compensation for metabolic acidosis, can mask underlying disturbances. A comprehensive evaluation of arterial blood gases, including pCO_2 and bicarbonate levels, is mandatory for accurately assessing acid–base status [66]. Additionally, serum and urinary anion gap measurements, though not routinely performed, play a key role in diagnosing high anion gap acidosis, particularly D-lactic acidosis. An elevated anion gap with normal L-lactate levels should prompt suspicion for D-lactic acidosis in patients with residual small bowel and colonic continuity [62].

Historically, the lack of standardized guidelines contributed to inconsistent monitoring practices across healthcare systems. However, recent recommendations from European Society for Clinical Nutrition and Metabolism (ESPEN) and American Society for Parenteral and Enteral Nutrition (ASPEN) now emphasize the importance of acid–base balance in SBS patients, promoting more proactive management [29, 67].

6.3.3 Consequences of Unrecognized Acid–Base Disturbance

Unrecognized acid–base disturbances in SBS can lead to serious complications affecting multiple organ systems. Persistent dysfunction contributes to bone demineralization and metabolic bone disease, increasing the risk of fractures and osteoporosis [68]. Additionally, impaired acid–base balance can negatively impact intestinal and cardiovascular function, further complicating overall health status [69]. Patients with an undiagnosed acid–base disturbance are also more susceptible to dehydration and electrolyte imbalances, particularly during acute illnesses or environmental stressors such as hot weather, which can exacerbate fluid losses and metabolic instability.

References

1. Forbes A. Nutritional support in gastrointestinal disease module 12.2 challenges in treating intestinal failure and short bowel syndrome. 2008. https://lllnutrition.com/mod_lll/TOPIC12/old_version/m122.htm. Accessed 10 Dec 2024.
2. Szczygiel B, Jonkers-Schuitema CF, Naber T. Basics in clinical nutrition: nutritional support in extensive gut resections (short bowel). E Spen Eur E J Clin Nutr Metab. 2010;5:e63–e8. https://doi.org/10.1016/j.eclnm.2009.06.021.
3. Chang EB, Leung PS. Intestinal water and electrolyte transport. The gastrointestinal system. Dordrecht: Springer Netherlands; 2014. p. 107–34. https://doi.org/10.1007/978-94-017-8771-0_5.
4. Kiela PR, Ghishan FK. Physiology of intestinal absorption and secretion. Best Pract Res Clin Gastroenterol. 2016;30:145–59. https://doi.org/10.1016/j.bpg.2016.02.007.
5. Gill RK, Alrefai WA, Borthakur A, Dudeja PK. Intestinal anion absorption. physiology of the gastrointestinal tract. Elsevier; 2012. p. 1819–47. https://doi.org/10.1016/B978-0-12-382026-6.00067-1.
6. Heitzmann D, Warth R. Physiology and pathophysiology of potassium channels in gastrointestinal epithelia. Physiol Rev. 2008;88:1119–82. https://doi.org/10.1152/physrev.00020.2007.
7. Ghishan FK, Kiela PR. Small intestinal ion transport. Curr Opin Gastroenterol. 2012;28:130–4. https://doi.org/10.1097/MOG.0b013e32834e7bc3.
8. Fuller PJ, Brennan FE, Burgess JS. Acute differential regulation by corticosteroids of epithelial sodium channel subunit and Nedd4 mRNA levels in the distal colon. Pflugers Arch. 2000;441:94–101. https://doi.org/10.1007/s004240000366.
9. Beubler E, Bukhave K, Rask-Madsen J. Significance of calcium for the prostaglandin E2-mediated secretory response to 5-hydroxytryptamine in the small intestine of the rat in vivo. Gastroenterology. 1986;90:1972–7. https://doi.org/10.1016/0016-5085(86)90269-6.
10. Nightingale J, Woodward JM, Small Bowel and Nutrition Committee of the British Society of Gastroenterology. Guidelines for management of patients with a short bowel. Gut. 2006;55(Suppl 4):iv1-12. https://doi.org/10.1136/gut.2006.091108.
11. Pironi L. Definitions of intestinal failure and the short bowel syndrome. Best Pract Res Clin Gastroenterol. 2016;30:173–85. https://doi.org/10.1016/j.bpg.2016.02.011.
12. Dukowicz AC, Lacy BE, Levine GM. Small intestinal bacterial overgrowth: a comprehensive review. Gastroenterol Hepatol (N Y). 2007;3:112–22.
13. Massironi S, Cavalcoli F, Rausa E, Invernizzi P, Braga M, Vecchi M. Understanding short bowel syndrome: current status and future perspectives. Dig Liver Dis. 2020;52:253–61. https://doi.org/10.1016/j.dld.2019.11.013.

14. Billiauws L, Maggiori L, Joly F, Panis Y. Medical and surgical management of short bowel syndrome. J Visc Surg. 2018;155:283–91. https://doi.org/10.1016/j.jviscsurg.2017.12.012.
15. Lakkasani S, Seth D, Khokhar I, Touza M, Dacosta TJ. Concise review on short bowel syndrome: etiology, pathophysiology, and management. World J Clin Cases. 2022;10:11273–82. https://doi.org/10.12998/wjcc.v10.i31.11273.
16. Klek S, Forbes A, Gabe S, Holst M, Wanten G, Irtun Ø, et al. Management of acute intestinal failure: a position paper from the European Society for Clinical Nutrition and Metabolism (ESPEN) Special Interest Group. Clin Nutr. 2016;35:1209–18. https://doi.org/10.1016/j.clnu.2016.04.009.
17. Rubin DC, Levin MS. Mechanisms of intestinal adaptation. Best Pract Res Clin Gastroenterol. 2016;30:237–48. https://doi.org/10.1016/j.bpg.2016.03.007.
18. Nightingale JMD, Lennard-Jones JE, Walker ER, Farthing M. Jejunal efflux in short bowel syndrome. Lancet. 1990;336:765–8. https://doi.org/10.1016/0140-6736(90)93238-K.
19. Ladefoged K, ØLgaard K. Fluid and electrolyte absorption and renin-angiotensin-aldosterone axis in patients with severe short-bowel syndrome. Scand J Gastroenterol. 1979;14:729–35. https://doi.org/10.3109/00365527909181945.
20. Ladefoged K, Olgaard K. Sodium homeostasis after small-bowel resection. Scand J Gastroenterol. 1985;20:361–9. https://doi.org/10.3109/00365528509091665.
21. Nightingale JMD. Management of patients with a short bowel. World J Gastroenterol. 2001;7:741. https://doi.org/10.3748/wjg.v7.i6.741.
22. Lennard-Jones JE. Oral rehydration solutions in short bowel syndrome. Clin Ther. 1990;12(Suppl A):129–37. discussion 138
23. Williams NS, Evans P, King RF. Gastric acid secretion and gastrin production in the short bowel syndrome. Gut. 1985;26:914–9. https://doi.org/10.1136/gut.26.9.914.
24. Buchman AL. Short bowel syndrome. In: Emad Qayed and Nikrad Shahnavaz, editors. Sleisenger & Fordtran's Gastrointestinal and Liver Disease. 11th ed. Philadelphia: Elsevier; 2021. p. 1720–1735.e4. ISBN: 9780323636599.
25. Fitzpatrick WJ, Zentler-Munro PL, Northfield TC. Ileal resection: effect of cimetidine and taurine on intrajejunal bile acid precipitation and lipid solubilisation. Gut. 1986;27:66–72. https://doi.org/10.1136/gut.27.1.66.
26. Billiauws L, Joly F. Emerging treatments for short bowel syndrome in adult patients. Expert Rev Gastroenterol Hepatol. 2019;13:241–6. https://doi.org/10.1080/17474124.2019.1569514.
27. Nystrom E, Bergquist W. Fluids and electrolytes. Adult short bowel syndrome. Elsevier; 2019. p. 27–43. https://doi.org/10.1016/B978-0-12-814330-8.00003-2.
28. Spiller RC, Trotman IF, Higgins BE, Ghatei MA, Grimble GK, Lee YC, et al. The ileal brake—inhibition of jejunal motility after ileal fat perfusion in man. Gut. 1984;25:365–74. https://doi.org/10.1136/gut.25.4.365.
29. Pironi L, Cuerda C, Jeppesen PB, Joly F, Jonkers C, Krznarić Ž, et al. ESPEN guideline on chronic intestinal failure in adults—update 2023. Clin Nutr. 2023;42:1940–2021. https://doi.org/10.1016/j.clnu.2023.07.019.
30. Ng DHL, Pither CAR, Wootton SA, Stroud MA. The 'not so short-bowel syndrome': potential health problems in patients with an ileostomy. Color Dis. 2013;15:1154–61. https://doi.org/10.1111/codi.12252.
31. Parrish CR, DiBaise JK. Managing the adult patient with short bowel syndrome. Gastroenterol Hepatol (N Y). 2017;13:600–8.
32. Ladefoged K. Intestinal and renal loss of infused minerals in patients with severe short bowel syndrome. Am J Clin Nutr. 1982;36:59–67. https://doi.org/10.1093/ajcn/36.1.59.
33. Kraft MD, Btaiche IF, Sacks GS, Kudsk KA. Treatment of electrolyte disorders in adult patients in the intensive care unit. Am J Health Syst Pharm. 2005;62:1663–82. https://doi.org/10.2146/ajhp040300.
34. Whang R, Whang DD, Ryan MP. Refractory potassium repletion. A consequence of magnesium deficiency. Arch Intern Med. 1992;152:40–5.
35. Sur M, Mohiuddin SS. Potassium. [updated 2024 Oct 5]. In: StatPearls [internet]. Treasure Island (FL): StatPearls Publishing; 2025.

36. Sinar DR, Bozymski EM, Blackshear JL. Effects of oral potassium supplements on upper gastrointestinal mucosa: multicenter clinical comparison of three formulations and placebo. Clin Ther. 1986;8:157–63.
37. Couture J, Létourneau A, Dubuc A, Williamson D. Evaluation of an electrolyte repletion protocol for cardiac surgery intensive care patients. Can J Hosp Pharm. 2013:66. https://doi.org/10.4212/cjhp.v66i2.1231.
38. Alscher M. Hyper- und Hypokaliämien—"the silent killer". DMW—Deutsche Medizinische Wochenschrift. 2016;141:1531–6. https://doi.org/10.1055/s-0042-109043.
39. Hanna S, Harrison M, Macintyre I, Fraser R. The syndrome of magnesium deficiency in man. Lancet. 1960;276:172–6. https://doi.org/10.1016/S0140-6736(60)91323-4.
40. Rude RK, Singer FR. Magnesium deficiency and excess. Annu Rev Med. 1981;32:245–59. https://doi.org/10.1146/annurev.me.32.020181.001333.
41. Nightingale JM, Lennard-Jones JE, Gertner DJ, Wood SR, Bartram CI. Colonic preservation reduces need for parenteral therapy, increases incidence of renal stones, but does not change high prevalence of gall stones in patients with a short bowel. Gut. 1992;33:1493–7. https://doi.org/10.1136/gut.33.11.1493.
42. Hessov I, Andersson H, Isaksson B. Effects of a low-fat diet on mineral absorption in small-bowel disease. Scand J Gastroenterol. 1983;18:551–4. https://doi.org/10.3109/00365528309181636.
43. Horton R, Biglieri EG. Effect of aldosterone on the metabolism of magnesium. J Clin Endocrinol Metab. 1962;22:1187–92. https://doi.org/10.1210/jcem-22-12-1187.
44. https://www.fda.gov/drugs/drugsafety/ucm245011.htm. n.d.
45. Kroll MH, Elin RJ. Relationships between magnesium and protein concentrations in serum. Clin Chem. 1985;31:244–6. https://doi.org/10.1093/clinchem/31.2.244.
46. Ab Rahim SN, Nordin N, Wan Omar WFA, Zulkarnain S, Kumar S, Sinha S, et al. The laboratory and clinical perspectives of magnesium imbalance. Cureus. 2023;15:e49835. https://doi.org/10.7759/cureus.49835.
47. Nightingale JMD. Physiology and problems of a short bowel. Intestinal failure. Cham: Springer International Publishing; 2023. p. 223–42. https://doi.org/10.1007/978-3-031-22265-8_16.
48. Schuette SA, Lashner BA, Janghorbani M. Bioavailability of magnesium diglycinate vs magnesium oxide in patients with ileal resection. J Parenter Enter Nutr. 1994;18:430–5. https://doi.org/10.1177/0148607194018005430.
49. Fukumoto S, Matsumoto T, Tanaka Y, Harada S-I, Ogata E. Renal magnesium wasting in a patient with short bowel syndrome with magnesium deficiency: effect of 1 α-hydroxyvitamin D_3 treatment*. J Clin Endocrinol Metab. 1987;65:1301–4. https://doi.org/10.1210/jcem-65-6-1301.
50. Smith LH, Fromm H, Hofmann AF. Acquired hyperoxaluria, nephrolithiasis, and intestinal disease. N Engl J Med. 1972;286:1371–5. https://doi.org/10.1056/NEJM197206292862601.
51. Tondapu P, Provost D, Adams-Huet B, Sims T, Chang C, Sakhaee K. Comparison of the absorption of calcium carbonate and calcium citrate after Roux-en-Y gastric bypass. Obes Surg. 2009;19:1256–61. https://doi.org/10.1007/s11695-009-9850-6.
52. Kenny CM, Murphy CE, Boyce DS, Ashley DM, Jahanmir J. Things we do for no reason™: calculating a "corrected calcium" level. J Hosp Med. 2021;16:499–501. https://doi.org/10.12788/jhm.3619.
53. Seidner DL. Parenteral nutrition-associated metabolic bone disease. J Parenter Enter Nutr. 2002:26. https://doi.org/10.1177/014860710202600511.
54. Brown KA, Dickerson RN, Morgan LM, Alexander KH, Minard G, Brown RO. A new graduated dosing regimen for phosphorus replacement in patients receiving nutrition support. J Parenter Enter Nutr. 2006;30:209–14. https://doi.org/10.1177/0148607106030003209.
55. Terlevich A, Hearing SD, Woltersdorf WW, Smyth C, Reid D, Mccullagh E, et al. Refeeding syndrome: effective and safe treatment with phosphates polyfusor. Aliment Pharmacol Ther. 2003;17:1325–9. https://doi.org/10.1046/j.1365-2036.2003.01567.x.
56. da Silva JSV, Seres DS, Sabino K, Adams SC, Berdahl GJ, Citty SW, et al. ASPEN consensus recommendations for refeeding syndrome. Nutr Clin Pract. 2020;35:178–95. https://doi.org/10.1002/ncp.10474.

57. Kestenbaum B, Drüeke TB. Disorders of calcium, phosphate, and magnesium metabolism. Comprehensive clinical nephrology. Elsevier; 2010. p. 130–48. https://doi.org/10.1016/B978-0-323-05876-6.00010-1.
58. Mehanna HM, Moledina J, Travis J. Refeeding syndrome: what it is, and how to prevent and treat it. BMJ. 2008;336:1495–8. https://doi.org/10.1136/bmj.a301.
59. Sheldon GF, Grzyb S. Phosphate depletion and repletion: relation to parenteral nutrition and oxygen transport. Ann Surg. 1975;182:683–9. https://doi.org/10.1097/00000658-197512000-00004.
60. Gennari FJ, Weise WJ. Acid-base disturbances in gastrointestinal disease. Clin J Am Soc Nephrol. 2008;3:1861–8. https://doi.org/10.2215/CJN.02450508.
61. Kato K, Sugiura S, Yano K, Fukuoka T, Itoh A, Nagino M, et al. The latent risk of acidosis in commercially available total parenteral nutrition (TPN) products: a randomized clinical trial in postoperative patients. J Clin Biochem Nutr. 2009;45:68–73. https://doi.org/10.3164/jcbn.08-260.
62. Stanciu S, De Silva A. Metabolic acidosis in short bowel syndrome: think D-lactic acid acidosis. BMJ Case Rep. 2018:bcr-2018-224221. https://doi.org/10.1136/bcr-2018-224221.
63. Dounousi E, Zikou X, Koulouras V, Katopodis K. Metabolic acidosis during parenteral nutrition: pathophysiological mechanisms. Indian J Crit Care Med. 2015;19:270–4. https://doi.org/10.4103/0972-5229.156473.
64. Donnino MW, Carney E, Cocchi MN, Barbash I, Chase M, Joyce N, et al. Thiamine deficiency in critically ill patients with sepsis. J Crit Care. 2010;25:576–81. https://doi.org/10.1016/j.jcrc.2010.03.003.
65. Nakasaki H, Ohta M, Soeda J, Makuuchi H, Tsuda M, Tajima T, et al. Clinical and biochemical aspects of thiamine treatment for metabolic acidosis during total parenteral nutrition. Nutrition. 1997;13:110–7. https://doi.org/10.1016/S0899-9007(96)00384-X.
66. Jones BJM. Acid-base disturbances. Intestinal failure. Cham: Springer International Publishing; 2023. p. 377–90. https://doi.org/10.1007/978-3-031-22265-8_25.
67. Ayers P, Adams S, Boullata J, Gervasio J, Holcombe B, Kraft MD, et al. A.S.P.E.N. Parenteral nutrition safety consensus recommendations. J Parenter Enter Nutr. 2014;38:296–333. https://doi.org/10.1177/0148607113511992.
68. Cunningham J, Fraher LJ, Clemens TL, Revell PA, Papapoulos SE. Chronic acidosis with metabolic bone disease. Am J Med. 1982;73:199–204. https://doi.org/10.1016/0002-9343(82)90179-6.
69. Mitch WE. Metabolic and clinical consequences of metabolic acidosis. J Nephrol. 2006;19(Suppl 9):S70–S5.

7 Refeeding Syndrome: Prevention, Diagnosis, and Treatment

Liliana Mirea

7.1 Definition

The refeeding syndrome is a life-threatening complication that describes the metabolic disturbances developing during the nutritional repletion of individuals who are significantly malnourished, or in a state of starvation [1, 2]. Patients with short bowel syndrome are at risk of refeeding syndrome because they often present with malnutrition due to their compromised ability to absorb nutrients.

7.2 Risk Factors

Refeeding syndrome may remain asymptomatic during the prodromal stage, so identifying high-risk patients is essential [3, 4].

One of the primary guidelines for evaluating and treating refeeding syndrome is the National Institute for Health and Care Excellence (NICE) guideline. This guideline identifies several risk factors for refeeding syndrome (Fig. 7.1), but has a low sensitivity and specificity, so clinicians should remain cautious regarding each risk factor [5, 6]. Other guidelines and criteria exist to identify and assess individuals at risk for refeeding syndrome, such as the American Society for Parenteral and Enteral Nutrition (ASPEN), the Short Nutritional Assessment Questionnaire (SNAQ), and the Global Leadership Initiative on Malnutrition (GLIM), but ongoing research is needed to validate their predictive capabilities [7].

L. Mirea (✉)
Faculty of Medicine, Carol Davila University of Medicine and Pharmacy, Bucharest, Romania

Anesthesiology and Intensive Care Clinic, Clinical Emergency Hospital, Bucharest, Romania

A. Trifan et al. (eds.), *Short Bowel Syndrome in Adults*, https://doi.org/10.1007/978-3-031-95848-9_7

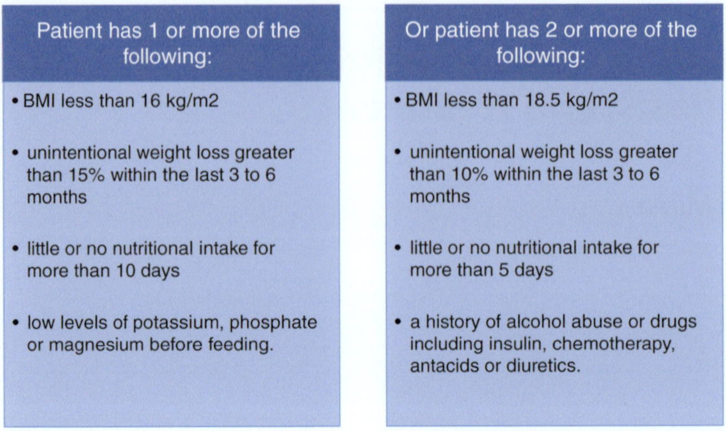

Fig. 7.1 NICE criteria

7.3 Pathophysiology

The key biochemical feature of refeeding syndrome is hypophosphatemia, but additional significant metabolic consequences such as fluid balance abnormalities, disrupted glucose metabolism, and specific vitamin deficiencies (thiamine deficiency), along with hypokalemia and hypomagnesemia, emphasize the complexity of this syndrome [3, 8].

As glucose levels rise, the body responds by increasing insulin production. The intake of glucose following a period of starvation inhibits gluconeogenesis due to the release of insulin [3]. This rise in insulin facilitates the movement of potassium and phosphorus into cells. This shift occurs partly because of the phosphorylation of glucose during glycolysis and also due to the direct activation of the sodium–potassium adenosine triphosphate (ATP) pump [5]. Overly large doses of glucose can result in hyperglycemia and its consequences, such as osmotic diuresis, dehydration, and metabolic acidosis [3].

Phosphorus is crucial for cellular function and performs numerous physiological roles, playing a central role in various cellular metabolic pathways, including glycolysis and oxidative phosphorylation (involving production of ATP) [8]. A depletion of phosphorus will lead to a reduction in the production of 2,3-diphosphoglycerate. This decrease causes a leftward shift in the oxygen–hemoglobin dissociation curve, which enhances hemoglobin's affinity for oxygen while reducing its release to the tissues. As a result, metabolically active tissues may become deprived of oxygen [5, 8]. The switch from catabolism to anabolism will cause, as mentioned before, a shift of potassium and magnesium into the cells. Magnesium, besides playing an important role as a cofactor for many enzymes, is also a cofactor for the sodium–potassium ATPase pump; therefore, uncorrected hypomagnesemia can impair potassium repletion. Potassium as the primary intracellular cation has crucial physiological functions, being responsible for maintaining the electrical cellular membrane potential [1, 8].

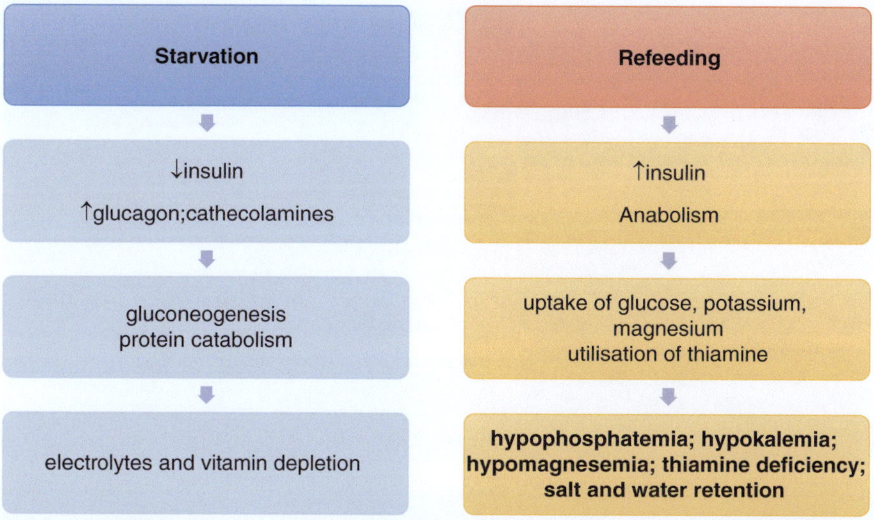

Fig. 7.2 Starvation and refeeding metabolic effects

Thiamine is a vital cofactor in glucose metabolism and facilitates the conversion of lactate to pyruvate. Following a period of starvation, the demand for thiamine increases, which will cause thiamine depletion and finally causing the accumulation of lactate [1, 5, 8].

The changes in carbohydrate metabolism significantly impact sodium and water balance. When carbohydrates are reintroduced, there is a rapid reduction in the renal excretion of sodium and water. A fluid repletion in these patients will lead to fluid overload [3] (Fig. 7.2).

7.4 Diagnosis

Hypophosphatemia has been employed as an indicator for refeeding syndrome, but ASPEN proposed that a decrease in any of the three electrolytes (phosphorus, potassium, and magnesium) may indicate a total-body deficit and necessitate monitoring or intervention. ASPEN classifies patients into three levels of severity: mild, moderate, and severe.

- Mild: A decrease in any one, two, or three of serum phosphorus, potassium, or magnesium levels by 10–20%.
- Moderate: A decrease in any one, two, or three of serum phosphorus, potassium, or magnesium levels by 20–30%.
- Severe: A decrease in any one, two, or three of serum phosphorus, potassium, or magnesium levels by more than 30%, or the presence of organ dysfunction resulting from these decreases or due to thiamine deficiency, occurring within 5 days of reintroducing calories [5, 7].

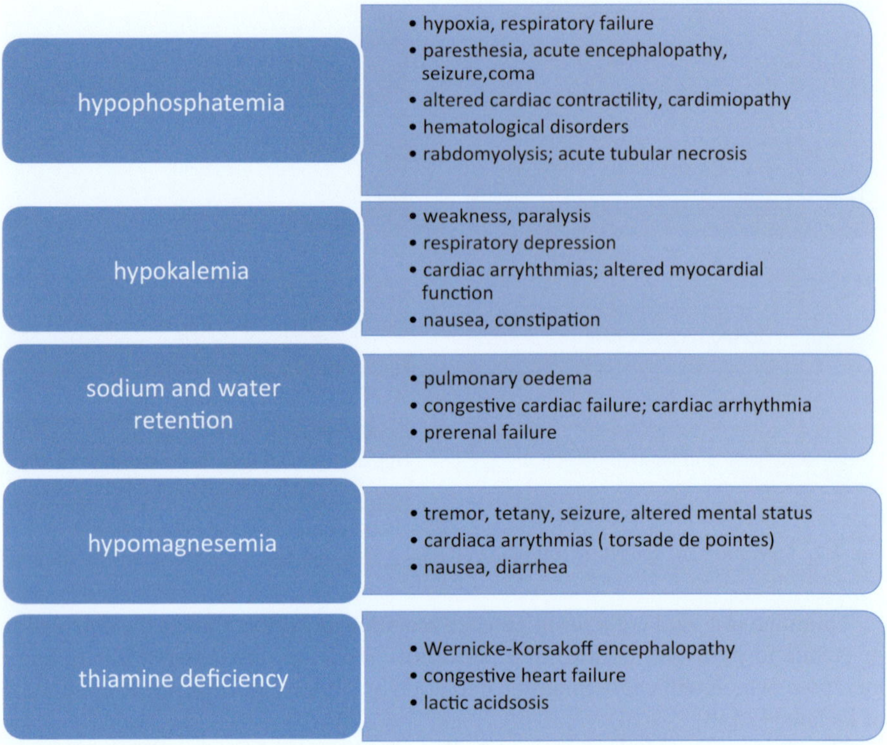

Fig. 7.3 Clinical manifestations of refeeding syndrome [1, 2, 8]

The refeeding syndrome can present with varying degrees of severity, ranging from clinically insignificant changes in electrolyte levels to severe depletion and the risk of end-organ failure. The clinical signs of refeeding syndrome are related to pre-existing electrolyte and vitamin deficiencies (Fig. 7.3), along with the resulting abnormalities that occur when nutrition support is initiated [1, 7].

7.5 Prevention and Management

The initial step in preventing refeeding syndrome is to anticipate its onset by monitoring some key parameters [9–11].

- Vital signs: regularly check the heart rate, blood pressure, oxygen saturation, temperature, and overall health.
- Fluid balance: monitor intake and output to detect signs of dehydration or fluid overload.
- Electrolyte levels: measure at least once daily for the first week. Crucial electrolytes include sodium, potassium, phosphorus, magnesium, and calcium. Regular checks help identify imbalances that can lead to complications.

- Electrocardiogram: continuously monitor to detect arrhythmias that may occur with electrolyte disturbances.
- Ventilatory function: assess respiratory rate and effort to identify any respiratory distress or failure.
- Blood gases: evaluate arterial blood gases to identify metabolic and respiratory disorders.
- Neurological status: observe for signs of confusion and other neurological symptoms indicative of electrolyte imbalances or vitamin deficiency.
- Weight: regularly track weight changes to detect fluid retention or loss, which can be critical during refeeding.
- Glycemic control: monitor blood glucose levels to avoid complications associated with hyperglycemia.

All guidelines advise that vitamin supplementation should be initiated right away, before and throughout the first 10 days of refeeding. It is also crucial to restore circulatory volume and to administer potassium, phosphate, calcium, and magnesium supplements unless baseline blood levels are elevated prior to refeeding [3, 10]. It is recommended to administer thiamine 200–300 mg intravenously or orally before feeding and a daily maintenance dose of 100 milligrams during nutritional support [9, 10].

Regarding the initiation of nutrition, several guidelines provide recommendations to prevent refeeding syndrome:

- The National Institute for Health and Care Excellence (NICE) recommends a maximum 10 and 5 kcal/kg/day in "extreme" cases and to gradually increase the nutritional intake to meet or exceed full requirements within 4–7 days [6].
- The Irish Society for Clinical Nutrition and Metabolism (IrSPEN) and the Clinical Nutrition Steering Group (CNSG) recommend in extreme risk 5 kcal/kg/day and in high risk 10 kcal/kg. In moderate risk patients, the IrSPEN suggests 20 kcal/kg, while the CNSG recommends to introduce at a maximum of 50% of requirements for the first 2 days [7].

It is recommended to provide electrolyte supplementation both before and during nutritional support. The daily requirements are as follows: potassium (2 to 4 mmol/kg/day), phosphate (0.3–0.6 mmol/kg/day), and magnesium (0.2 mmol/kg/day intravenously or 0.4 mmol/kg/day orally) [1, 2, 10]. Regarding the macronutrients, the following distribution is recommended: 50–60% carbohydrates, 30–40% fat, and 15–20% protein [10].

The fluid balance is another important parameter to monitor. The fluids should be restricted to amounts sufficient to maintain renal function, with zero fluid balance, while maintaining normal urine output. Patients typically require 20–25 ml/kg/day during the initial phase, and then, adjustments are made according to the fluid balance. To limit the edema formation, a sodium restriction can be taken into consideration (<1 mmol/kg/day) [2, 10, 12].

In summary, patients at risk of refeeding syndrome require an interdisciplinary approach and daily evaluations to ensure optimal management.

References

1. Kraft MD, Btaiche IF, Sacks GS. Review of the refeeding syndrome. Nutr Clin Pract. 2005;20(6):625–33.
2. Stanga Z, Brunner A, Leuenberger M, Grimble RF, Shenkin A, Allison SP, et al. Nutrition in clinical practice-the refeeding syndrome: illustrative cases and guidelines for prevention and treatment. Eur J Clin Nutr [Internet]. 2008;62(6):687–94.
3. Mehanna HM, Moledina J, Travis J. Refeeding syndrome: what it is, and how to prevent and treat it. Br Med J [Internet]. 2008;336(7659):1495–8.
4. Xie Y, Zhu W, Li N, Li J. Short bowel syndrome presenting with re-feeding syndrome in a Han Chinese patient: a case report. J Med Case Rep. 2012;6:1.
5. Persaud-Sharma D, Saha S, Trippensee AW. Refeeding syndrome [internet]. PubMed. Treasure Island, FL: StatPearls Publishing; 2022.
6. National Institute for Health and Care Excellence. Nutrition support for adults: or Nutrition support for adults: oral al nutrition support, enter nutrition support, enteral tube feeding al tube feeding and parenteral nutrition al nutrition Clinical guideline [Internet]. 2017.
7. da Silva JSV, Seres DS, Sabino K, Adams SC, Berdahl GJ, Citty SW, et al. ASPEN consensus recommendations for refeeding syndrome. Nutr Clin Pract [Internet]. 2020;35(2):178–95.
8. Crook MA, Hally V, Panteli JV. The importance of the refeeding syndrome. Nutrition. 2001;17(7–8):632–7.
9. Sobotka L. Basics in clinical nutrition: refeeding syndrome. e-SPEN, Eur E J Clin Nutr Metab. 2010;5(3):e146–7.
10. Sobotka L. Basics in clinical nutrition. Prague: Galén; 2019.
11. Singer P, Blaser AR, Berger MM, Calder PC, Casaer M, Hiesmayr M, et al. ESPEN practical and partially revised guideline: clinical nutrition in the intensive care unit. Clin Nutr [Internet]. 2023;42(9):1671–89.
12. Reber E, Friedli N, Vasiloglou MF, Schuetz P, Stanga Z. Management of refeeding syndrome in medical inpatients. J Clin Med [Internet]. 2019;8(12):2202.

8 Cholelithiasis and Nephrolithiasis in Short Bowel Syndrome

Liana Gheorghe and Carmen Ester

8.1 Introduction

Short bowel syndrome (SBS) is a condition that results from the surgical removal or congenital absence of a significant portion of the small intestine, leading to malabsorption and a range of metabolic disturbances. Patients with SBS present an increased risk for both cholelithiasis and nephrolithiasis due to the altered absorption of fluids, electrolytes, and nutrients caused by the shortened intestinal tract. Both conditions are classified as late complications of significant small bowel resection. There are many mechanisms that lead to the formation of gallstones and kidney stones in affected patients and are linked to the difficulties in the absorption of bile salts, fat, and oxalates, as well as microbiota changes and modifications in fluid balance.

8.1.1 Cholelithiasis

Following ileal resection, the enterohepatic circulation of bile salts is disrupted. The subsequent loss of bile salts surpasses the liver's compensatory capacity for increased synthesis, leading to a decline in bile salt concentration within the bile. Reducing chenodeoxycholate levels promotes increased cholesterol secretion, rendering the bile lithogenic. Clinically, this condition has been associated with a higher incidence of gallstone formation. Another possible mechanism is bile stasis due to the diminished enteric hormonal stimulation of gallbladder contractions, which may lead to biliary stasis and accumulation of biliary sludge.

L. Gheorghe · C. Ester (✉)
Carol Davila University of Medicine and Pharmacy, Bucharest, Romania

Center for Digestive Diseases and Liver Transplant, Fundeni Clinical Institute, Bucharest, Romania

A. Trifan et al. (eds.), *Short Bowel Syndrome in Adults*,
https://doi.org/10.1007/978-3-031-95848-9_8

8.1.2 Nephrolithiasis

Hyperoxaluria is observed in patients who have undergone ileal resection and those with short bowel syndrome following distal small bowel resection. This condition arises due to enhanced colonic absorption of oxalate, a process facilitated by the presence of bile salts in the colon. Hyperoxaluria contributes to renal calculi formation, with reduced citrate intake further exacerbating the risk. Management strategies include adherence to a low-oxalate diet and administration of cholestyramine to bind bile salts, while citrate supplementation helps prevent stone formation.

A low-oxalate diet typically excludes foods such as cocoa, tea, and coffee while also limiting the intake of citrus beverages, tomatoes, and certain fruits [1].

8.2 Pathophysiology of Cholelithiasis in Short Bowel Syndrome

Gallstones can cause life-threatening complications, including cholecystitis (commonly associated with larger stones >10 mm), obstructive jaundice (often due to multiple stones), pancreatitis (typically caused by smaller stones), and small bowel obstruction. In rare cases, gallstones may contribute to the development of gallbladder carcinoma or cholangiocarcinoma. Larger gallstones and their presence in high numbers are more likely to be symptomatic. Pigment gallstones are more frequent in patients with SBS than cholesterol ones, although a contribution of cholesterol in forming this type of stones is often cited [2].

8.3 Bile Acid Malabsorption and Gallstone Formation

Cholelithiasis in SBS is primarily driven by bile acid malabsorption, which occurs when the reabsorption of bile salts in the terminal ileum is compromised due to surgical resection. Bile salts are essential for the solubilization of cholesterol in bile, and when these salts are not adequately reabsorbed, their concentration in bile decreases. This leads to the precipitation of cholesterol, forming cholesterol gallstones.

The relevant factors contributing to cholelithiasis in SBS include: reduced enterohepatic circulation (bile acids are normally reabsorbed in the ileum and transported back to the liver, but especially when there is ileum resection, bile acid reabsorption is impaired, resulting in cholesterol-supersaturated bile), decreased bile salt availability (reduced absorption of bile acids leads to a smaller available bile salt pool, which diminishes the emulsification of dietary fats and impairs digestion), and delayed gallbladder emptying (in patients with SBS, there is a modified gastrointestinal motility that leads to impaired gallbladder contraction and stasis, further increasing the risk of gallstone formation).

Patients with intestinal failure (IF) who require prolonged parenteral support for over 5 years exhibit a progressively increased susceptibility to cholelithiasis, with a prevalence of 38% after two decades [3].

In contrast, of the 10–15% of people who are diagnosed with gallstones in the general population in the UK, only 1–4% develop symptoms, and fewer than 1% require surgical intervention annually, with Western Europe, in particular, the UK leading in the number of cases and an increasing global level of gallstone-associated disease over the past 30 years [4].

8.4 Risk Factors for Cholelithiasis in SBS

1. Extent of ileal resection: The more extensive the resection, particularly of the ileum, the greater the risk of bile acid malabsorption and gallstone formation.
2. Use of parenteral nutrition: Many SBS patients require long-term parenteral nutrition, with a bypass effect on the gastrointestinal tract and delayed gallbladder emptying.
3. Weight loss: Rapid weight loss due to malabsorption is experienced by a significant number of SBS patients, which can alter bile composition and increase the likelihood of gallstone formation. Interfering factors can be increased secretion of hormones that contribute to gallbladder wall relaxation (such as pancreatic polypeptide and somatostatin) or diminished secretion of hormones contributing to contractility, such as cholecystokinin [5].
4. Intestinal microbiota: Bacterial overgrowth can affect the deconjugation of bile acids, making them less effective at solubilizing cholesterol and further increasing the risk of cholelithiasis. The release of bile salt hydrolases by the gut microbiota and their capacity to produce an increased amount of secondary bile acids (directly and by slowing transit time) predispose to gallstone formation [6].
5. High caloric intake and higher administration of parenteral lipids: Although routine prophylactic cholecystectomy is not recommended, performing an incidental cholecystectomy during abdominal surgery conducted for other indications may be a reasonable approach for patients with asymptomatic cholelithiasis [7].
6. Medication: Medications such as opiates and anticholinergics reduce gallbladder contractility. Narcotics decrease the flow through the sphincter of Oddi, and anticholinergics increase bile stasis. Also, loperamide and octreotide (used for high-output stomas) have been shown to reduce postprandial gallbladder contractility [8].
7. Presence of Crohn's disease: Gallstones are often found in patients with ileitis, more than in those with ileocolitis or colitis [9]. If the distal ileum loses function, the enterohepatic circulation of bile salts is disrupted. However, some studies suggest that gallstone formation is connected to the length of the disease and previous surgery rather than the resection site.

8.5 Clinical Manifestations of Cholelithiasis

Patients with cholelithiasis may remain asymptomatic, or they may present with classic symptoms of biliary colic, including:

- right upper quadrant abdominal pain, which typically occurs after meals and can radiate to the right shoulder or back.
- nausea and vomiting are common in symptomatic gallstone disease.
- complications: If gallstones obstruct the bile ducts, patients can develop cholecystitis, cholangitis, or pancreatitis, presenting with fever, jaundice, and severe abdominal pain.

Treatment-related cholecystitis was recently described in a patient with preexisting cholelithiasis who was treated with glucagon-like peptide-2 (GLP-2) analogs (teduglutide) [10]. Given its inhibitory effect on gallbladder contraction, teduglutide may contribute to gallstone-related complications. The histopathological finding of mucosal hyperplasia suggests an additional mechanism for gallbladder dysfunction.

In this regard, prophylactic cholecystectomy in SBS patients with known gallstones before initiating GLP-2 therapy might be attempted. This approach could help mitigate the risk of cholecystitis and its associated complications. Future studies could further evaluate the benefits of this preventive strategy in high-risk patients.

8.6 Nephrolithiasis Epidemiology

As early as 1972, patients with ileal resection were proved to be at increased risk of hyperoxaluria, and later, patients undergoing jejunoileal bypass for obesity were proved to have an increased risk of developing renal stones [11]. A large study comprising 2323 patients with inflammatory bowel disease (IBD) proved an increased risk of kidney stones and malabsorption symptoms in patients undergoing surgery. Also, risk factors for nephrolithiasis in patients with IBD were different from the ones in the general population: low serum bicarbonate level, high disease activity, and the use of certain drugs (ciprofloxacin, metronidazole, steroids, and immunomodulators). The decolonization of the intestinal tract from *Oxalobacter formigenes* (an oxalate-fermenting bacterium) is frequently associated with hyperoxaluria and kidney stones [12].

8.7 Pathophysiology of Nephrolithiasis in Short Bowel Syndrome

8.7.1 Oxalate Malabsorption and Kidney Stone Formation

Nephrolithiasis in SBS is most commonly associated with hyperoxaluria, which results from altered fat absorption. In the normal intestine, calcium binds to oxalate, preventing its absorption. However, fat malabsorption occurs in SBS, especially with significant ileal resection, and free fatty acids in the intestine bind to calcium. This leaves oxalate unbound and more freely absorbed by the colon, leading to elevated urinary oxalate levels and the formation of calcium oxalate stones.

Calcium oxalate is not easily soluble, with a solubility of approximately 7 mg/L at 37 °C in a simple solution. Urine is a highly complex solution containing matter that is both an inhibitor and promoter of crystallization. For example, citrate and pyrophosphate reduce calcium availability by forming soluble complexes with calcium; magnesium forms a soluble complex with oxalate; and Tamm–Horsfall glycoprotein, along with other glycosaminoglycans, inhibits various phases of calcium oxalate stone formation.

Under normal conditions, urine is supersaturated with calcium oxalate. However, crystal formation does not typically occur freely in solution but rather by deposition on existing surfaces, such as tubular casts, sodium urate or uric acid crystals, or cellular debris.

Uric acid, a weak acid with a pKa of 5.75, is highly insoluble in its undissociated form, with a solubility limit of 100 mg/L. Urate salts are significantly more soluble, so urine pH is the most critical factor influencing the solubility of uric acid. High urine concentration and low urinary pH are significant risk factors for uric acid stone formation.

8.7.2 Contributing Factors to Nephrolithiasis

The main factors that promote nephrolithiasis in SBS patients include:

1. ***Fat malabsorption.*** The loss of the small intestine's absorptive surface leads to steatorrhea. Free fatty acids bind to calcium, leaving oxalate unbound and more readily absorbed in the colon (Fig. 8.1).

   Fat, a significant calorie source, is the most difficult nutrient to digest and absorb. Excess fat in some patients with SBS may exacerbate steatorrhea and diarrhea, resulting in substantial nutrient and water loss. Furthermore, in the patient with a remaining colon segment, too much fat can displace calcium from oxalate, allowing the unbound oxalate to be absorbed in the colon.

   When there is not enough hydration, enhanced oxalate absorption may induce oxalate nephropathy. Restriction in dietary fat is key in the SBS patient with a remaining colon, severe steatorrhea, and/or a history of oxalate nephrolithiasis.

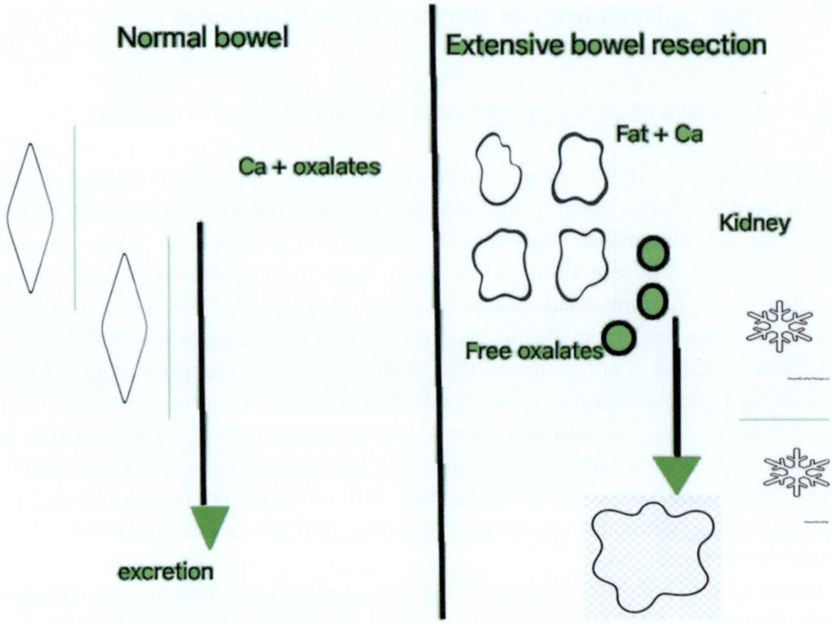

Fig. 8.1 Oxalate excretion in normal bowel vs. extensive bowel resection

Restricting oxalate in patients with a history of kidney stones is also important as long as the clinician ensures the patient is adequately hydrated [13].

2. ***Hyperoxaluria.*** If oxalate absorption is increased in the colon, elevated urinary oxalate levels will be observed, predisposing patients to calcium oxalate stone formation.
3. ***Dehydration.*** Malabsorption of fluids and electrolytes is frequent in SBS patients, resulting in concentrated urine and thus promoting crystallization of the stone-forming salts.
4. ***Changes in urinary pH.*** In some cases, metabolic acidosis may develop due to loss of bicarbonate in the stool, and this mechanism can lead to acidification of the urine, predisposing to the formation of stones.
5. ***Low magnesium in urine.*** Magnesium is essential in inhibiting calcium oxalate crystal formation, with the contribution of citrate. If there is impaired magnesium absorption, a low magnesium concentration in urine will be observed, and prolonged use of proton pump inhibitors will further enhance this condition [14].
6. ***Intestinal microbiota.*** A low population of *Oxalobacter formigenes* in the gut microbiome increases urinary oxalate excretion with a higher risk of recurrent nephrolithiasis, even in individuals without gastrointestinal disorders [15].

8.8 Risk Factors for Nephrolithiasis in SBS

1. Extent of bowel resection: Patients with more extensive resections, particularly those affecting the ileum, have a higher risk of fat malabsorption and oxalate hyperabsorption.
2. Dehydration: Chronic dehydration and concentrated urine are common in SBS and contribute to stone formation.
3. Dietary sources of oxalate: High oxalate-containing food (like spinach or beetroot) is not familiar in diets and can vary with cultivation, season, and method of cooking (boiling reduces soluble oxalate). Wheat bran has a moderate to high concentration of oxalate as does black pepper, but the quantity consumed is relevant [16].
4. Hypocitraturia: Citrate is key for inhibiting calcium oxalate crystallization in the urine, leading to a significant risk for developing kidney stones. The leading causes are reduced glomerular filtration and acidosis [17].

In a recent study of patients with SBS, the incidence of urolithiasis was 24%, with 54.5% presenting clinical symptoms and 13.5% needing urgent decompression of the obstructed kidney. The main component of renal stones is calcium oxalate monohydrate/dihydrate [18].

SBS patients with a colon in continuity are at an increased risk for oxaluria and nephrolithiasis. In cases of fat malabsorption, calcium preferentially binds to unabsorbed fatty acids, leaving free oxalate available for colonic absorption. This oxalate is then filtered by the kidneys, where it binds with calcium, leading to oxalate nephrolithiasis and progressive obstructive nephropathy.

8.9 Clinical Manifestations of Nephrolithiasis

Patients with nephrolithiasis may present with:

- Flank pain: Severe, colicky pain radiating from the back to the lower abdomen or groin is a hallmark of kidney stones.
- Microscopic or macroscopic hematuria.
- Dysuria, urgency, and frequency can occur when stones are in the lower urinary tract.
- If obstruction of the ureters occurs—hydronephrosis or urinary tract infections.

8.10 Diagnosis of Cholelithiasis and Nephrolithiasis in SBS

8.10.1 Diagnostic Tools for Cholelithiasis

- Ultrasound: Abdominal ultrasound is the gold standard for detecting gallstones. It is noninvasive, widely available, and highly sensitive for detecting stones in the gallbladder.
- Hepatobiliary iminodiacetic acid (HIDA) scan: If gallbladder function is impaired without visible stones, a HIDA scan may be used to assess it.
- Magnetic resonance cholangiopancreatography (MRCP): This is a noninvasive imaging technique used to evaluate the biliary tree for gallstones or biliary obstruction.

8.10.2 Diagnostic Tools for Nephrolithiasis

- Urinalysis: This may reveal hematuria, an acidic or alkaline pH, and crystals that suggest the type of stone. A 24-hour urine collection can assess oxalate, calcium, and citrate levels.
- Imaging: Noncontrast helical computed tomography (CT) is the preferred imaging modality for detecting kidney stones due to its high sensitivity and specificity.
- Ultrasound: Renal ultrasound can detect stones, particularly in patients with concerns about radiation exposure, but it is less sensitive than CT.

8.11 Differential Diagnosis in Nephrolithiasis

The three types of primary hyperoxalurias are autosomal recessive inherited disorders with different phenotypes (type 1 has the most severe phenotype). Nowadays, testing for mutations can clarify the diagnosis [19].

8.12 Management of Cholelithiasis and Nephrolithiasis in SBS

8.12.1 Management of Cholelithiasis

In patients with asymptomatic gallstones, conservative management is recommended, as the risk of complications is low.

In those with symptomatic gallstones, cholecystectomy is the treatment of choice. Sphincterotomy may be performed in high-risk patients. Complications such as bile leak might compromise the intestinal anastomosis and prolong the parenteral nutrition administration [20].

Promoting oral intake in order to stimulate gallbladder contraction and avoid bile stasis is complemented by the use of bile acid-binding agents like ursodeoxycholic acid to reduce cholesterol saturation in bile. Nonsteroidal anti-inflammatory drugs (NSAIDs) may prevent gallstone formation by a prokinetic effect caused by the presence of different types of eicosanoids in the gallbladder wall, thus promoting the production of prokinetic molecules like leukotrienes or prostaglandins. It is noted that this effect is not seen in non-SBS patients [21].

8.12.2 Management of Nephrolithiasis

The management of nephrolithiasis in patients with SBS involves a multifaceted approach, including hydration, dietary adjustments, supplementation, medications, and, when necessary, surgical intervention. Key strategies include the following:

- **Adequate hydration**: It is the cornerstone of nephrolithiasis prevention in SBS. Patients should be encouraged to drink enough fluids to maintain a urine output of at least 2 liters per day.
- **Calcium supplementation**: Oral calcium supplements can bind oxalate in the gut, reducing oxalate absorption and the risk of kidney stone formation. Typically, 800–1200 mg/day, in divided doses not exceeding 500 mg, is used [22].
- **Dietary modifications**: To reduce the risk of hyperoxaluria, patients should avoid high-oxalate foods and maintain a diet rich in calcium. A low-fat diet can also help mitigate fat malabsorption and oxalate absorption (Table 8.1).
- **Medications:** Potassium citrate may be used to alkalinize the urine and reduce stone formation, particularly in patients with metabolic acidosis. Another strategy involves using cholestyramine to bind oxalate found in the gut lumen [13].
- **Kidney stones**: Recommendation for surgery—if renal colic is present, conservative treatment should be applied and give the chance for decompression, but urgent surgery is needed if there is an infection of the obstructed kidney or if there is obstruction of solitary kidney/bilateral obstruction and it is impossible to

Table 8.1 Food and beverages to avoid—high in oxalate

Fruits	Apricots, blackberries, cherries, currants, figs	Pears, grapes, raw oranges, plums, rhubarb	Strawberries, tangerines, lemons, limes, orange peels
Vegetables	Sweet potatoes, parsley, raw red cabbage, celery	Eggplant, endive, mustard greens, spinach, kale	Green peppers, tomatoes, tomato soup or juice, vegetable soup, white corn
Nuts	Almonds, cashews, peanuts	Peanut butter	Nut butters
Beverages	Chocolate-containing beverages	Cocoa, cola	Tea, instant coffee
Starches	Grits, bran cereal	Whole wheat bread	French fries
Other	Tofu, soy products	Black olives	Vegetable soup with the above vegetables, pepper (>1 tsp. per day)
Alcohol	Draft beer		

control pain. If the stones do not pass, several therapies can be offered, such as lithotripsy, ureteroscopy, or percutaneous nephrolithotomy.

8.13 Conclusions

Cholelithiasis and nephrolithiasis are common late complications of short bowel syndrome, driven by bile salt malabsorption, fat malabsorption, hyperoxaluria, and metabolic disturbances. Preventive care should focus on optimizing hydration, dietary modifications, and targeted supplementation to reduce the risk of developing stones. Early recognition and personalised management can limit complications, improve quality of life, and protect longterm organ function.

References

1. Morton AR, Iliescu EA, Wilson JW. Nephrology: 1. Investigation and treatment of recurrent kidney stones. CMAJ. 2002;166(2):213–8. PMID: 11829004; PMCID: PMC99277
2. Shabanzadeh DM. Incidence of gallstone disease and complications. Curr Opin Gastroenterol. 2018;34(2):81–9. https://doi.org/10.1097/MOG.0000000000000418.
3. Sanders G, Kingsnorth AN. Gallstones. BMJ. 2007;335(7614):295–9. https://doi.org/10.1136/bmj.39267.452257.AD. PMID: 17690370; PMCID: PMC1941876
4. Li ZZ, Guan LJ, Ouyang R, Chen ZX, Ouyang GQ, Jiang HX. Global, regional, and national burden of gallbladder and biliary diseases from 1990 to 2019. World J Gastrointest Surg. 2023;15(11):2564–78. https://doi.org/10.4240/wjgs.v15.i11.2564. PMID: 38111771; PMCID: PMC10725539
5. Johansson C, Kollberg B, Efendic S, Uvnäs-Wallensten K. Effects of graded doses of somatostatin on gallbladder emptying and pancreatic enzyme output after oral glucose in man. Digestion. 1981;22(1):24–31. https://doi.org/10.1159/000198591.
6. Hu H, Shao W, Liu Q, Liu N, Wang Q, Xu J, Zhang X, Weng Z, Lu Q, Jiao L, Chen C, Sun H, Jiang Z, Zhang X, Gu A. Gut microbiota promotes cholesterol gallstone formation by modulating bile acid composition and biliary cholesterol secretion. Nat Commun. 2022;13(1):252. https://doi.org/10.1038/s41467-021-27758-8. PMID: 35017486; PMCID: PMC8752841
7. Pak M, Lindseth G. Risk factors for cholelithiasis. Gastroenterol Nurs. 2016;39(4):297–309. https://doi.org/10.1097/SGA.0000000000000235. PMID: 27467059; PMCID: PMC8802735
8. Appleton ND, Lal S, Carlson GL, Shaw S, Stevens P, Peristerakis I, Soop M. Cholelithiasis and related morbidity in chronic intestinal failure: a longitudinal cohort study from a national specialized centre. J Gastrointest Surg. 2019;23(10):2002–6. https://doi.org/10.1007/s11605-018-3979-3. Epub 2018 Oct 15. PMID: 30324401; PMCID: PMC6773818
9. Hutchinson R, Tyrrell PN, Kumar D, Dunn JA, Li JK, Allan RN. Pathogenesis of gall stones in Crohn's disease: an alternative explanation. Gut. 1994;35(1):94–7. https://doi.org/10.1136/gut.35.1.94. PMID: 8307459; PMCID: PMC1374640
10. Goto Y, Masumoto K, Jimbo T, Sasaki T, Tanaka Y, Shirane K. Cholecystitis following the initiation of glucagon-like peptide-2 analogue for short bowel syndrome: a case report. Nutr Clin Pract. 2024;39(5):1247–50. https://doi.org/10.1002/ncp.11159. Epub 2024 May 26
11. O'Leary JP, Thomas WC Jr, Woodward ER. Urinary tract stone after small bowel bypass for morbid obesity. Am J Surg. 1974;127(2):142–7. https://doi.org/10.1016/0002-9610(74)90150-0.
12. Fagagnini S, Heinrich H, Rossel JB, Biedermann L, Frei P, Zeitz J, Spalinger M, Battegay E, Zimmerli L, Vavricka SR, Rogler G, Scharl M, Misselwitz B. Risk factors for gallstones

and kidney stones in a cohort of patients with inflammatory bowel diseases. PLoS One. 2017;12(10):e0185193. https://doi.org/10.1371/journal.pone.0185193. PMID: 29023532; PMCID: PMC5638235
13. Parrish CR, DiBaise JK. Managing the adult patient with short bowel syndrome. Gastroenterol Hepatol (N Y). 2017;13(10):600–8. PMID: 29230136; PMCID: PMC5718176
14. Perazella MA. Proton pump inhibitors and hypomagnesemia: a rare but serious complication. Kidney Int. 2013;83(4):553–6. https://doi.org/10.1038/ki.2012.462.
15. Siener R, Bangen U, Sidhu H, Hönow R, von Unruh G, Hesse A. The role of Oxalobacter formigenes colonization in calcium oxalate stone disease. Kidney Int. 2013;83(6):1144–9. https://doi.org/10.1038/ki.2013.104. Epub 2013 Mar 27
16. Attalla K, De S, Monga M. Oxalate content of food: a tangled web. Urology. 2014;84(3):555–60. https://doi.org/10.1016/j.urology.2014.03.053.
17. Rudman D, Dedonis JL, Fountain MT, Chandler JB, Gerron GG, Fleming GA, Kutner MH. Hypocitraturia in patients with gastrointestinal malabsorption. N Engl J Med. 1980;303(12):657–61. https://doi.org/10.1056/NEJM198009183031201.
18. Rudziński M, Ławiński M, Gradowski Ł, Antoniewicz AA, Słodkowski M, Bedyńska S, Kostro J, Singer P. Kidney stones are common in patients with short-bowel syndrome receiving long-term parenteral nutrition: a predictive model for urolithiasis. JPEN J Parenter Enteral Nutr. 2022;46(3):671–7. https://doi.org/10.1002/jpen.2133. Epub 2021 Jun 11
19. Cochat P, Rumsby G. Primary hyperoxaluria. N Engl J Med. 2013;369(7):649–58. https://doi.org/10.1056/NEJMra1301564. Erratum in: N Engl J Med. 2013 Nov 28;369(22):2168
20. Fort JM, Azpiroz F, Casellas F, Andreu J, Malagelada JR. Bowel habit after cholecystectomy: physiological changes and clinical implications. Gastroenterology. 1996;111(3):617–22. https://doi.org/10.1053/gast.1996.v111.pm8780565.
21. O'Donnell LJ, Wilson P, Guest P, Catnach SM, McLean A, Wickham JE, Fairclough PD. Indomethacin and postprandial gallbladder emptying. Lancet. 1992;339(8788):269–71. https://doi.org/10.1016/0140-6736(92)91333-4.
22. Nightingale JM. The medical management of intestinal failure: methods to reduce the severity. Proc Nutr Soc. 2003;62(3):703–10. https://doi.org/10.1079/PNS2003283. PMID: 14692605

9 D-Lactate Encephalopathy in Patients with Short Bowel Syndrome

Liliana Mirea and Ioana Marina Grintescu

9.1 Introduction

The gut microbiota plays a crucial role in the production of both D-lactate and L-lactate. The balance between these enantiomers is determined by the presence of specific lactate dehydrogenases in the bacterial flora. Different bacterial species generate varying amounts of D- and L-lactate, influenced by their relative abundance and activity [1].

Some species of *Lactobacillus* produce an enzyme called racemase, which has the ability to convert one enantiomer into another. Racemases catalyze the reactions that reverse the chiral configuration of a compound, such as converting D-lactate into L-lactate and vice versa [1, 2].

For a long time, it was believed that humans could not metabolize D-lactate into pyruvate due to the lack of D-lactate dehydrogenase. However, recent research has identified the enzyme D-2-hydroxyacid dehydrogenase (found in the liver and kidneys), which can metabolize D-lactate. D-lactic acid can also be formed through the glyoxylate pathway by ingesting fermented foods (such as wine, beer, tomatoes, etc.) (Fig. 9.1) [3].

L. Mirea (✉) · I. M. Grintescu
Faculty of Medicine, Carol Davila University of Medicine and Pharmacy, Bucharest, Romania

Anesthesiology and Intensive Care Clinic, Clinical Emergency Hospital, Bucharest, Romania
e-mail: ioana.grintescu@rospen.ro

A. Trifan et al. (eds.), *Short Bowel Syndrome in Adults*,
https://doi.org/10.1007/978-3-031-95848-9_9

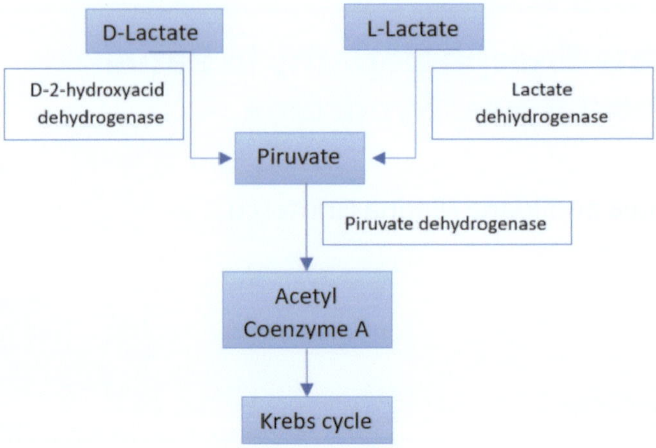

Fig. 9.1 Lactate metabolism

9.2 Pathophysiology

Short bowel syndrome is strongly linked with D-lactic acidosis. The precise mechanism of D-lactic acidosis in short bowel syndrome is not fully elucidated. The intestinal surface responsible for absorption is reduced, leading to an increased flow of undigested carbohydrates reaching the colon, where they undergo fermentation by the gut microbiota, generating organic acids, including short-chain fatty acids and lactate (Fig. 9.2) [4].

In a low pH environment, acid-resistant bacteria thrive, thereby perpetuating the cycle of acid production. *Lactobacillus* species (such as *Lactobacillus acidophilus*, *Lactobacillus fermentum*, *Lactobacillus plantarum*, and *Lactobacillus salivarius*) along with D-lactate-producing bifidobacteria are present in significant quantities in patients with short bowel syndrome. Research has indicated that there can be an increase of up to 60% in D-lactate-producing bacteria among these patients [1].

Organic acids generated during colonic fermentation can be divided into two groups: those that result in pyruvate as a metabolic byproduct (such as lactate and propionate) and those that do not (such as acetate and butyrate). The latter are converted into acetyl coenzyme A (acetyl-CoA) and subsequently oxidized into ketone bodies or fatty acids [3].

In the context of D-lactic acidosis, the presence of organic acids that do not generate pyruvate (such as acetate and butyrate) can impact the body's acid–base balance. Bacterial fermentation produces enantiomers of lactate and acetate, with acetate being essential for the formation of acetyl-CoA. Excessive production of acetyl-CoA initiates a negative feedback mechanism that reduces the activity of pyruvate dehydrogenase, the enzyme responsible for converting pyruvate into acetyl-CoA. As a result, this leads to an accumulation of pyruvate, which, through a similar negative feedback mechanism, decreases the activity of D-2-hydroxyacid dehydrogenase, ultimately causing a buildup of D-lactate (Fig. 9.3) [1–3].

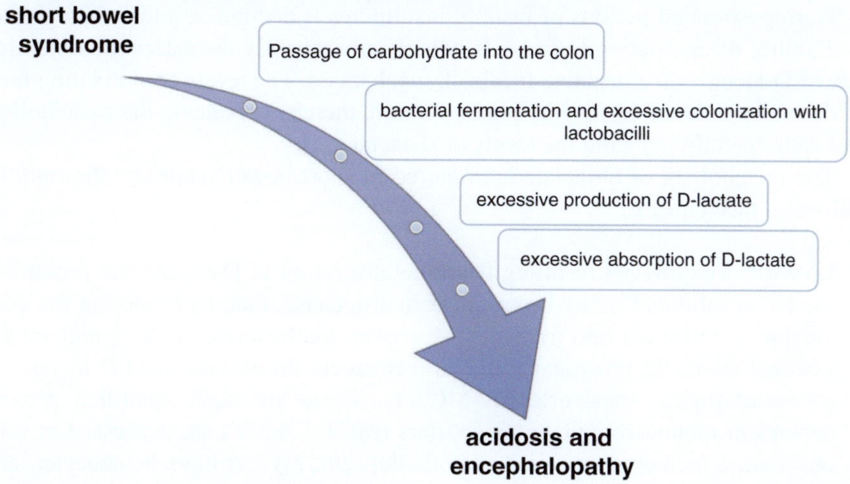

Fig. 9.2 D-lactic acidosis

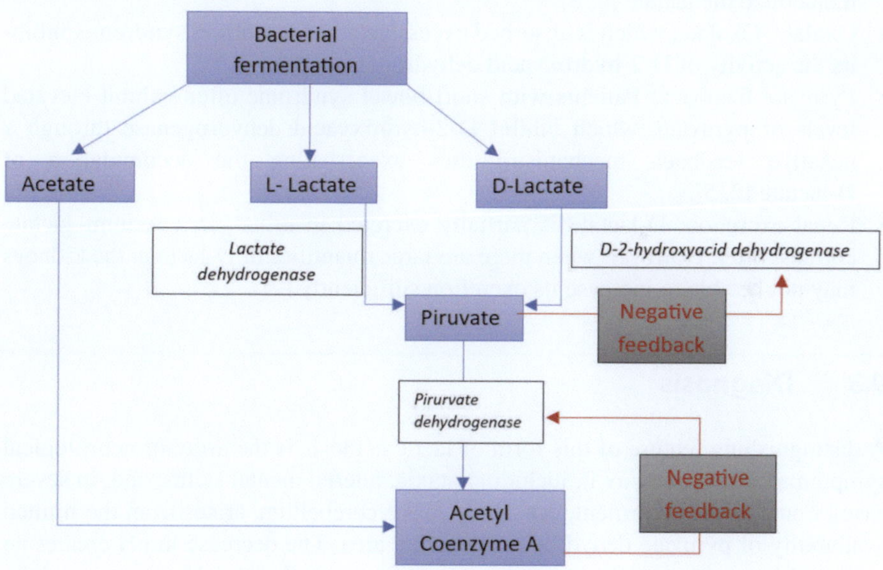

Fig. 9.3 D-lactate metabolism in short bowel syndrome

During extended periods of fasting, insulin levels decline, resulting in a greater availability of circulating fatty acids, which subsequently decreases the oxidation rate of D-lactate via a negative feedback mechanism. The levels of circulating fatty acids can be reduced by insulin administration, thereby enhancing their catabolism and consequently reducing the levels of D-lactate [3].

The metabolism of D-lactate is impaired in short bowel syndrome through the following mechanisms:

- Low pH: The low pH resulting from the absorption of D-lactate and protons in the colon inhibits D-2-hydroxyacid dehydrogenase, thereby hindering the conversion of D-lactate into pyruvate. Moreover, the formation of a significant pH gradient across the intestinal epithelium enhances the absorption of D-lactate via monocarboxylate transporter 1 (MCT-1). There are eight identified proton-dependent monocarboxylate transporters (MCTs). MCTs are expressed in various tissues, including the retina, endothelial cells, myocardium, hepatocytes, and nervous tissue [5].
- Activity of D-2-hydroxyacid dehydrogenase: Excessive production of D-lactate can cause the enzyme to become saturated, restricting its ability to effectively metabolize the lactate [2, 6].
- Oxalate: Oxalate, which is absorbed excessively in short bowel syndrome, inhibits the activity of D-2-hydroxyacid dehydrogenase [1].
- Pyruvate feedback: Patients with short bowel syndrome often exhibit elevated levels of pyruvate, which inhibit D-2-hydroxyacid dehydrogenase through a negative feedback mechanism, thus exacerbating the accumulation of D-lactate [2, 5].
- Renal excretion: D-lactate is partially excreted in urine via a sodium–lactate cotransporter. However, when there are large quantities of D-lactate, the kidneys may not be able to increase its excretion sufficiently [2].

9.3 Diagnosis

A distinguishing feature of this form of lactic acidosis is the array of neurological symptoms that accompany it, including ataxia, altered mental status, and, in severe cases, coma. The impairment, especially in the cerebellum, arises from the limited availability of pyruvate dehydrogenase in that area. The decrease in pH creates an unfavorable environment for enzymatic reactions, including those catalyzed by pyruvate dehydrogenase. Consequently, this leads to a reduced production of acetyl coenzyme A, which in turn disrupts neurotransmitter synthesis. Additionally, the organic acids produced in the colon may act as false neurotransmitters, resulting in severe neurological manifestations [1, 5, 7].

The diagnosis can be difficult to establish because measuring D-lactate levels in the blood requires specialized tests that are not commonly available in clinical practice. Therefore, clinicians should suspect D-lactic acidosis in patients with short bowel syndrome who exhibit neurological symptoms (such as dysarthria,

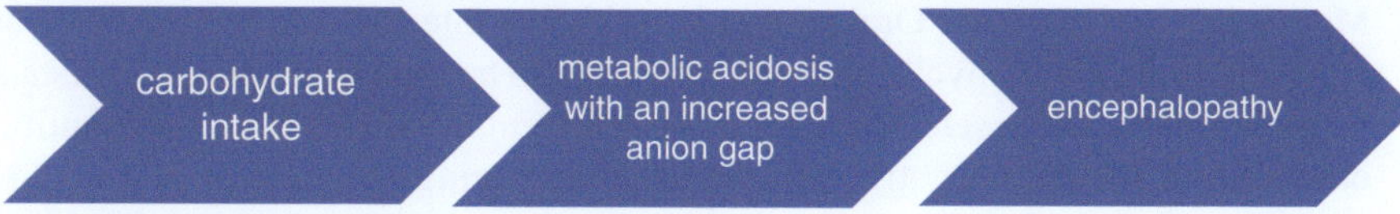

Fig. 9.4 D-lactic acidosis characteristics

ataxia, gait disturbances, headaches, and nystagmus) that typically arise after carbohydrate intake and can last from a few hours to several days (Fig. 9.4). These symptoms may even appear several years after the diagnosis of short bowel syndrome has been established. When serum D-lactate measurement is possible, a level of 3 mmol/L or higher confirms the diagnosis of D-lactic acidosis. However, it is worth noting that D-lactate levels do not always correlate with the clinical presentation [1, 2, 5].

The analysis of the acid–base profile indicates a metabolic acidosis with an elevated anion gap, characterized by a delta–delta ratio ranging from 1 to 2. It is noted that the rise in the anion gap is less than anticipated due to the more efficient renal excretion of D-lactate in comparison to L-lactate [1].

D-lactic acidosis exhibits distinct characteristics compared to L-lactic acidosis in terms of changes in the anion gap and serum bicarbonate levels. The increase in the anion gap observed in D-lactic acidosis tends to be disproportionately smaller than the decrease in serum bicarbonate concentration. This phenomenon can be explained by the more efficient urinary excretion of D-lactate [2]. Thus, D-lactic acidosis can lead to both metabolic acidosis with an increased anion gap and hyperchloremic metabolic acidosis. Additionally, an increase in urinary anion gap is observed. This context carries a risk of misdiagnosing renal tubular acidosis in patients presenting with hyperchloremic acidosis and an elevated urinary anion gap. In such cases, calculating the excretion of NH_4^+ using the urinary osmolarity gap will show higher values in D-lactic acidosis compared to renal tubular acidosis [1–3]. The loss of intestinal absorption capacity in short bowel syndrome results in various nutritional deficiencies, such as thiamine deficiency, which can lead to neurological symptoms, thereby contributing to the pathogenesis of D-lactic acidosis [3, 8].

Electroencephalogram monitoring in patients at risk of D-lactic acidosis can facilitate the early detection of encephalopathy and guide suitable interventions. However, it is important to note that the changes observed are nonspecific [1, 3].

9.4 Treatment

The treatment for D-lactic acidosis focuses on the following principles:

- Correction of metabolic acidosis: This includes rehydration, electrolyte replacement, and intravenous administration of sodium bicarbonate. Supplementing with calcium may be helpful in managing D-lactic acidosis, as it aids in increasing the intestinal pH [1, 5, 9].

- Modification of gut flora: Oral antibiotics with low intestinal absorption (such as metronidazole, clindamycin, and vancomycin) can be used to target acid-resistant bacteria and facilitate selective alteration of the gut flora. However, these antibiotics may also have negative effects by encouraging the growth of resistant organisms that produce D-lactate. Evidence supporting the use of probiotics is currently inconclusive [1, 3, 5, 7].
- Hemodialysis: In severe cases, hemodialysis may be employed to quickly remove D-lactate from the body [2, 8].
- Monitoring and correction of nutrient deficiencies: It is crucial to address any micro- and macronutrient deficiencies that often accompany short bowel syndrome [8].
- Surgical intervention: Surgical options may be considered to enhance intestinal function and can include procedures such as intestinal lengthening, bowel resection, colonic interposition, or small intestine transplantation [10].
- Other therapeutic approaches: Experimental strategies, still under investigation, include the use of bioengineered artificial intestines or fecal microbiota transplantation [11, 12].

References

1. Kowlgi NG, Chhabra L. D-lactic acidosis: an underrecognized complication of short bowel syndrome. Gastroenterol Res Pract. 2015;2015:1–8.
2. Remund B, Yılmaz B, Sokollik C. D-lactate: implications for gastrointestinal diseases. Children (Basel). 2023;10(6):945.
3. Vella A, Farrugia G. D-lactic acidosis: pathologic consequence of saprophytism. Mayo Clin Proc. 1998;73(5):451–6.
4. Khrais A, Ali H, Choi S, Ahmed A, Ahlawat S. D-lactic acidosis in short bowel syndrome. Cureus [Internet]. 2022; [cited 2025 Feb 18]; Available from: https://pmc.ncbi.nlm.nih.gov/articles/PMC9240996/
5. Kang KP, Lee S, Kang SK. D-lactic acidosis in humans: review of update. Electrolyte & Blood Press. 2006;4(1):53.
6. de Vrese M, Koppenhoefer B, Barth CA. D-lactic acid metabolism after an oral load of dl-lactate. Clin Nutr. 1990;9(1):23–8.
7. Planas-Vilaseca A, Guerrero-Pérez F, Marengo AP, Lopez-Urdiales R, Virgili-Casas N. D-lactic acidosis: a rare cause of metabolic acidosis. Endocrinología y Nutrición (English Edition). 2016;63(8):433–4.
8. Sobotka L. Basics in clinical nutrition. Prague: Galén; 2019.
9. Caldarini MI, Pons S, D'Agostino D, Depaula JA, Greco G, Negri G, et al. Abnormal fecal flora in a patient with short bowel syndrome. Dig Dis Sci. 1996;41(8):1649–52.
10. Iyer KR. Surgical management of short bowel syndrome. J Parenter Enter Nutr. 2014;38(1_suppl):53S59S.
11. Davidovics ZH, Vance K, Etienne N, Hyams JS. Fecal transplantation successfully treats recurrent D-lactic acidosis in a child with short bowel syndrome. J Parenter Enter Nutr. 2015;41(5):896–7.
12. Martin LY, Ladd MR, Werts A, Sodhi CP, March JC, Hackam DJ. Tissue engineering for the treatment of short bowel syndrome in children. Pediatr Res [Internet]. 2017;83(1–2):249–57. [cited 2019 Dec 10]. Available from: https://www.ncbi.nlm.nih.gov/pmc/articles/PMC6002962/

Metabolic Bone Disease in Short Bowel Syndrome: Diagnosis and Management

10

Ionuț Adrian Saizu and Liana Gheorghe

10.1 Introduction

Intestinal failure (IF) occurs when the gut can no longer maintain nutrition and hydration without external supplementation, and it is classified based on its duration [1]. Short bowel syndrome (SBS), the most common cause of chronic intestinal failure, results from a reduced absorptive area in the small intestine due to surgical resection (e.g., Crohn's disease, trauma, malignancy, radiation, or mesenteric ischemia), or congenital defects [1]. In adults, SBS is defined as having less than 200 cm of small bowel remaining, while in children it is defined as having less than 25% of the normal intestinal length for their age [2]. After resection, the remaining bowel undergoes adaptation—structural and functional changes that boost its absorptive capacity, a critical step toward regaining full intestinal function. Additionally, "functional SBS" describes cases where bowel function is impaired despite sufficient length (e.g., Crohn's disease or rapid intestinal transit) [1].

Metabolic bone disease (MBD) encompasses conditions characterized by a widespread reduction in bone density and strength. This decline in bone mineral density (BMD) leads to osteopenia, osteoporosis, or osteomalacia, conditions which can be linked to prolonged administration of parenteral nutrition (PN) in patients with IF. The bone turnover consists of the process whereby osteoclasts resorb old bone and osteoblasts form new tissue to repair and reinforce the structure against mechanical stress. The majority of remodeling is done by the trabecular bone (28%), and the process is regulated by factors such as parathyroid hormone (PTH), vitamin D, and the concentrations of calcium (Ca), magnesium (Mg), and phosphorus (P) [3].

I. A. Saizu (✉) · L. Gheorghe
Carol Davila University of Medicine and Pharmacy, Bucharest, Romania

Center for Digestive Diseases and Liver Transplant, Fundeni Clinical Institute, Bucharest, Romania

A. Trifan et al. (eds.), *Short Bowel Syndrome in Adults*,
https://doi.org/10.1007/978-3-031-95848-9_10

An estimated 40% to 100% of adults receiving long-term PN may develop some degree of bone demineralization, but the true incidence of MBD in both adult and pediatric patients with chronic intestinal failure remains unknown [5–7]. While the exact causes of PN-associated MBD remain unclear, traditional risk factors are the main reasons for MBD rather than IF. Female sex, older age, low sunlight exposure, physical inactivity, smoking and alcohol consumption, chronic inflammation (e.g., Crohn's disease), and use of corticosteroids or long-term anticoagulants are the general causes for MBD in patients with IF/PN. Vitamin and mineral deficiencies (e.g., vitamin D) are directly related with malabsorption. The presence of toxic contaminants in PN solutions, like acetate, which can lead to calcium loss in urine, or excessive sodium or amino acids, can lead as well to MBD [8].

MBD can develop as a complication in patients on long-term PN therapy, but as reported by longitudinal studies, this condition can affect even patients who never underwent PN. In this aspect, MBD is posing as a significant challenge for clinicians in managing patients with IF [9].

10.2 Etiopathogenesis

MBD in home parenteral nutrition (HPN) patients arises from multiple interrelated factors that contribute to bone demineralization, impaired remodeling, and increased fracture risk. Nutritional deficiencies and imbalances, parenteral nutrition-related factors, metabolic and endocrine disorders, underlying disease-related factors, and use of medication-induced bone loss (e.g., corticosteroids, long-term heparin use, and immunosuppressants) are considered mainstays in MBD pathophysiology.

10.2.1 Bone Disease and Calcium–Phosphorus Balance in Parenteral Nutrition

Calcium and phosphorus, essential for bone structure, are primarily stored in the skeleton, and their deficiency can cause bone erosion, impaired growth, and increased fracture risk, particularly in pediatric patients [4]. A negative calcium balance is a key factor in bone disease among HPN patients, resulting from insufficient calcium intake and increased urinary calcium loss, leading to bone demineralization and weakening [10, 11]. Ensuring adequate calcium and phosphorus supplementation in PN is challenging due to calcium–phosphate precipitation, influenced by high mineral concentrations, low amino acid levels, elevated temperatures, increased pH, and prolonged infusion times [4, 12–14]. This issue is particularly critical in neonates, who have higher mineral requirements but limited fluid intake, making precise PN formulation and solubility monitoring essential for maintaining bone health [4, 12, 15]. A Ca–P solubility curve is used to determine the maximum concentrations of calcium and phosphate that can be safely mixed in a parenteral nutrition (PN) solution without forming precipitates. By using solubility curves, clinical pharmacists and nutrition specialists can optimize PN composition, ensuring adequate calcium and phosphorus delivery while minimizing precipitation risks [4, 16].

10.2.2 Urinary Calcium Excretion and Hypercalciuria

Excessive protein intake in HPN increases urinary calcium excretion, leading to a negative calcium balance [17]. Studies indicate a dose-dependent relationship between amino acid intake and urinary calcium loss, showing that higher protein intake correlates with increased calcium excretion [18, 19]. Additionally, high-protein loads in PN solutions contribute to metabolic acidosis, which reduces renal calcium resorption, further exacerbating calcium loss and increasing the risk of bone demineralization [7, 18, 20].

HPN patients, known as cyclic PN patients, exhibit higher urinary calcium excretion, with levels increasing by up to 80% compared to those on continuous PN [21]. This effect is likely due to the rapid infusion rate of cyclic PN, which accelerates calcium filtration and excretion. However, the overall impact may be mitigated by reduced calcium losses during the hours when PN is not being administered.

10.2.3 Metabolic Acidosis and Bone Loss

Chronic metabolic acidosis in long-term HPN patients can disrupt vitamin D metabolism and compromise the bone buffering system, leading to MBD [4]. Conditions such as SBS, renal disease, and bacterial overgrowth can elevate D-lactic acid levels, further contributing to osteomalacia and an increased risk of fractures [22].

10.2.4 Aluminum Contamination

Aluminum toxicity disrupts bone metabolism by reducing PTH secretion and impairing vitamin D metabolism, which can lead to bone pain and fractures [23]. In the early 1980s, aluminum contamination in PN solutions was a significant cause of MBD and osteomalacia, particularly in infants [24, 25]. However, regulatory changes implemented since 2004 by the US Food and Drug Administration (FDA) have significantly reduced aluminum levels in PN formulations, leading to a decline in the prevalence of aluminum-related metabolic bone disease [26].

10.2.5 Vitamins D and K Deficiencies

Vitamin D plays a crucial role in calcium homeostasis by enhancing both intestinal absorption and renal reabsorption of calcium and phosphorus. It also plays a role in skeletal integrity by inducing osteoclast formation and bone resorption [27]. A deficiency in vitamin D can lead to osteomalacia in adults and rickets in children, particularly in individuals with malabsorption syndromes or liver and renal failure [28]. Otherwise, vitamin D requirements are minimal in HPN patients and seem to be not greater than the recommended dose for patients on a normal diet. Hypercalcemia can be caused by vitamin D toxicity, making this a concern in HPN patients. While excessive vitamin D supplementation in HPN has been linked to MBD, complete discontinuation is not recommended due to the risk of deficiency and its impact on bone metabolism [1, 4, 29].

Similarly, vitamin K is essential for osteocalcin, a key protein involved in bone mineralization. Deficiencies can arise from alteration of the colonic flora (e.g., antibiotic use), fat malabsorption, or PN dependency, leading to reduced BMD and an increased risk of fractures [30, 31].

10.2.6 Fluoride and MBD

Fluoride plays a complex role in bone metabolism, with effects that depend on dose, duration of exposure, and individual bone health status. At physiological levels, fluoride contributes to bone mineralization by stimulating osteoblast activity, potentially increasing bone mass and trabecular bone density [32]. Some studies suggest a positive correlation between fluoride exposure and lumbar spine BMD in HPN patients, likely due to its effect on trabecular bone formation [33]. However, excessive fluoride intake can lead to skeletal fluorosis, characterized by abnormal bone hardening, increased fragility, and impaired bone quality. High fluoride levels may also contribute to mineralization defects, reducing bone strength and increasing fracture risk, particularly in cortical bone such as the femoral neck [34].

10.2.7 Medications and Bone Disease

Certain medications significantly impact bone health by disrupting bone formation, calcium metabolism, and mineral density. Corticosteroids (e.g., prednisone) suppress osteoblast activity, decrease calcium absorption, and increase urinary calcium excretion, leading to bone loss and increased fracture risk [35, 36]. Additionally, the long-term use of warfarin has been linked to reduced BMD, particularly in children [37–39].

Other drugs, including methotrexate, cyclosporine, and heparin, have been associated with osteopenia, further compromising bone strength [40–42].

10.2.8 Concomitant Diseases and Bone Health

Patients requiring PN due to conditions such as inflammatory bowel disease (IBD), cancer, and malabsorption disorders face an increased risk of bone disease. Individuals with IBD are particularly vulnerable to higher fracture rates, often resulting from malnutrition, chronic inflammation, and prolonged corticosteroid use. Malabsorption disorders, including Crohn's disease, celiac disease, and short bowel syndrome, further contribute to calcium and vitamin D deficiencies, leading to bone demineralization and increased fracture susceptibility [43–49].

10.3 Clinical Presentation

MBD is a significant concern for patients receiving prolonged parenteral nutrition (PN), as it can lead to osteomalacia, osteopenia, or osteoporosis. Proper monitoring and management strategies, including nutritional optimization and supplementation, are essential to mitigate these effects and maintain bone health.

Osteomalacia is a condition characterized by the softening of bones due to defective bone mineralization of the newly formed organic matrix, usually caused by a deficiency of vitamin D, calcium, or phosphate. Most patients are asymptomatic, but osteomalacia can lead to bone pain and muscle weakness. In adults, osteomalacia is the equivalent of rickets in children [28].

Osteopenia is a disorder characterized by lower-than-normal bone mineral density (BMD), but not low enough to be classified as osteoporosis. The decrease in bone mineralization reduces bone mass, leading to osteopenia. It indicates weakened bones with an increased risk of fractures but is often asymptomatic. Osteoporosis is characterized by decreased bone mineral density (BMD) and deterioration of the normal architecture of bone, leading to increased bone fragility and a higher risk of atraumatic fractures [4, 50, 51].

MBD in long-term PN can present as asymptomatic, bone pain (mainly in the spine and lower joints), or fractures with minimal trauma or even atraumatic. Pironi et al. highlighted that 33% of these patients exhibited MBD in the spine and hip regions, 50% in the femoral neck, and 24% had experienced previous fractures. Additionally, a significant negative correlation was found between the duration of HPN and bone mineral density (BMD), indicating that longer HPN duration is associated with lower BMD [6].

A crucial point is that biochemical markers of bone metabolism may either appear normal or display only slight abnormalities, so early detection can be cumbersome. The laboratory results—including hypercalcemia, hypocalcemia, hypercalciuria, normal 25-hydroxyvitamin D with low 1,25-dihydroxyvitamin D, elevated alkaline phosphatase, and low to normal PTH—suggest disruptions in calcium and vitamin D metabolism.

10.4 Diagnosis

The diagnosis of MBD in patients receiving long-term HPN should be based on a combination of bone densitometry scanning and biochemical assessments [29, 52, 53].

Given the increased risk of osteoporosis and bone fragility, it is crucial to identify and address general risk factors that may negatively impact bone health. These include chronic inflammation, infections, medication effects, and other underlying disease-related factors. By proactively managing these risks, the progression of bone deterioration can be minimized. In this aspect, regular screening and monitoring should be integrated into the care plan for all HPN patients, with periodic bone densitometry scans and biochemical evaluations [1, 29, 52, 53]. This comprehensive approach supports early intervention, prevention of complications, and improved long-term bone health in this vulnerable population.

Dual-energy X-ray absorptiometry (DEXA) is used to assess the advancement of MBD by diagnosing osteopenia and osteoporosis. DEXA is considered the gold standard for bone mineral density (BMD) assessment due to its high precision, speed, and reliability, making it essential for both diagnosis and follow-up in metabolic bone disease management. DEXA operates by using two X-ray beams at different energy levels to differentiate between bone and soft tissue. The system measures the attenuation of each beam as it passes through the body, allowing for precise calculation of bone mineral density. Low-energy X-rays are absorbed more by bone, while high-energy X-rays penetrate soft tissues. The difference in X-ray absorption is used to quantify bone mineral content (g/cm^2). DEXA is a low-radiation dose procedure and does not require contrast agents, making it safe for repeated assessments [54–57]. The low-dose radiations are used to determine BMD of the lumbar spine, femoral neck, and radius [58].

BMD of an individual is compared to a reference group of young, gender-matched adults. Deviations from the reference mean are expressed in standard deviations (SDs), known as the T-score (mean BMD value of young adult reference mean) or Z-score (mean BMD value of age-, sex-, and ethnicity-matched healthy control), which is used to classify osteoporosis and fracture risk [8]. The T-score in DEXA compares an individual's bone mineral density (BMD) to that of a young, healthy adult, helping diagnose osteoporosis and fracture risk, while the Z-score compares BMD to age-matched peers, identifying abnormal bone loss and potential secondary causes of osteoporosis, especially in younger individuals [59]. According to the World Health Organization (WHO), DEXA can differentiate normal tissue, osteopenia, and osteoporosis using the T-score. A T-score of ≥ -1 SD is considered normal, a T-score between -1 and -2.5 SDs indicates osteopenia, and a T-score of ≤ -2.5 SDs is diagnostic of osteoporosis [4, 60]. According to the European Society for Clinical Nutrition and Metabolism (ESPEN), BMD should be measured at starting HPN and then yearly [1, 29]. For individuals with normal DEXA scan results, follow-up assessments are typically conducted every 1 to 3 years to monitor bone health [4, 60]. The risk of fractures increases significantly with decreasing BMD, with studies estimating a 1.4 to 1.6 times higher fracture risk for every 1 SD reduction in BMD Z-score [61]. Pironi et al., in a in a cross-sectional multicenter study, showed that the BMD Z-score appeared predictive of fracture risk, and factors such as age at HPN initiation and BMI were major factors associated with BMD Z-scores [6].

The biochemical evaluation of metabolic bone disease (Table 10.1) involves measuring, every 4 months, serum levels of key minerals such as calcium (Ca), phosphorus (P), and magnesium (Mg), along with the optional assessment of their

Table 10.1 Diagnosis and monitoring protocol for metabolic bone disease in patients on home parenteral nutrition for chronic intestinal failure

Bone mineral density (DEXA)	At starting HPN, then yearly
Serum Ca, Mg, P	Every 4 months; additional as per clinical need
Urinary Ca, Mg, P	Every 4 months; additional as per clinical need
Serum 25-hydroxyvitamin D, PTH, bone turnover markers	Yearly; additional as per clinical need
Serum 1,25-dihydroxyvitamin D	If vitamin D toxicity is suspected
Serum aluminum and micronutrients	If clinical suspicion
Bone biopsy (+/− double tetracycline labeling)	For differential diagnosis of osteomalacia and osteoporosis

Abbreviations: *DEXA* dual-energy X-ray absorptiometry, *PTH* parathyroid hormone, *HPN* home parenteral nutrition

24-h urinary excretion [29, 62, 63]. Additionally, every 12 months, it includes serum and/or urinary markers of bone turnover, such as bone formation markers—osteocalcin, bone-specific alkaline phosphatase (BSAP), and procollagen type I N-terminal propeptide (P1NP)—and bone resorption markers—C-terminal telopeptide of type I collagen (CTX) and N-terminal telopeptide (NTX) [29, 64]. Furthermore, it assesses plasma concentrations of parathyroid hormone (PTH), 25-hydroxyvitamin D, yearly, and, if necessary, 1,25-dihydroxyvitamin D, when vitamin D toxicity is suspected [29]. Monitoring serum fluoride levels is essential to prevent excess accumulation, which may exacerbate MBD or lead to fluorosis-related complications [21, 32].

According to ESPEN, patients with MBD due to HPN should follow preventive strategies similar to those recommended for the general population. Additionally, it is essential to address underlying disease-related factors, such as infections and chronic inflammation, to minimize bone deterioration and maintain overall metabolic stability [29].

Moreover, biological tests for concomitant diseases (e.g., Crohn's disease, celiac disease, etc.) should always be considered in order to evaluate their activity status or the response to treatment. Addressing underlying disease-related factors, such as infections and chronic/acute inflammation, is essential for managing overall health and preventing complications.

A tetracycline-labeled bone biopsy is a specialized technique used to evaluate bone metabolism and mineralization. It involves a minimally invasive technique using a cannulated drill to obtain iliac crest bone samples. Similarly, it requires administering tetracycline antibiotics, which bind to newly forming bone and fluoresce under ultraviolet (UV) light, allowing for the evaluation of bone turnover and mineralization rates. The procedure includes administering two doses of tetracycline, followed by a bone biopsy from the iliac crest. Under fluorescence microscopy, tetracycline appears as fluorescent bands, with the spacing between them indicating bone formation rates. This method is particularly useful in diagnosing osteoporosis, osteomalacia, renal osteodystrophy, and other metabolic bone diseases [65].

Colazo et al. concluded that tetracycline-labeled bone biopsies are underutilized in diagnosing metabolic bone diseases. The procedure, which involves a minimally invasive technique using a cannulated drill to obtain iliac crest bone samples, was found to be well tolerated with minimal complications. The biopsies provided high-quality specimens that facilitated accurate histological diagnoses, leading to treatment modifications in the majority of cases. Patients who underwent biopsy-guided treatment adjustments demonstrated significant improvements in bone mineral density (BMD) as measured by dual-energy X-ray absorptiometry (DEXA), following the intervention. The authors advocate for the inclusion of tetracycline-labeled bone biopsies in the diagnostic and therapeutic management of select patients with metabolic bone diseases, despite advancements in noninvasive imaging and biomarker analysis.

Although invasive, it provides direct histological evidence of bone health and is more precise than serum biomarkers in detecting subtle metabolic bone disorders. It is primarily used when standard imaging or biochemical markers are inconclusive, helping to refine diagnoses and treatment strategies for patients with unexplained fractures or complex bone diseases [8] (Table 10.1).

10.5 Treatment

The management of bone metabolic disease in patients on HPN is determined by etiopathogenesis and includes general and lifestyle recommendations, addressing underlying causes, optimizing nutrition, and medical treatment.

10.5.1 General and Lifestyle Recommendations

To promote optimal bone health, it is advisable to engage in regular low-impact physical exercise. Ensuring adequate exposure to sunlight is important as well, as it facilitates production of vitamin D. In areas with limited sunlight, the use of UVB-emitting devices might be considered to maintain sufficient vitamin D levels. Maintaining a balanced diet rich in protein and calories supports overall nutritional status, which is vital for bone maintenance.

Incorporating dairy products into the diet can provide a good source of calcium. Additionally, it is recommended to cease cigarette smoking and limit alcohol consumption, as these habits can negatively impact bone density. For women in the perimenopausal and postmenopausal stages, estrogen replacement therapy may be beneficial in preserving bone mass—leading to a significant reduction in vertebral and nonvertebral fractures [66]. However, careful consideration should be given, especially to those with an increased risk of venous thrombosis [67].

10.5.2 Optimizing Parenteral Nutrition Formula

The ESPEN practical guidelines for clinical nutrition in chronic intestinal failure recommend, as a first step in treating BMD, to optimize the parenteral nutrition regimens by ensuring adequate supplementation of vitamin D, calcium, and phosphate [68]. The usual dose of vitamin D (e.g., cholecalciferol and ergocalciferol) added in PN formula for adult patients with intestinal failure is 200 IU/d, while doses for children are higher ranging up to 400 IU/d [4]. Thompson et al. found that 68% of patients with HPN were deficient, and 27% were insufficient in vitamin D levels, recommending vitamin supplementation in all these patients, but close monitoring is advised due to its toxicity risk. Studies reported corrections of hypercalcemia, hypercalciuria, and osteomalacia following the withdrawal of vitamin D [9, 69–71]. Adequate calcium (10–15 mmol/day) and phosphorus (10–40 mmol/day) should be included in PN to prevent deficiency and maintain bone mineralization. The Ca–P solubility curve helps determine the maximum safe concentrations of calcium and phosphate in PN to prevent precipitation [4, 16]. Vitamin K is included routinely as well in PN at a daily dose of 150 μg through intravenous (IV) multivitamin preparations [72, 73]. Aluminum levels within PN solution should be less than 25 μg/L according to FDA amendment. Protein levels of PN admixtures should not exceed 1.5 g/kg/d to avoid metabolic acidosis and hypercalciuria, and acetate amount should be adjusted as well to maintain normal serum bicarbonate [4]. Other PN-related factors that should be taken into account are fluid volume to maintain fluid balance, infusion rate (i.e., slow perfusion rate may reduce hypercalciuria), and sodium levels (i.e., hypercalciuria may be induced by high levels of urinary sodium) [8].

The ESPEN guidelines advocate for a timely management of general risk factors for osteoporosis, along with addressing potential negative influences on bone health, such as chronic inflammation, infections, medications, other disease-related factors, and prevention and treatment of metabolic acidosis, in all patients receiving long-term HPN [68]. Oral supplementation of calcium and magnesium plays a supportive role, being essential for bone mineralization, preventing osteoporosis and fracture risk. For adults, oral calcium supplementation typically ranges from 1000 to 1500 mg per day, especially when PN calcium content is insufficient, while oral magnesium supplementation often ranges from 300 to 600 mg per day or 12–24 mmol/day, depending on the individual's deficiency status [8, 74].

10.5.3 Pharmacologic Treatment

The aim of pharmacologic treatment of BMD in patients with HPN is to reduce the incidence of fracture (e.g., hip and spine).

Bisphosphonates, such as zoledronic acid and alendronate, are effective antiresorptive agents commonly used in osteoporosis patients at high risk of fractures. However, long-term use requires careful monitoring to prevent adynamic bone disease. Antiresorptive agents' mechanism is based on modifying calcium metabolism, inhibiting osteoclast action by reducing recruitment of osteoclast precursor, inducing apoptosis of osteoclasts, and inhibiting bone marrow cell differentiation [75, 76]. The effects of these actions are represented by bone strength improvements, preservation of bone structure, and prevention of additional bone loss. Most bisphosphonates are taken orally.

However, patients with SBS and HPN experience poor intestinal absorption due to intestinal failure and malabsorption. In this aspect, medications like clodronate and pamidronate, which are IV forms of antiresorptive agents, are the therapeutic options in patients with intestinal failure and HPN. Pamidronate IV improves the T-score of spine, hip, and lumbar sacral DEXA [77–79]. Bisphosphonates effectively treat bone loss but can have side effects that require monitoring.

Common issues include gastrointestinal discomfort, such as heartburn, dyspepsia, and even mucosal injury [80]. Osteonecrosis of the jaw (ONJ) is a rare but serious complication, mainly in cancer patients receiving high doses [81]. Long-term use may also lead to atypical femur fractures with minimal trauma. Hypocalcemia is another concern, requiring calcium and vitamin D supplementation. Some patients, particularly those on intravenous bisphosphonates, may experience flu-like symptoms such as fever and muscle pain. Additionally, high-dose intravenous therapy can affect kidney function, requiring caution in those with renal disease [82].

PTH analogs, like teriparatide, a subcutaneously administered anabolic agent, are beneficial for treating low bone turnover osteoporosis, particularly in cases that do not respond to bisphosphonates [83]. Denosumab, a receptor activator of nuclear factor kappa-B ligand (RANKL) inhibitor, is another option for severe osteoporosis, but ensuring adequate calcium and vitamin D levels is crucial to prevent hypocalcemia. Denosumab is an effective treatment for minimizing bone loss, particularly in cancer patients. Its subcutaneous administration offers convenience, and it lacks renal toxicity or acute-phase reactions [84].

10.6 Conclusion

MBD is a common complication in chronic intestinal failure, especially in patients on long-term home parenteral nutrition HPN. It results from nutritional deficiencies, PN-related factors, metabolic disturbances, comorbidities, and certain medications, leading to osteopenia, osteoporosis, or osteomalacia.

Diagnosis combines regular DEXA with biochemical monitoring, and sometimes bone biopsy. Management includes lifestyle measures, optimizing PN composition, correcting metabolic imbalances, and using pharmacologic treatments such as bisphosphonates, PTH analogues, or denosumab.

A proactive, individualized strategy is essential to prevent fractures, maintain bone strength, and improve long-term outcomes.

References

1. Pironi L, Arends J, Baxter J, et al. ESPEN endorsed recommendations. Definition and classification of intestinal failure in adults. Clin Nutr. 2015;34(2):171–80. https://doi.org/10.1016/j.clnu.2014.08.017.
2. Merritt RJ, Cohran V, Raphael BP, et al. Intestinal rehabilitation programs in the Management of Pediatric Intestinal Failure and Short Bowel Syndrome. J Pediatr Gastroenterol Nutr. 2017;65(5):588–96. https://doi.org/10.1097/MPG.0000000000001722.
3. Manolagas SC. Corticosteroids and fractures: a close encounter of the third cell kind. J Bone Miner Res. 2000;15(6):1001–5. https://doi.org/10.1359/jbmr.2000.15.6.1001.
4. Ferrone M, Geraci M. A review of the relationship between parenteral nutrition and metabolic bone disease. Nutr Clin Pract. 2007;22(3):329–39. https://doi.org/10.1177/0115426507022003329.
5. Cohen-Solal M, Baudoin C, Joly F, et al. Osteoporosis in patients on long-term home parenteral nutrition: a longitudinal study. J Bone Miner Res. 2003;18(11):1989–94. https://doi.org/10.1359/jbmr.2003.18.11.1989.
6. Pironi L, Morselli Labate AM, Pertkiewicz M, et al. Prevalence of bone disease in patients on home parenteral nutrition. Clin Nutr. 2002;21(4):289–96. https://doi.org/10.1054/clnu.2002.0548.
7. Hurley DL, McMahon MM. Long-term parenteral nutrition and metabolic bone disease. Endocrinol Metab Clin N Am. 1990;19(1):113–31.
8. Pironi L, Sasdelli AS. Bone and joint disease. In: Intestinal failure. Springer; 2023. p. 425–33. https://doi.org/10.1007/978-3-031-22265-8_28.
9. Shike M, Harrison JE, Sturtridge WC, et al. Metabolic bone disease in patients receiving long-term total parenteral nutrition. Ann Intern Med. 1980;92(3):343–50. https://doi.org/10.7326/0003-4819-92-3-343.
10. Koo WW, Sherman R, Succop P, et al. Fractures and rickets in very low birth weight infants: conservative management and outcome. J Pediatr Orthop. 1989;9(3):326–30.
11. Koo WWK, Tsang RC, Succop P, Krug-Wispe SK, Babcock D, Oestreich AE. Minimal vitamin D and high calcium and phosphorus needs of preterm infants receiving parenteral nutrition. J Pediatr Gastroenterol Nutr. 1989;8(2):225–33. https://doi.org/10.1097/00005176-198902000-00017.
12. Dunham B, Marcuard S, Khazanie PG, Meade G, Craft T, Nichols K. The solubility of calcium and phosphorus in neonatal total parenteral nutrition solutions. J Parenter Enter Nutr. 1991;15(6):608–11. https://doi.org/10.1177/0148607191015006608.
13. Poole RL, Rupp CA, Kerner JA. Calcium and phosphorus in neonatal parenteral nutrition solutions. J Parenter Enter Nutr. 1983;7(4):358–60. https://doi.org/10.1177/0148607183007004358.
14. Niemiec PW, Vanderveen TW. Compatibility considerations in parenteral nutrient solutions. Am J Hosp Pharm. 1984;41(5):893–911.
15. Fitzgerald KA, MacKay MW. Calcium and phosphate solubility in neonatal parenteral nutrient solutions containing TrophAmine. Am J Hosp Pharm. 1986;43(1):88–93.
16. Anderson C, Eggert L, Fitzgerald K, Jackson D, Farr F. Calcium and phosphate solubility curve equation for determining precipitation limits in compounding parenteral nutrition. Hosp Pharm. 2022;57(6):779–85. https://doi.org/10.1177/00185787221104367.
17. Kim Y, Linkswiler HM. Effect of level of protein intake on calcium metabolism and on parathyroid and renal function in the adult human male. J Nutr. 1979;109(8):1399–404. https://doi.org/10.1093/jn/109.8.1399.
18. De Vernejoul MC, Messing B, Modrowski D, Bielakoff J, Buisine A, Miravet L. Multifactorial low remodeling bone disease during cyclic total parenteral nutrition. J Clin Endocrinol Metab. 1985;60(1):109–13. https://doi.org/10.1210/jcem-60-1-109.
19. Bengoa J, Sitrin M, Wood R, Rosenberg I. Amino acid-induced hypercalciuria in patients on total parenteral nutrition. Am J Clin Nutr. 1983;38(2):264–9. https://doi.org/10.1093/ajcn/38.2.264.

20. Goodman AD, Lemann J, Lennon EJ, Relman AS. Production, excretion, and net balance of fixed acid in patients with renal acidosis*. J Clin Invest. 1965;44(4):495–506. https://doi.org/10.1172/JCI105163.
21. Wood R, Bengoa J, Sitrin M, Rosenberg I. Calciuretic effect of cyclic versus continuous total parenteral nutrition. Am J Clin Nutr. 1985;41(3):614–9. https://doi.org/10.1093/ajcn/41.3.614.
22. Karton MA, Rettmer R, Lipkin EW, Ott SM, Chait A. D-lactate and metabolic bone disease in patients receiving long-term parenteral nutrition. JPEN J Parenter Enteral Nutr. 1989;13(2):132–5. https://doi.org/10.1177/0148607189013002132.
23. Goodman WG, Henry DA, Horst R, Nudelman RK, Alfrey AC, Coburn JW. Parenteral aluminum administration in the dog: II. Induction of osteomalacia and effect on vitamin D metabolism. Kidney Int. 1984;25(2):370–5. https://doi.org/10.1038/ki.1984.26.
24. Ott SM, Maloney NA, Klein GL, et al. Aluminum is associated with low bone formation in patients receiving chronic parenteral nutrition. Ann Intern Med. 1983;98(6):910–4. https://doi.org/10.7326/0003-4819-98-6-910.
25. Klein G, Alfrey A, Miller N, et al. Aluminum loading during total parenteral nutrition. Am J Clin Nutr. 1982;35(6):1425–9. https://doi.org/10.1093/ajcn/35.6.1425.
26. Willhite CC, Karyakina NA, Yokel RA, et al. Systematic review of potential health risks posed by pharmaceutical, occupational and consumer exposures to metallic and nanoscale aluminum, aluminum oxides, aluminum hydroxide and its soluble salts. Crit Rev Toxicol. 2014;44(sup4):1–80. https://doi.org/10.3109/10408444.2014.934439.
27. Bar-Shavit Z, Teitelbaum SL, Reitsma P, et al. Induction of monocytic differentiation and bone resorption by 1,25-dihydroxyvitamin D3. Proc Natl Acad Sci. 1983;80(19):5907–11. https://doi.org/10.1073/pnas.80.19.5907.
28. Driscoll RH, Meredith SC, Sitrin M, Rosenberg IH. Vitamin D deficiency and bone disease in patients with Crohn's disease. Gastroenterology. 1982;83(6):1252–8.
29. Cuerda C, Pironi L, Arends J, et al. ESPEN practical guideline: clinical nutrition in chronic intestinal failure. Clin Nutr. 2021;40(9):5196–220. https://doi.org/10.1016/j.clnu.2021.07.002.
30. Maillard C, Berruyer M, Serre CM, Dechavanne M, Delmas PD. Protein-S, a vitamin K-dependent protein, is a bone matrix component synthesized and secreted by osteoblasts. Endocrinology. 1992;130(3):1599–604. https://doi.org/10.1210/endo.130.3.1531628.
31. Conly JM, Stein K, Worobetz L, Rutledge-Harding S. The contribution of vitamin K2 (menaquinones) produced by the intestinal microflora to human nutritional requirements for vitamin K. Am J Gastroenterol. 1994;89(6):915–23.
32. Nielsen FH. Micronutrients in parenteral nutrition: boron, silicon, and fluoride. Gastroenterology. 2009;137(5):S55–60. https://doi.org/10.1053/j.gastro.2009.07.072.
33. Hallanger Johnson JE, Kearns AE, Doran PM, Khoo TK, Wermers RA. Fluoride-related bone disease associated with habitual tea consumption. Mayo Clin Proc. 2007;82(6):719–24.
34. Nagendra L, Kapoor N, Bhattacharya S Metabolic bone disease in the tropics. .; 2000.
35. Reid IR, Ibbertson HK. Evidence for decreased tubular reabsorption of calcium in glucocorticoid-treated asthmatics. Horm Res. 1987;27(4):200–4. https://doi.org/10.1159/000180820.
36. LoCascio V, Bonucci E, Imbimbo B, et al. Bone loss in response to long-term glucocorticoid therapy. Bone Miner. 1990;8(1):39–51. https://doi.org/10.1016/0169-6009(91)90139-q.
37. Rosen HN, Maitland LA, Suttie JW, Manning WJ, Glynn RJ, Greenspan SL. Vitamin K and maintenance of skeletal integrity in adults. Am J Med. 1993;94(1):62–8. https://doi.org/10.1016/0002-9343(93)90121-5.
38. Pauli RM, Lian JB, Mosher DF, Suttie JW. Association of congenital deficiency of multiple vitamin K-dependent coagulation factors and the phenotype of the warfarin embryopathy: clues to the mechanism of teratogenicity of coumarin derivatives. Am J Hum Genet. 1987;41(4):566–83.
39. Fiore CE, Tamburino C, Foti R, Grimaldi D. Reduced axial bone mineral content in patients taking an oral anticoagulant. South Med J. 1990;83(5):538–42. https://doi.org/10.1097/00007611-199005000-00013.

40. Cvetkovic M, Mann GN, Romero DF, et al. The deleterious effects of long-term cyclosporine a, cyclosporine G, and FK506 on bone mineral metabolism in vivo. Transplantation. 1994;57(8):1231–7. https://doi.org/10.1097/00007890-199404270-00016.
41. Sambrook PN, Kelly PJ, Keogh AM, et al. Bone loss after heart transplantation: a prospective study. J Heart Lung Transplant. 1994;13(1 Pt 1):116–20. discussion 121
42. Gnudi S, Butturini L, Ripamonti C, Avella M, Bacci G. The effects of methotrexate (MTX) on bone. A densitometric study conducted on 59 patients with MTX administered at different doses. Ital J Orthop Traumatol. 1988;14(2):227–31.
43. Silvennoinen JA, Karttunen TJ, Niemela SE, Manelius JJ, Lehtola JK. A controlled study of bone mineral density in patients with inflammatory bowel disease. Gut. 1995;37(1):71–6. https://doi.org/10.1136/gut.37.1.71.
44. Compston J. Osteoporosis in inflammatory bowel disease. Gut. 2003;52(1):63–4. https://doi.org/10.1136/gut.52.1.63.
45. Bregni G, Beck B. Toward targeted therapies in Oesophageal cancers: an overview. Cancers (Basel). 2022;14(6) https://doi.org/10.3390/cancers14061522.
46. Schoon EJ, Blok BM, Geerling BJ, Russel MG, Stockbrügger RW, Brummer RM. Bone mineral density in patients with recently diagnosed inflammatory bowel disease. Gastroenterology. 2000;119(5):1203–8. https://doi.org/10.1053/gast.2000.19280.
47. Mazure R, Vazquez H, Gonzalez D, et al. Bone mineral affection in asymptomatic adult patients with celiac disease. Am J Gastroenterol. 1994;89(12):2130–4.
48. Vestergaard P. Fracture risk in patients with celiac disease, Crohn's disease, and ulcerative colitis: a Nationwide follow-up study of 16,416 patients in Denmark. Am J Epidemiol. 2002;156(1):1–10. https://doi.org/10.1093/aje/kwf007.
49. Kärnsund S, Lo B, Bendtsen F, Holm J, Burisch J. Systematic review of the prevalence and development of osteoporosis or low bone mineral density and its risk factors in patients with inflammatory bowel disease. World J Gastroenterol. 2020;26(35):5362–74. https://doi.org/10.3748/wjg.v26.i35.5362.
50. Seidner DL. Parenteral nutrition-associated metabolic bone disease. J Parenter Enter Nutr. 2002;26(5S):S37. https://doi.org/10.1177/014860710202600511.
51. Griscom NT, Jaramillo D. "Osteoporosis," "Osteomalacia," and "Osteopenia.". Am J Roentgenol. 2000;175(1):268–9. https://doi.org/10.2214/ajr.175.1.1750268b.
52. Diamanti A, Bizzarri C, Basso MS, et al. How does long-term parenteral nutrition impact the bone mineral status of children with intestinal failure? J Bone Miner Metab. 2010;28(3):351–8. https://doi.org/10.1007/s00774-009-0140-0.
53. Siepler J. Principles and strategies for monitoring home parenteral nutrition. Nutr Clin Pract. 2007;22(3):340–50. https://doi.org/10.1177/0115426507022003340.
54. Messina C, Albano D, Gitto S, et al. Body composition with dual energy X-ray absorptiometry: from basics to new tools. Quant Imaging Med Surg. 2020;10(8):1687–98. https://doi.org/10.21037/qims.2020.03.02.
55. Blake GM, Fogelman I. Dual energy X-ray absorptiometry and its clinical applications. Semin Musculoskelet Radiol. 2002;06(3):207–18. https://doi.org/10.1055/s-2002-36718.
56. DeVita MV, Stall SH. Dual-energy X-ray absorptiometry: a review. J Ren Nutr. 1999;9(4):178–81. https://doi.org/10.1016/S1051-2276(99)90030-4.
57. Blake GM, Fogelman I. Technical principles of dual energy X-ray absorptiometry. Semin Nucl Med. 1997;27(3):210–28. https://doi.org/10.1016/S0001-2998(97)80025-6.
58. Lipkin EW. Metabolic bone disease in the long-term parenteral nutrition patient. Clin Nutr. 1995;14:65–9. https://doi.org/10.1016/S0261-5614(95)80287-8.
59. Sheu A, Diamond T. Diagnostic tests: bone mineral density: testing for osteoporosis. Aust Prescr. 2016;39(2):35–9. https://doi.org/10.18773/austprescr.2016.020.
60. Kanis JA, Kanis JA. Assessment of fracture risk and its application to screening for postmenopausal osteoporosis: synopsis of a WHO report. Osteoporos Int. 1994;4(6):368–81. https://doi.org/10.1007/BF01622200.
61. Kanis JA. Diagnosis of osteoporosis and assessment of fracture risk. Lancet. 2002;359(9321):1929–36. https://doi.org/10.1016/S0140-6736(02)08761-5.

62. Seibel MJ. Biochemical markers of bone turnover: part I: biochemistry and variability. Clin Biochem Rev. 2005;26(4):97–122.
63. Romero Barco CM, Manrique Arija S, Rodríguez PM. Biochemical markers in osteoporosis: usefulness in clinical practice. Reumatología Clínica (English Edition). 2012;8(3):149–52. https://doi.org/10.1016/j.reumae.2011.05.004.
64. Hlaing TT, Compston JE. Biochemical markers of bone turnover—uses and limitations. Ann Clin Biochem: Int J Lab Med. 2014;51(2):189–202. https://doi.org/10.1177/0004563213515190.
65. Colazo JM, Quirion J, Judice AD, et al. Utility of iliac crest tetracycline-labelled bone biopsy in osteoporosis and metabolic bone disease: an evaluation of 95 cases over a period of 25 years. Bone Rep. 2023;19:101715. https://doi.org/10.1016/j.bonr.2023.101715.
66. Gambacciani M, Levancini M. Featured editorial hormone replacement therapy and the prevention of postmenopausal osteoporosis. Menopausal Review. 2014;4:213–20. https://doi.org/10.5114/pm.2014.44996.
67. Abou-Ismail MY, Citla Sridhar D, Nayak L. Estrogen and thrombosis: a bench to bedside review. Thromb Res. 2020;192:40–51. https://doi.org/10.1016/j.thromres.2020.05.008.
68. Pironi L, Arends J, Bozzetti F, et al. ESPEN guidelines on chronic intestinal failure in adults. Clin Nutr. 2016;35(2):247–307. https://doi.org/10.1016/j.clnu.2016.01.020.
69. Shike M, Sturtridge WC, Tam CS, et al. A possible role of vitamin D in the genesis of parenteral-nutrition-induced metabolic bone disease. Ann Intern Med. 1981;95(5):560–8. https://doi.org/10.7326/0003-4819-95-5-560.
70. Verhage AH, Cheong WK, Allard JP, Jeejeebhoy KN. Increase in lumbar spine bone mineral content in patients on long-term parenteral nutrition without vitamin D supplementation. J Parenter Enter Nutr. 1995;19(6):431–6. https://doi.org/10.1177/0148607195019006431.
71. Vieth R. The mechanisms of vitamin D toxicity. Bone Miner. 1990;11(3):267–72. https://doi.org/10.1016/0169-6009(90)90023-9.
72. Lennon C, Davidson KW, Sadowski JA, Mason JB. The vitamin K content of intravenous lipid emulsions. J Parenter Enter Nutr. 1993;17(2):142–4. https://doi.org/10.1177/0148607193017002142.
73. Camilo ME, Jatoi A, O'Brien M, et al. Bioavailability of phylloquinone from an intravenous lipid emulsion. Am J Clin Nutr. 1998;67(4):716–21. https://doi.org/10.1093/ajcn/67.4.716.
74. Tridimas A, Padidela R, Bassett J, et al. Reducing metabolic bone disease burden in intestinal failure children on home parenteral nutrition. JPGN Rep. 2023;4(4):e368. https://doi.org/10.1097/PG9.0000000000000368.
75. Hughes DE, Wright KR, Uy HL, et al. Bisphosphonates promote apoptosis in murine osteoclasts in vitro and in vivo. J Bone Miner Res. 1995;10(10):1478–87. https://doi.org/10.1002/jbmr.5650101008.
76. Carano A, Teitelbaum SL, Konsek JD, Schlesinger PH, Blair HC. Bisphosphonates directly inhibit the bone resorption activity of isolated avian osteoclasts in vitro. J Clin Invest. 1990;85(2):456–61. https://doi.org/10.1172/JCI114459.
77. Raman M, Aghdassi E, Baun M, et al. Metabolic bone disease in patients receiving home parenteral nutrition: a Canadian study and review. J Parenter Enter Nutr. 2006;30(6):492–6. https://doi.org/10.1177/0148607106030006492.
78. Pastore S, Londero M, Barbieri F, Di Leo G, Paparazzo R, Ventura A. Treatment with pamidronate for osteoporosis complicating long-term intestinal failure. J Pediatr Gastroenterol Nutr. 2012;55(5):615–8. https://doi.org/10.1097/MPG.0b013e31825f1c7d.
79. Haderslev KV, Tjellesen L, Sorensen HA, Staun M. Effect of cyclical intravenous clodronate therapy on bone mineral density and markers of bone turnover in patients receiving home parenteral nutrition. Am J Clin Nutr. 2002;76(2):482–8. https://doi.org/10.1093/ajcn/76.2.482.
80. Yamamoto K, Kishino M, Nakamura S, Tokushige K. Symptoms and upper gastrointestinal mucosal injury associated with bisphosphonate therapy. Intern Med. 2019;58(8):1049–56. https://doi.org/10.2169/internalmedicine.1271-18.
81. Shane E, Goldring S, Christakos S, et al. Osteonecrosis of the jaw: more research needed. J Bone Miner Res. 2006;21(10):1503–5. https://doi.org/10.1359/jbmr.060712.

82. Kennel KA, Drake MT. Adverse effects of bisphosphonates: implications for osteoporosis management. Mayo Clin Proc. 2009;84(7):632–8. https://doi.org/10.1016/S0025-6196(11)60752-0.
83. Leder BZ. Parathyroid hormone and parathyroid hormone-related protein analogs in osteoporosis therapy. Curr Osteoporos Rep. 2017;15(2):110–9. https://doi.org/10.1007/s11914-017-0353-4.
84. Raje N, Yee. Denosumab, a RANK ligand inhibitor, for the management of bone loss in cancer patients. Clin Interv Aging. Published online September. 2012;7:331. https://doi.org/10.2147/CIA.S14566.

Intestinal Failure-Associated Liver Disease

11

Speranța Iacob and Liana Gheorghe

11.1 Introduction

11.1.1 Definition

Intestinal failure (IF)-associated liver disease (IFALD) is a spectrum of liver dysfunction that arises as a complication in individuals with chronic intestinal failure (IF) type III, due to prolonged dependence on parenteral nutrition (PN), although it can also occur in patients with prolonged type II IF who require extended parenteral support [1, 2]. The term “IFALD” has replaced the older terminology of parenteral nutrition-associated liver disease (PNALD), as endorsed by the European Society for Clinical Nutrition and Metabolism (ESPEN) [2, 3], reflecting the multifactorial nature of the condition beyond PN alone.

IFALD encompasses a spectrum of liver dysfunction, including cholestasis, steatosis, steatohepatitis, and progressive fibrosis, which can ultimately lead to cirrhosis and end-stage liver disease. The disease is diagnosed when liver injury occurs in the absence of other primary parenchymal liver pathology, hepatotoxic factors, or biliary obstruction [4–6].

11.1.2 Epidemiology

The prevalence of IFALD varies depending on the population studied, duration of PN, and underlying health conditions. Overall, IFALD is more prevalent in pediatric

S. Iacob (✉) · L. Gheorghe
Carol Davila University of Medicine and Pharmacy, Bucharest, Romania

Center for Digestive Diseases and Liver Transplant, Fundeni Clinical Institute, Bucharest, Romania

A. Trifan et al. (eds.), *Short Bowel Syndrome in Adults*,
https://doi.org/10.1007/978-3-031-95848-9_11

patients compared to adults. However, IFALD reveals a concerning prevalence among both pediatric and adult populations.

In pediatric population, the incidence of IFALD ranges from 40% to 60%, with neonates exhibiting the highest prevalence, reaching up to 85% [5, 7, 8]. This higher susceptibility in neonates is associated with conditions like short bowel syndrome (SBS), prematurity, and prolonged PN use [8, 9]. Mortality rates can reach up to 40% among children with established IFALD, making it a leading indication for intestinal transplantation [10].

The prevalence of IFALD in adults is lower, ranging from 15% to 40%. Factors contributing to this lower prevalence include differences in underlying diseases, shorter PN duration, and better tolerance to PN [5, 6]. A 6-year follow-up study of 90 adults receiving home PN revealed that 50% developed persistent IFALD [11]. A prospective 1-year study indicated that IFALD-cholestasis and IFALD-fibrosis may resolve during the initial phase of PN, while IFALD-steatosis tends to persist [12].

IFALD remains a critical concern due to its potential progression to liver fibrosis, cirrhosis, and increased mortality, with 3.6–8.8% of deaths among PN-dependent patients with benign underlying diseases attributable to IFALD [13].

11.2 Etiology and Risk Factors

The development of IFALD is multifactorial, influenced by prolonged PN, intestinal failure, infections, nutritional imbalances, and systemic factors.

Long-term PN is a primary contributor to IFALD. However, PN is essential for individuals with intestinal failure; however, both nutrient toxicity and deficiency are key contributors to the development of IFALD in adults and children.

11.2.1 Nutrient Toxicity

Excessive intake of specific nutrients can overwhelm the liver's metabolic capacity, leading to hepatotoxicity. In both adult and pediatric populations, excessive energy intake and glucose overload (exceeding 7 mg/kg/min) can disrupt hepatic metabolism, promoting lipogenesis and hepatic steatosis. Additionally, soybean-based lipid emulsions (LEs) administered at doses greater than 1 g/kg/day are associated with the accumulation of phytosterols—plant-derived sterols, when administered intravenously, accumulate in hepatocytes due to limited gastrointestinal absorption, impair bile flow and contribute to cholestasis. Soybean oil-based LEs (SOLEs) and safflower oil-based LEs are rich in ω-6 polyunsaturated fatty acids (PUFAs) and low in ω-3 PUFAs. SOLE has a linoleic acid (LA) to α-linolenic acid (ALA) ratio of 7:1, while safflower oil-based LE contains more LA and less ALA than SOLE [14]. Additionally, soybean oil contains γ-tocopherol, a less bioavailable form of vitamin E. Continuous PN infusion over 24 h, common in adults, exacerbates hepatic stress by bypassing the natural circadian rhythm of nutrient metabolism. Moreover, an overload of trace elements, such as copper and manganese, can accumulate in the liver, further aggravating hepatocellular injury [5, 6, 15, 16].

11.2.2 Nutrient Deficiency

Nutrient deficiencies in PN can impair critical metabolic processes, weakening the liver's antioxidant defenses and contributing to IFALD. In adults, deficiencies in choline, carnitine, methionine, taurine, essential fatty acids, and vitamins C and E compromise lipid metabolism and increase oxidative stress. In pediatric patients, the lack of choline—a vital nutrient for lipid metabolism—combined with essential amino acid deficiencies disrupts protein synthesis and liver function. Furthermore, prolonged periods without enteral nutrition (EN) and extended dependence on PN limit gut stimulation, impairing bile flow and exacerbating cholestasis [5, 6, 17, 18].

Prolonged PN use directly correlates with liver dysfunction, as shown by Fitzgibbons et al. [19], who observed biopsy-proven liver fibrosis in children with short bowel syndrome. Liver enzyme abnormalities are found in 25–100% of PN patients [20].

In both populations, balancing nutrient intake is crucial for preventing IFALD, emphasizing the importance of individualized PN regimens that minimize nutrient excess while ensuring sufficient intake of essential nutrients.

11.2.3 Patient-Related Factors

Patient-related factors play a significant role in the development of IFALD, with differences observed between adults and pediatric populations. These factors can be categorized as IF-related and systemic-related.

1. In both adults and children, **IF-related factors** primarily arise from compromised intestinal function and dysbiosis [21, 22].

Adults:

- Lack of oral feeding and prolonged fasting reduce enteral stimulation, impairing bile flow and promoting cholestasis.
- Conditions such as short bowel syndrome (SBS) and small bowel bacterial overgrowth (SBBO) lead to malabsorption and increased translocation of endotoxins and bacteria [11].
- Disruptions in the gut microbiome, suppression of Paneth cell bactericidal responses, and decreased IgA secretion weaken the mucosal immunity.
- Alterations in bile acid metabolism, loss of gut hormone stimulation, and reduced fibroblast growth factor 19 (FGF19) levels contribute to impaired hepatic metabolism [23, 24].

Children:

- Pediatric patients face additional risk factors, including congenital abnormalities such as gastroschisis and intestinal atresia, which disrupt normal gastrointestinal function.
- Prolonged PN and reduced enteral intake lead to intestinal and biliary stasis, while SBS with stoma further limits nutrient absorption and increases the risk of intestinal dysbiosis [11].
- Similar to adults, children also experience small bowel bacterial overgrowth, alterations in bile acid metabolism, and impaired gut hormone stimulation, all of which contribute to IFALD development [25, 26].

2. **Systemic-Related Factors,** Including Infections, Metabolic Disturbances, and Genetic Predispositions, Further Exacerbate IFALD Risk in both Populations

Adults:

- Central line-associated bloodstream infections and sepsis are common complications of PN, leading to systemic inflammation and liver injury.
- The use of hepatotoxic agents, such as alcohol, certain medications (antibiotics, antifungal agents, immunosuppressants, and opioids), and viral hepatitis, can directly impair liver function, increasing susceptibility to IFALD [27, 28].
- Genetic predispositions such as NOD2 mutations may increase the risk of extensive intestinal resection or impair intestinal adaptation, contributing to the development of IFALD [29].

Children:

- Prematurity and low birth weight are critical risk factors in neonates, as immature liver function makes them more vulnerable to metabolic disturbances.
- Early initiation of PN, often required in neonatal intensive care units, increases the risk of cholestasis and liver injury.
- Recurrent infections, frequent sepsis, and exposure to medications that affect liver metabolism can accelerate IFALD progression [27, 28].
- Genetic predispositions (genetic variations affecting farnesoid X receptor (FXR) signaling; genetic mutations in coxsackie and adenovirus receptor-like membrane protein; loss-of-function mutation in the filamin gene—associated with congenital short bowel syndrome) further contribute to the risk of liver dysfunction in pediatric patients [30, 31].

In both adults and children, patient-related factors are crucial in the pathogenesis of IFALD, with IF-related factors primarily arising from compromised intestinal function and systemic-related factors involving infections and metabolic disturbances. While both populations share common risk factors such as SBS, SBBO, and prolonged PN, children face additional challenges related to prematurity, congenital abnormalities, and early PN exposure, highlighting the need for tailored management approaches to mitigate IFALD risk.

11.3 Predictive Biomarkers in IFALD

Accurate biomarkers are essential for the early detection and management of IFALD. Recent studies emphasize the significance of plasma citrulline, FGF19, and the MESIF score in assessing both intestinal function and liver health.

Plasma citrulline serves as a reliable indicator of intestinal absorptive capacity and correlates with liver function in patients with intestinal failure. As citrulline is synthesized primarily by enterocytes, low plasma levels signal compromised intestinal function, which often coexists with hepatic dysfunction. In a cohort of patients with chronic intestinal failure (CIF), low plasma citrulline was identified as an independent predictor of chronic cholestasis, emphasizing its role in IFALD monitoring [32, 33].

Fibroblast growth factor 19 (FGF19), produced in the ileum in response to bile acid absorption, is crucial for regulating bile acid synthesis and maintaining liver health. In IFALD, disruption of enterohepatic circulation leads to reduced FGF19 levels, impairing bile acid homeostasis and contributing to cholestatic liver injury [24]. A single-center study of 135 adults with CIF demonstrated that low FGF19 levels were independently associated with chronic cholestasis and reduced survival. Additionally, low FGF19 was linked to increased portal inflammation, fibrosis, and impaired intestinal barrier function, further exacerbating liver injury. The activation of FXR-FGF19 signaling has shown therapeutic potential in mitigating IFALD, with experimental models highlighting its role in reducing hepatic inflammation and promoting liver repair [34].

Model for end-stage intestinal failure (MESIF) score is a composite prognostic tool designed to predict survival in adult patients with CIF. Developed by Koelfat et al. [34], this scoring system integrates three key variables: plasma citrulline, serum FGF19, and the frequency of PN infusions. The MESIF formula is as follows: **MESIF score = (12.05 × citrulline) + (12.09 × FGF19) + (3.29 × weekly PN infusions).** Scores range from 3 to 47, with risk categories defined as follows:

- **Low risk:** ≤20 (5-year survival rate: 80%).
- **Intermediate risk:** 20–40 (5-year survival rate: 58%).
- **High risk:** >40 (5-year survival rate: 14%).

This scoring system offers a comprehensive assessment of both intestinal and liver health, aiding clinicians in identifying patients at higher risk of IFALD-related complications and those who may benefit from closer monitoring or intestinal transplantation.

Other Emerging Biomarkers:

- **Extracellular Vesicles (EVs):** EVs carrying molecular signatures of liver injury show potential as noninvasive biomarkers for early IFALD diagnosis and monitoring [35].
- **Bilirubin Levels:** Elevated bilirubin, particularly conjugated bilirubin, remains a key indicator of cholestasis and liver dysfunction in IFALD, complementing the predictive value of FGF19 and liver stiffness measurements [36].

Plasma citrulline, serum FGF19, and the MESIF score are crucial biomarkers for assessing IFALD risk and guiding clinical management. Among these, FGF19 stands out for its dual role in predicting cholestasis and overall survival. The MESIF score, by combining intestinal and liver health indicators, offers a practical tool for risk stratification and treatment planning. Continued research into additional biomarkers, such as extracellular vesicles, promises to further enhance the early diagnosis and management of IFALD, ultimately improving patient outcomes.

11.4 Clinical Manifestations

11.4.1 Early Symptoms of IFALD

The initial clinical manifestations of IFALD often include jaundice, hepatomegaly, splenomegaly, elevated liver enzymes, particularly alkaline phosphatase and bilirubin, and general fatigue [4, 37]. Elevated liver enzymes, including alanine aminotransferase (ALT) and aspartate aminotransferase (AST), serve as biomarkers for liver injury and dysfunction, with studies indicating that these elevations can occur within weeks of initiating PN [9, 15].

11.4.2 Progression to Advanced Disease

As IFALD progresses, patients may develop more severe symptoms indicative of advanced liver disease, such as ascites, portal hypertension, and hepatic encephalopathy, as a consequence of liver fibrosis and cirrhosis [37, 38]. The progression of IFALD is often insidious, with many patients exhibiting abnormal liver function tests long before the onset of overt clinical symptoms [37]. Histopathological studies have shown that liver damage can progress from steatosis and cholestasis to fibrosis and ultimately cirrhosis, significantly increasing morbidity and mortality risks [39, 40]. In pediatric populations, the rapid progression to cirrhosis can occur in cases of ultra-short bowel syndrome, underscoring the urgency of monitoring liver function in these patients [29]. Furthermore, the management of IFALD has evolved, with recent studies highlighting the effectiveness of fish oil lipid emulsions in reversing liver damage and improving liver function. However, despite advancements in treatment, many patients on long-term PN continue to exhibit elevated liver enzymes and histologic abnormalities, indicating that ongoing monitoring and intervention are essential to prevent the progression to end-stage liver disease [37, 41].

11.5 Diagnosis

IFALD lacks standardized diagnostic criteria, making early detection and intervention crucial for improving patient outcomes.

11.5.1 Role of Routine Liver Function Tests (LFTs) in IFALD Monitoring

Routine LFTs remain the cornerstone of IFALD surveillance. Elevated levels of bilirubin, alkaline phosphatase, and transaminases often signal liver dysfunction, with cholestasis being one of the earliest manifestations of IFALD. Studies indicate that LFT abnormalities can appear as early as 2 weeks after PN initiation, underscoring the need for frequent monitoring. Furthermore, declining serum albumin and thrombocytopenia may indicate advanced hepatic fibrosis or cirrhosis, necessitating more comprehensive liver assessment [19, 25].

11.5.2 Imaging Modalities for Noninvasive Liver Assessment

Beyond biochemical markers, imaging plays a critical role in assessing liver health in IFALD patients:

- **Ultrasound**: It is widely used for detecting hepatomegaly, biliary sludge, and gallbladder abnormalities.
- **Magnetic Resonance Imaging (MRI)**: MRI, particularly quantitative MRI, has emerged as a promising tool for evaluating liver steatosis and fibrosis. Proton density fat fraction (PDFF) measurements reliably quantify hepatic fat accumulation in IFALD steatosis [38, 42].
- **FibroScan (Transient Elastography [TE])**: It measures liver stiffness and correlates with fibrosis severity. Liver stiffness exceeding 6.5 kPa was independently associated with IFALD-cholestasis, with an area under the receiver operating characteristic curve (AUROC) of 0.714. However, its accuracy may be limited in patients with PN-associated cholestasis [43].
- **Two-Dimensional Shear Wave Elastography (2D-SWE)**: **2D-SWE** demonstrates potential in differentiating moderate/severe fibrosis from mild disease, with AUROC values exceeding 0.80 [44].

11.5.3 Emerging Noninvasive Biomarkers for IFALD Detection

Recent research has introduced several biomarkers and imaging techniques that improve early detection and monitoring of IFALD:

- **Serum Fibroblast Growth Factor 19 (FGF19)**: Being a crucial regulator of bile acid metabolism, FGF19 levels are significantly reduced in IFALD patients with cholestasis. A study involving 203 patients reported that serum FGF19 $\leq$ 107 pg/mL was an independent predictor of IFALD-cholestasis, with an AUROC of 0.810, indicating strong diagnostic accuracy [43].
- **FibroScan** [37, 45]: Alongside FGF19, liver stiffness measured via FibroScan demonstrated predictive value, with liver stiffness values exceeding 6.5 kPa independently associated with IFALD-cholestasis.
  - In patients with short bowel syndrome (SBS) receiving long-term PN, those with a small bowel length <100 cm had significantly higher liver stiffness values (6.1 kPa vs. 4.7 kPa; $p = 0.028$), suggesting a higher risk of fibrosis.
  - In pediatric populations, a combined algorithm using TE and AST levels accurately classified liver fibrosis severity, with a TE cutoff of 11.3 kPa and AST $\geq$40 U/L providing an 88.1% accuracy.
- **Liver Maximum Capacity (LiMAx) Test**: LiMAx test measures cytochrome P450 1A2 activity and demonstrated higher sensitivity in detecting early liver dysfunction compared to FibroScan and standard liver tests. In a longitudinal study, LiMAx values continuously decreased from baseline to 24 months in patients requiring stable PN [44].
- **Fibrosis (FIB)-4 Index**: FIB-4 index is originally developed for chronic viral hepatitis and NAFLD, correlates with fibrosis severity in IFALD, and may serve as a screening tool, especially when combined with imaging techniques.
- **Enhanced Liver Fibrosis (ELF) Score**: Comprising hyaluronic acid, TIMP-1, and PIIINP, the ELF score offers a non-invasive alternative for fibrosis assessment, although further validation in IFALD is required.
- **Indocyanine Green (ICG) Clearance Test**: It reflects hepatic excretory capacity and correlates with fibrosis progression. ICG clearance was significantly reduced in advanced IFALD, highlighting its utility as a noninvasive marker of liver function.

This combination of serum biomarkers (FGF19, ELF score, and FIB-4), imaging tools (FibroScan and LiMAx), and liver function tests (ICG clearance) represents a comprehensive approach to early IFALD detection, enabling timely interventions and reducing the need for invasive liver biopsies.

11.5.4 Liver Biopsy: Gold Standard for Diagnosis

Despite advancements in noninvasive diagnostics, liver biopsy remains the gold standard for confirming IFALD, particularly in cases where laboratory and imaging findings are inconclusive. Histopathological features [47] include the following:

- Phase 1 IFALD: cholestasis, bile ductular proliferation, portal bile plugs, and periportal fibrosis.
- Phase 2 IFALD: persistent fibrosis and steatosis following PN discontinuation.
- Progression to cirrhosis: reported in up to 18% of pediatric patients with long-term PN dependence.

There is an urgent need for a consensus definition of IFALD that integrates biochemical markers, imaging, and novel serum biomarkers. Future research should focus on validating non-invasive diagnostic algorithms that combine LFTs, FGF19, transient elastography, and MRI-based fibrosis assessment. Developing risk stratification models to identify high-risk IFALD patients early, enabling preemptive interventions such as modified lipid formulations in PN.

11.6 Prevention Strategies and Management

Nutritional management is a cornerstone in the prevention and treatment of IFALD, particularly in patients reliant on prolonged PN.

Optimizing the composition of PN is essential to minimize the risk of liver dysfunction. Strategies include careful adjustment of macronutrient ratios, particularly the reduction of lipid intake, which has been associated with cholestasis and liver injury. The incorporation of fish oil-based emulsions has emerged as a promising alternative to traditional lipid emulsions.

These omega-3 fatty acid-rich emulsions are less hepatotoxic and can improve liver function by promoting the secretion of bile acids and reducing inflammation [48, 49].

Moreover, preventing overfeeding is crucial, as excess caloric intake can exacerbate liver injury and contribute to the development of steatosis. Regular monitoring of energy expenditure and adjusting PN accordingly can help achieve optimal nutritional status.

11.6.1 Enteral Feeding Strategies

Maximizing enteral nutrition is another vital strategy in the management of patients with IFALD. Whenever feasible, even partial enteral feeding can significantly reduce the reliance on PN, thereby decreasing the risk of liver complications. Enteral feeding promotes gut integrity, enhances nutrient absorption, and stimulates bile flow, which can mitigate cholestasis. Enteral nutrition activates the farnesoid X receptor (FXR) and induces FGF19, crucial for regulating bile acid synthesis and reducing cholestasis [23, 49]. Studies have shown that patients who receive early enteral nutrition exhibit improved outcomes, including reduced rates of IFALD and shorter durations of PN dependence. Implementing a stepwise approach to increase enteral intake, starting with small volumes and gradually escalating, can facilitate tolerance and optimize nutritional delivery.

11.6.2 Lipid-Sparing Strategies

The transition from conventional lipid emulsions to omega-3 fatty acid-based emulsions is a critical lipid-sparing strategy in the management of IFALD. Fish oil-based emulsions provide essential fatty acids that are less likely to accumulate in the liver and have demonstrated hepatoprotective effects. Clinical trials have reported significant improvements in liver function parameters, including reductions in bilirubin and transaminase levels, following the switch to omega-3 fatty acid-based emulsions. Moreover, fish oil emulsions are rich in vitamin E, which acts as an antioxidant, reducing oxidative stress and inflammation. This shift not only aids in liver health but also supports overall nutritional status, making it a valuable intervention in the management of IFALD [46, 48].

11.6.3 Managing Infections

Preventing catheter-related bloodstream infections (CRBSIs) is paramount in patients receiving PN, as sepsis can significantly worsen IFALD. Implementing strict aseptic techniques during catheter insertion and maintenance, along with regular monitoring for signs of infection, is essential. Additionally, the use of antimicrobial-coated catheters and adherence to evidence-based guidelines for catheter care can further reduce the incidence of CRBSIs.

11.6.4 Medical Interventions

Several medical treatments have shown promise in improving liver health in patients with IFALD.

Ursodeoxycholic acid (UDCA) is a hydrophilic bile acid used to treat cholestasis in IFALD patients by improving bile flow and reducing liver inflammation. UDCA works by replacing toxic hydrophobic bile acids with less cytotoxic hydrophilic bile acids, promoting bile secretion and reducing hepatic inflammation. Studies indicate that UDCA is effective in both adults and children, with doses ranging from 10 to 20 mg/kg/day divided into two doses [50]. In adults with IFALD, UDCA has been shown to improve liver function tests, including reductions in bilirubin, ALT and gamma-glutamyl transferase (GGT) levels. In pediatric populations, a pilot study of seven children demonstrated the resolution of jaundice, hepatomegaly, and normalization of laboratory values within 1–2 weeks of UDCA administration [5]. Discontinuation of UDCA led to a relapse in liver enzyme elevation, which resolved upon re-initiation of the treatment. In very-low-birth-weight infants, UDCA treatment shortened the course of cholestasis and reduced peak serum bilirubin levels compared to historical controls.

While UDCA is generally well-tolerated, potential side effects include diarrhea, which can be problematic for patients with short bowel syndrome [50]. Therefore, careful dose titration and monitoring are essential to minimize side effects while optimizing therapeutic benefits. Given its ability to improve bile flow and reduce cholestasis, UDCA remains a cornerstone in the management of IFALD.

Furthermore, antioxidants may play a role in mitigating oxidative stress, which is a contributing factor to liver injury in IFALD. Research has suggested that supplementation with antioxidants, such as vitamin E and selenium, may help improve liver function and reduce inflammation. Glucagon-like peptide-2 (GLP-2) analogs, such as teduglutide, glepaglutide, and apraglutide, have shown potential in improving intestinal absorption, reducing PN dependence, and supporting liver health [5, 51]. These medical interventions should be considered as adjuncts to nutritional management and other therapeutic strategies.

11.6.5 Surgical Interventions

For patients with short bowel syndrome, surgical interventions may be necessary to reduce PN dependence and prevent IFALD [6, 49]. Procedures such as bowel lengthening (e.g., serial transverse enteroplasty and Bianchi procedure) or autologous gastrointestinal reconstructive procedures can increase the absorptive capacity of the intestine, reducing the need for PN. Additionally, restoring bowel continuity can improve enterohepatic circulation and bile flow, further mitigating the risk of cholestasis. In cases of advanced IFALD with liver failure, intestinal transplantation, with or without liver transplantation (LT), may be required. Early referral to specialized intestinal rehabilitation and transplant centers can improve outcomes by optimizing patient management and timing of transplantation.

11.7 Transplantation

11.7.1 Isolated Liver Transplantation

Liver transplantation (LT) is a critical intervention for patients with end-stage IFALD, particularly when conventional nutritional and medical therapies fail to maintain liver function. Progressive liver disease with liver failure (coagulopathy, elevated bilirubin) and portal hypertension despite optimization of PN, recurrent bloodstream infections, or severe metabolic derangements further warrant transplantation [9, 52]. In cases of ultra-short bowel syndrome, where the risk of rapid progression to cirrhosis is high, early referral is crucial to optimize outcomes and prevent irreversible liver damage [39], as emphasized by updated consensus guidelines [53]. Isolated LT is a viable option for children with short bowel syndrome (SBS) and IFALD who demonstrate potential for intestinal adaptation. Key criteria for isolated LT include progressive IFALD, ≥50 cm of functional bowel without an intact ileocecal valve, or ≥ 30 cm with an intact valve, and the ability to tolerate 50% of daily energy intake enterally for 4 weeks with satisfactory growth [54, 55]. However, children with dysmotile bowel or recurrent infections should be considered for combined liver–intestine transplantation unless dysmotility resolves with minimal infection frequency. In cases involving advanced fibrosis or venous thrombosis, combined transplantation is often necessary to improve survival and long-term outcomes [56].

11.7.2 Intestinal and Multivisceral Transplantation

Intestinal transplantation (IT) is indicated when PN becomes unsustainable due to loss of central venous access, life-threatening infections, or advanced IFALD. The 5-year survival rate for isolated IT is 65%, compared to 22% for multivisceral transplantation [57], with pediatric recipients demonstrating better outcomes. Recent guidelines highlight invasive intra-abdominal desmoids, acute intestinal infarction with hepatic failure, and progressive IFALD as primary indications for transplantation [53]. Beyond improving survival, IT also significantly enhances quality of life, reducing the burden of PN dependence and promoting greater social integration [58].

11.7.3 Outcomes and Quality of Life (QoL) after Transplantation

Significant advancements in surgical techniques and postoperative care have improved outcomes for patients undergoing liver transplantation for IFALD, enabling substantial recovery of liver function and improved QoL [53, 59]. Compared to PN, IT offers rehabilitative benefits, including psychological, emotional, and social improvements that persist long-term [58, 60]. Studies indicate that patients experience an enhanced ability to eat, travel, and engage in daily activities as early as 3 months post-IT, with benefits sustained over time despite potential financial pressures [60]. For patients with both liver and intestinal failure, combined transplantation is recommended to address the complexity of managing these conditions. Continued research and advancements in clinical practice will further refine transplantation criteria and enhance long-term outcomes for this vulnerable population.

References

1. Deutsch L, Cloutier A, Lal S. Advances in chronic intestinal failure management and therapies. Curr Opin Gastroenterol. 2020;36:223–9.
2. Pironi L, Arends J, Bozzetti F. ESPEN guidelines on chronic intestinal failure in adults. Clin Nutr. 2017;36:619.
3. Fleming CR, Remington M. Intestinal failure. In: Hill GL, editor. Nutrition and the surgical patient. Edinburgh: Churchill Livingstone; 1981. p. 323.
4. Bond A, Huijbers A, Pironi L. Diagnosis and management of intestinal failure-associated liver disease in adults. Aliment Pharmacol Ther. 2019;50(6):640–53. https://doi.org/10.1111/apt.15432.
5. Zafirovska M, Zafirovski A, Kozjek N. Current insights regarding intestinal failure-associated liver disease. Nutrients. 2023;15(14):3169. https://doi.org/10.3390/nu15143169.

6. Fousekis F, Mitselos I, Christodoulou D. New insights into intestinal failure–associated liver disease. Saudi J Gastroenterol. 2021;27(1):3–12. https://doi.org/10.4103/sjg.sjg_551_20.
7. Huff K, Breckler F, Cruse W. Pediatric SMOFlipid therapy: patient response and safety concerns. JPEN J Parenter Enteral Nutr. 2020;45(4):792–9. https://doi.org/10.1002/jpen.1929.
8. Khalaf R, Ford S. Intestinal failure-associated liver disease in the neonatal ICU. Curr Opin Pediatr. 2022;34(2):184–90. https://doi.org/10.1097/mop.0000000000001105.
9. Nandivada P, Fell G, Gura K. Lipid emulsions in the treatment and prevention of PN-associated liver disease. Am J Clin Nutr. 2016;103(2):629S–34S. https://doi.org/10.3945/ajcn.114.103986.
10. Willis TC, Carter BA, Rogers SP. High rates of mortality and morbidity in infants with PN-associated cholestasis. JPEN J Parenter Enteral Nutr. 2010;34:32–7.
11. Cavicchi M, Beau P, Crenn P. Prevalence of liver disease in home PN patients. Ann Intern Med. 2000;132:525–32.
12. Sasdelli AS, Guidetti M, Pazzeschi C. IFALD in adult patients: a one-year study. Nutrition. 2019;65:2.
13. Dibb M, Soop M, Teubner A. Survival and nutritional dependence on home PN. Clin Nutr. 2017;36:570–6.
14. Secor JD, Yu L, Tsikis S. Managing IFALD: current strategies. Expert Opin Drug Saf. 2021;20:307–20.
15. Nandivada P, Carlson S, Chang M. Treatment of PN-associated liver disease. Adv Nutr. 2013;4(6):711–7.
16. Madnawat H, Welu A, Gilbert E. Mechanisms of PN-associated liver and gut injury. Nutr Clin Pract. 2019;35(1):63–71.
17. Fundora J, Aucott SW. IFALD in neonates. Neoreviews. 2020;21:e591–9.
18. Villafranca J, Guindo M, Sanz E. Cyclic PN and liver dysfunction. Nutr J. 2017;16(1)
19. Fitzgibbons S, Jones B, Hull M. PN-associated liver fibrosis in children. J Pediatr Surg. 2010;45(1):95–9.
20. Park H, Lee S, Jung S. PN-associated liver disease in adults. JPEN J Parenter Enteral Nutr. 2020;45(3):643–8.
21. Wang Y, Liu Y, Gao B. Untargeted metabolomics reveal PN-associated alterations in pediatric SBS. Meta. 2022;12(7):600. https://doi.org/10.3390/metabo12070600.
22. Denton C, Price A, Friend J. Role of the gut–liver axis in PN-associated injury. Children. 2018;5(10):136. https://doi.org/10.3390/children5100136.
23. Manithody CS, Van Nispen J, Murali V. Bile acids and gut microbiota in PN injury. J Hum Nutr. 2020;4(1):286. https://doi.org/10.36959/487/286.
24. van Erpecum KJ, Schaap FG. Intestinal failure and FGF19 in IFALD. J Hepatol. 2015;62(6):1231–3. https://doi.org/10.1016/j.jhep.2015.03.012.
25. Mutanen A, Nissinen MJ, Lohi J. Serum plant sterols and liver injury in pediatric IF. Am J Clin Nutr. 2014;100:1085–94.
26. Wang Y, Chen S, Yan W. Congenital short-bowel syndrome in China. JPEN J Parenter Enteral Nutr. 2021;45(5):1009–15. https://doi.org/10.1002/jpen.1974.
27. Rosseel Z, Cortoos P, Jonckheer J. PN, sepsis, heart failure, and liver test disturbances. Nutrients. 2023;15(11):2612. https://doi.org/10.3390/nu15112612.
28. Choi S, Lee K, Choi J. Prognostic factors in PN-dependent pediatric IF. Pediatr Gastroenterol Hepatol Nutr. 2016;19(1):44. https://doi.org/10.5223/pghn.2016.19.1.44.
29. Schäffler H, Schneider N, Hsieh CJ. NOD2 mutations and IF in absence of Crohn's disease. Clin Nutr. 2013;32(6):1029–35. https://doi.org/10.1016/j.clnu.2013.02.014.
30. Koelfat KVK, Visschers RGJ, Hodin CM. FXR agonism protects against IFALD. J Clin Transl Res. 2017;3(3):318–27.
31. Wang Y, Chen S, Yan W. Congenital short-bowel syndrome: clinical and genetic presentation. JPEN J Parenter Enteral Nutr. 2021;45(5):1009–15. https://doi.org/10.1002/jpen.1974.
32. Bailly-Botuha C, Colomb V, Thioulouse E. Plasma citrulline reflects enterocyte mass in SBS. Pediatr Res. 2009;65(5):559–63. https://doi.org/10.1203/PDR.0b013e31819986da.
33. Saitoh W, Takada S, Hirao J. Plasma citrulline as a biomarker for intestinal injury. Toxicol Lett. 2018;295:416–23. https://doi.org/10.1016/j.toxlet.2018.07.009.

34. Koelfat KVK, Huijbers A, Schaap FG. Citrulline and FGF19 predict cholestasis and poor survival in IF. Am J Clin Nutr. 2019;109(6):1620–9. https://doi.org/10.1093/ajcn/nqz036.
35. Wang L, Tang H, Li S. Extracellular vesicles as biomarkers in liver failure. Front Immunol. 2023;14:1116518. https://doi.org/10.3389/fimmu.2023.1116518.
36. Ramírez-Mejía MM, Castillo-Castañeda SM, Pal SC. Bilirubin's role in liver disease. J Clin Transl Hepatol. 2024;12(11):939–48. https://doi.org/10.14218/JCTH.2024.00156.
37. Huijbers A, Koggel L, Bronkhorst C. Noninvasive assessments of IFALD. JPEN J Parenter Enteral Nutr. 2019;43(5):615–26. https://doi.org/10.1002/jpen.1524.
38. Huijbers A, Wanten G, Dekker H. Hepatic steatosis assessment in home PN patients. JPEN J Parenter Enteral Nutr. 2017;42(4):778–85. https://doi.org/10.1177/0148607117711667.
39. Ueno T, Takase K, Deguchi K. Early detection of liver fibrosis using M2BPGi in IF patients. Pediatr Surg Int. 2022;38(12):1807–13. https://doi.org/10.1007/s00383-022-05240-w.
40. Huard G, Fiel M, Moon J. Advanced liver fibrosis in adults undergoing ITx. JPEN J Parenter Enteral Nutr. 2018;42(7):1195–202. https://doi.org/10.1002/jpen.1148.
41. Fligor S, Tsikis S, Hirsch T. Inflammation drives pathogenesis of early IFALD. Sci Rep. 2024;14(1):4240. https://doi.org/10.1038/s41598-024-54675-9.
42. Fragkos KC, Picasso Bouroncle MC, Kumar S. Serum scoring and MRI in IFALD: a feasibility study. Nutrients. 2020;12(7):2151. https://doi.org/10.3390/nu12072151.
43. Xiao Y, Maitiabula G, Wang H. Predictive value of serum FGF19 and liver stiffness in IFALD. Clin Nutr ESPEN. 2024;59:89–95. https://doi.org/10.1016/j.clnesp.2023.11.008.
44. Blüthner E, Pape UF, Stockmann M. Non-invasive liver function assessment in IF patients. Nutrients. 2020;12(5):1217. https://doi.org/10.3390/nu12051217.
45. Knop V, Neuberger SC, Marienfeld S. IFALD in SBS patients: evaluation by transient elastography. Nutrition. 2019;63-64:134–40. https://doi.org/10.1016/j.nut.2019.02.001.
46. Tabone T, Mooney P, Donnellan C. Challenges in screening and diagnosing IFALD. Nutr Clin Pract. 2024;39(5):1003–25. https://doi.org/10.1002/ncp.11116.
47. Naini BV, Lassman CR. TPN therapy and liver injury: a histopathologic study. Hum Pathol. 2012;43(6):826–33. https://doi.org/10.1016/j.humpath.2011.07.008.
48. Sharkey L, BIFA Committee. BAPEN/BIFA guidelines on the diagnosis and management of IFALD 2022.
49. Wichman BE, Nilson J, Govindan S. Mechanisms for PN-associated liver disease. Nutr Clin Pract. 2022;37(2):265–73.
50. Raphael BP, Duggan C. Prevention and treatment of IFALD in children. Semin Liver Dis. 2012;32(4):341–7.
51. Diamanti A, Lezo A, D'Antiga L. Teduglutide in pediatric IF: SIGENP statement. Dig Liver Dis. 2022;54:1320–7.
52. Hakimian D, Wall E, Herlitz J. Parenteral fish oil lipid emulsion in adults. Eur J Clin Nutr. 2024;78(9):796–800. https://doi.org/10.1038/s41430-024-01462-4.
53. Kaufman SS, Avitzur Y, Beath SV. Indications for ITx: consensus in 2019. Transplantation. 2020;104(5):937–46. https://doi.org/10.1097/TP.0000000000003065.
54. Taha AM, Sharif K, Johnson T. Outcomes of isolated LT for SBS and IFALD. J Pediatr Gastroenterol Nutr. 2012;54(4):547–51. https://doi.org/10.1097/MPG.0b013e31823f42e7.
55. Dell-Olio D, Beath SV, de Ville de Goyet J. Isolated LT in infants with SBS: outcomes and factors. J Pediatr Gastroenterol Nutr. 2009;48(3):334–40. https://doi.org/10.1097/mpg.0b013e31818c6099.
56. Bryan NS, Russell SC, Ozler O. Pediatric ITx in the modern era. J Pediatr Gastroenterol Nutr. 2024;79(2):278–89. https://doi.org/10.1002/jpn3.12274.
57. Ramisch D, Rumbo C, Echevarria C. Long-term outcomes of ITx and MVTx in Argentina. Transplant Proc. 2016;48(2):457–62. https://doi.org/10.1016/j.transproceed.2015.12.066.
58. Pironi L, Sasdelli AS. Current insights into ITx indications. Curr Opin Organ Transplant. 2021;26(2):186–91. https://doi.org/10.1097/MOT.0000000000000846.
59. Dimopoulou A, Dimopoulou D, Zavras N. Ileal bypass for pruritus relief in PFIC. Folia Med (Plovdiv). 2023;65(1):183–5. https://doi.org/10.3897/folmed.65.e73628.
60. Ambrose T, Holdaway L, Smith A. Impact of ITx on quality of life. Clin Nutr. 2020;39(6):1958–67. https://doi.org/10.1016/j.clnu.2019.08.023.

Insights into Nutritional Management of Short Bowel Syndrome: Nutritional Assessment and Diet Considerations

12

Mihaela Ghioca, Roxana Vadan, Daria Ana Arina Gheorghe, and Liana Gheorghe

12.1 Nutritional Assessment

Short bowel patients are inherently at risk of malnutrition and cannot survive without nutritional oral, enteral and intravenous support. Repeated evaluation of the nutritional status is required to assure the need and adequacy of nutritional intervention.

Nutritional assessment of these patients is complex, comprising general tools, common to other diseases (dietary intake, anthropometric measurements, body composition and functional assessment) but also elements particular to short bowel syndrome (SBS; specific deficiencies that can be anticipated, being secondary to the loss of specific absorptive parts of the intestine).

12.1.1 Measurement of Ingestion and Excretion of Nutrients

Oral dietary intake is evaluated through 24-h recall and 2- to 3-day diet records. Relaying on a single-day recall may not accurately reflect dietary patterns so at least a three day recall (two weekdays and one weekend day) is more precise. Symptoms that impair food intake must be specifically asked for dysgeusia, nausea, vomiting, bloating and diarrhoea. Also, a thorough medication history can identify potential side effects that impair food intake.

Stool assessment by 24-h stool colection with evaluation of stool volume, consistency, of the presence of undigested food can be of use in grading the severity of malabsorption and is especially important for stoma patients. The amount and type

M. Ghioca (✉) · R. Vadan · D. A. A. Gheorghe · L. Gheorghe
Carol Davila University of Medicine and Pharmacy, Bucharest, Romania

Center for Digestive Diseases and Liver Transplant, Fundeni Clinical Institute, Bucharest, Romania

A. Trifan et al. (eds.), *Short Bowel Syndrome in Adults*,
https://doi.org/10.1007/978-3-031-95848-9_12

of fluid that the patient is allowed to drink is determined by the volume of the output (e.g. restriction of hypotonic fluids and intake of electrolyte fluids are recommended in high output fistulas).

Urinary output by collecting the 24-h urine is an indicator not only of kidney function but also of hydration status. It improves with better absorption of water and electrolytes. It is desired that diuresis is at least 1 l urine/day with a urinary sodium less than 20 mmol/l [1].

12.1.2 Nutrition-Focused Physical Exam (NFPE)

NFPE is the head-to-toe examination focused on the diagnosis of malnutrition, dehydration and physical signs of micronutrient deficiencies.

Clinically malnutrition manifests by loss of body fat and muscle mass.

Subjective assessment of fat reserves is done visually at orbital level, triceps level and thoracic cage (the space between the ribs).

The physical signs of muscle mass depletion are protruding bones (acromion, clavicle and patella) and reduced muscle mass appreciated at the following sites: hand interosseous muscles (loss of muscle results in depressed area between fingers), temporalis muscle, deltoid muscle, supraclavicular muscle, quadriceps muscle and gastrocnemius muscle.

Dehydration can be diagnosed clinically by poor skin turgor, dry mucosae (dry conjunctiva, dry mouth) and slow capillary refill.

Clinical signs and several symptoms of vitamin and mineral deficiencies are listed in Table 12.1.

12.1.3 Objective Measurements of Nutritional Status

12.1.3.1 Anthropometric Measurements

Weight, height and body mass index (BMI) are routinely measured in each patient. The more in-depth anthropometric measurements are useful since BMI do not accurately reflect nutritional status in SBS patients, but their use is conditioned by local protocols and availability. Also, anthropometry is time consuming and even if it uses objective measurements, of nutritional status, it is operator dependent.

Skinfold thickness is an indirect measure of subcutaneous adipose tissue. It can be measured using skinfold callipers at various sites (triceps, pectoral, subcapsular, abdomen, suprailiac and thigh).

Skeletal muscle mass is measured by midarm muscle circumference (MAMC), arm muscle area (AMA), mid-upper arm circumference (MUAC) and calf circumference (CC). Values can be expressed as percentage of standard (available from reference charts) to define the severity of loss (adequate, marginal, depleted, wasted) or as cut-off values, determined for specific populations.

Table 12.1 Clinical signs and symptoms of nutritional deficits [2]

Vitamin or mineral	Clinical signs and symptoms of deficiency
B1(thiamine)	Mental changes (apathy, decreased short-term memory, irritability, confusion), cognitive deficits, congestive heart failure
B2 (riboflavin)	Seborrheic dermatitis, cheilosis, angular stomatitis
B3 (niacin)	Pellagra: Pigmented rash or brown discolouration of sun exposed skin; neurological symptoms: Depression, apathy, headache, loss of memory
B5 (pantothenic acid)	Deficit very rare. Postural hypotension, tachycardia, vertigo
B6 (pyridoxine)	Microcytic anaemia, seborrheic dermatitis, stomatitis, glossitis, depression and confusion
B7 (biotin)	Dermatitis, alopecia, ataxia
B9 (folic acid)	Megaloblastic anaemia, pancytopenia, glossitis, shallow oral ulcers, angular stomatitis, neuropsychiatric manifestation (difficulty in concentrating, irritability, headache)
B12 (cobalamin)	Megaloblastic anaemia, low WBC count, low platelet count, glossitis, dementia; paraesthesia
C (ascorbic acid)	Scaly, dry and brownish skin; oedema; purpura; easy bruising; dry and friable; corkscrew hair; swollen, bleeding gums; loss of teeth; depression
A	Night blindness, Bitot's spots, foamy conjunctiva, xerophthalmia
D	Osteomalacia (bone deformities, pain), tetanic spasms
E	Peripheral neuropathy, ataxia, skeletal myopathy, retinopathy
K	Increased prothrombin time, impaired clotting, prolonged bleeding, osteoporosis
Iron	Microcytic anaemia
Copper	Microcytic anaemia, neutropenia, osteoporosis, hair depigmentation, ataxia
Chromium	Hyperglycaemia, glycosuria, insulin resistance, peripheral neuropathy
Zinc	Skin rash of face, hands, feet and groins; alopecia, blunting of taste and smell; and delayed wound healing
Selenium	Cardiomyopathy, skeletal muscle myopathy

12.1.3.2 Dual-Energy X-Ray Absorptiometry (DXA)

Dual-energy X-ray absorptiometry (DXA) is generally used to appreciate bone mineral density, but it can also evaluate the soft tissue compartment: fat and lean mass overall (total body fat and total body muscle). Fat-free mass (FFM) is determined using DXA, and fat-free mass index (FFMI) is calculated by dividing fat-free mass by height squared. It has been shown that FFMI cut-off values for predicting low muscle mass are <18 kg/m^2 in men and <15 kg/m^2 in women [3].

Also, fat and lean mass in specific body parts such as legs, arms and torso can be measured using DXA. Appendicular skeletal muscle index (ASMI) can be calculated: the appendicular muscle (that refers to muscles of the legs and arms) is standardized by the patient's height. ASMI values calculated using DXA are considered reference values (gold standard) due to the accuracy of the method and are used to define sarcopenia: <7 kg/m^2 in males and <5.4 kg/m^2 in females [4].

12.1.3.3 Imaging Studies (Computed Tomography [CT], Magnetic Resonance Imaging [MRI], Ultrasound [US])

Using cross-sectional imaging, CT scans and MRI, the skeletal muscle area can be assessed at various levels. There is an association between the skeletal muscle area at the level of lumbar L3 vertebra and the overall skeletal muscle mass of the body. Skeletal muscle index (SMI) can be calculated using anatomical landmarks and dedicated software (SMI = skeletal muscle cross-sectional area (cm^2)/height^2 (m^2)) and is an objective measure of sarcopenia. The level of twelfth thoracic vertebra could also be used, and another muscle mass indicator is the area of psoas muscle.

Ultrasound (US) is widely available, not expensive, can be repeated easily and can be utilised for bedside measurements. It measures muscle thickness and cross-sectional area at various sites: thigh, calf, upper arm and musculus rectus abdominis. It is operator dependent and needs standardization regarding the degree of compressibility of the skin at measurement site. Also, cut-off values for sarcopenia are not yet determined in specific patient populations.

12.1.3.4 Bioelectrical Impedance Analysis (BIA): Single-Frequency (SF)-BIA, Multi-Frequency (MF)-BIA, Bioimpedance Spectroscopy (BIS), Bioelectrical Impedance Vector Analysis (BIVA)

Bioelectrical impedance analysis (BIA), single-frequency (SF)-BIA or multi-frequency (MF)-BIA, is a method that evaluates body composition and is largely available. BIA can be used in outpatient settings in patients with SBS-intestinal failure (IF) [5]. It is based on the electrical conductivity of various tissues, and it estimates muscle mass indirectly. Advanced MF-BIA techniques has the ability to measure impedance and resistance separately across five different cylinders within the human body which allows for whole and segmental (legs, arms and trunk) FFM analysis. Conventional BIA can be inaccurate if the patient has fluid retention; in this situation, phase angle (PA) and bioimpedance spectroscopy (BIS) can be used.

Phase angle (PA) is a parameter derived from BIA that reflects the integrity of cell membrane, higher values being related to better cell function. Phase angle is directly associated with lean mass and muscle mass in different age-groups and is used to define sarcopenia with specific cut-off values for various populations. Phase angle significantly predicted number of readmissions, length of hospital stay and mortality in patients with intestinal failure on long-term parenteral nutrition, while fat-free mass index only predicted mortality [6].

BIS is similar to BIA but uses 256 frequencies (as compared with 2–4 for BIA) and can quantify: body water, intracellular and extracellular fluid, fat free mass, fat mass and phase angle. Bioelectrical impedance vector analysis (BIVA) uses graphical vectors to analyse BIA data and presents the advantage that it allows information to be obtained simultaneously about changes in tissue hydration or soft tissue mass, independent of body weight. It has been suggested that BIVA may represent a better predictor of nutritional status for analysis and interpretation of body composition in patients with short bowel syndrome [7].

As stated earlier, BMI in patients with SBS underestimates the presence and the degree of low muscle mass [8]. A retrospective study performed at a tertiary referral centre for chronic intestinal failure patients that investigated body composition using BIA in a large cohort of 147 home parenteral nutrition (HPN) patients, one-third of them having SBS, showed that although the BMI appeared normal, half of the patients had high fat mass and two-thirds had low FFMI [6]. Also, only 10% of patients had all nutrition parameters within normal range (BMI and FFMI and FM), whereas 90% of patients had at least one parameter of body composition outside of the reference range. In this study, 34% of patients were malnourished according to Global Leadership Initiative on Malnutrition (GLIM) criteria [9].

12.1.3.5 Functional Status Assessment

Muscle strength is a measure of functional loss, and in most cases, it is an indicator of the presence of sarcopenia. Can be determined by using a dynamometer—handgrip strength: with the dominant arm bent at 90°; two or three measurements are done with 10–15 s rest period between the tests. It depends on the willingness of the patient to correctly perform the test (can be falsely low). When detected, low muscle strength must trigger the evaluation of muscle mass, regardless of clinical circumstances.

Sarcopenia is defined by low levels of muscle strength, low muscle quantity and/or quality and low physical performance and is a very important prognostic factor. Sarcopenia has been associated with reduced quality of life, increased hospitalizations, high hospitalization costs and increased risk of mortality. In patients with intestinal failure, the prevalence of sarcopenia is high, reaching 72.7% (95% CI; 59.3 to 83.0) compared to 34.5% (95% CI; 23.3 to 47.8) in those with intestinal insufficiency only [10].

When measured by European Working Group on Sarcopenia in Older People (EWGSOP) criteria in patients with chronic intestinal failure, the prevalence of sarcopenia was 59% (11). This prevalence did not change after 12 weeks of home-based individualized exercise sessions. But the risk of sarcopenia (assessed by SARC-F, a five-item questionnaire recommended for sarcopenia screening) was significantly reduced (from 38.8% at baseline to 29.0% after exercise [$p < 0.001$]). Also, a statistically significant increase in muscle mass ($p = 0.017$), muscle mass index ($p = 0.016$) and handgrip strength ($p = 0.019$) was observed after the exercise intervention which underscores the importance of regular physical activity for SBS patients [11].

12.1.4 Laboratory Evaluation of Nutritional Deficits

Serum parameters that can be deficient in SBS patients and need to be periodically measured are listed in Table 12.2. The frequency of screening for deficiencies is dictated by the clinical particularities of each case, being dependent mostly on the type of surgical resection and on the time elapsed from the surgery, more frequently in the early phases and at longer intervals in chronic, stable, HPN patients.

Table 12.2 Biochemical assessment

Basic biochemical parameters	Specific biochemical parameters
Hemoleucogram	Vitamins A, D, E, and B12; folic acid
Glucose	Iron, total iron binding capacity, ferritin
Urea, creatinine	Cu, Zn, se, Mn
Total protein, albumin	D-lactate
ALT, AST, FA, bilirubin	
INR	
Na, K, Mg, phosphate	
Cholesterol, triglycerides	
CRP	

Abbreviations: CRP, C-reactive protein

The European Society for Parenteral and Enteral Nutrition (ESPEN) recommends that in clinically stable patients on long-term HPN the following measurements can be done at all scheduled visits: body weight, body composition and hydration status, energy and fluid balance, and also biochemistry (haemoglobin, ferritin, albumin, C-reactive protein, electrolytes, venous blood gas analysis or serum bicarbonates, kidney function tests, liver function tests and glucose). In patients on long-term HPN, clinical signs and symptoms and biochemical indexes of vitamin and trace element deficiency or toxicity should be evaluated at least once per year [12].

In conclusion, nutritional assessment of short bowel syndrome patients is complex but of utmost importance in preventing and correcting nutritional deficiencies and improving the prognosis and quality of life for these patients.

12.2 Diet Considerations

12.2.1 Introduction

SBS is a malabsorptive condition secondary to a significant resection of the small intestine, which can cause malnutrition, dehydration and micronutrient deficiencies [13].

Given the classification into three groups of SBS patients (Group 1, end-jejunostomy; Group 2, jejunocolic anastomosis; and Group 3, jejunoileocolic anastomosis) [14], the management of this condition consists of dietary interventions that must be individualized into specific nutrient needs [15].

The management of malabsorption secondary to SBS is thus dependent on the degree of severity [16].

Regarding fluids intake and diet, general recommendations for patients with SBS include the following:

- Refrain from consuming water without food.
- Drink the majority of the liquids between meals.

- Drink liquids slowly.
- Restrict hypotonic fluids.
- Oral rehydration solutions that contain salt and carbohydrates are indicated [14].
- Consume small, balanced in nutrient meals, regularly throughout the day—a number of 6–8 meals/day is recommended.
- Adding salt to the diet is indicated in patients with a colon in continuity.
- Increase the amount of food consumed.
- Patients with colon should adopt a diet rich in complex carbohydrates (such as pasta, rice, potato and bread).
- Limit osmotically active sweeteners, as they may trigger diarrhoea; there is no need to always avoid lactose, unless there is a clear relationship between lactose ingestion and increase of diarrhoea, with a documented intolerance [12].
- Every meal and snack should contain a high-quality protein.
- Patients without a colon should refrain from consuming fat and patients with a colon should limit to less than 30% of fat consuming; oils with essential fatty acids, such as walnut, soy and sunflower, are indicated.
- Patients with a colon should limit oxalate consumption [16, 17].

Diet interventions pose an important role in the intestinal adaptation and symptom attenuation. The main purpose is to increase food consumption in order to maximize nutrient and fluid absorption, maintain an adequate urine output and decrease diarrhoea [17].

Energy absorption is dependent on the extent of intestinal resection; thus, patients with SBS have a tendency to have hyperphagia and to consume more than required in order to maintain proper nutrition; therefore, there is the indication to consume 6–8 small meals/day [17, 18].

Complex carbohydrates should consist 50–60% of energy intake in patients with a colon in continuity and 40–50% in patients without a colon, and those found in pasta, rice, cereal, potatoes and bread are generally well accepted. Also, patients without a colon should restrict sucrose and fructose; likewise, patients with a colon in continuity should limit them, because they can exacerbate the osmotic diarrhoea [18].

Given the malnutrition status, all patients with SBS may include in the diet increased levels of *proteins*, such as eggs, fish, chicken, turkey, beef and pork, consisting 20% of energy intake. A study on seven patients with end-jejunostomies that were fed with a peptide-based formula or an isocaloric and isonitrogenous polymeric formula found that there were no differences in nitrogen, fat, energy, carbohydrate, electrolyte, mineral or fluid absorption [19]. Cosnes et al. demonstrated that nitrogen absorption was improved by the use of peptide-based diet in a small study that evaluated six patients with 90–150 cm of remnant jejunum and end-jejunostomy [20].

Also, in a study published by Byrne et al. on 41 patients with SBS receiving parenteral nutrition, 30 g/day of oral glutamine added to the diet have reduced parenteral requirements, with a maintained effect obtained when combining diet, glutamine and growth hormone [21].

A diet consisting of *fat* in 20–30% of total calories in patients with a colon in continuity and 30–40% in patients without a colon will enhance the palatability of the diet, with an improvement in the number of calories absorbed [18]. Compared to a diet with regular long-chain triglycerides (LCTs) and given the fact that medium-chain triglycerides (MCTs) are rapidly decomposed, without the need of bile salts, and are easily absorbed through the intestinal mucosa and carried to the liver via portal vein, patients with a colon in continuity should benefit from a high content of MCT that provides a slight advantage in overall energy absorption (approximately 1.5 Mj/day). Also, replacement of LCT diet with MCT requires monitoring of potential deficiency in essential fatty acids and fat-soluble vitamins [12].

A diet with unabsorbed long-chain fatty acids may accelerate diarrhoea and steatorrhoea and decrease water and sodium absorption, forming complexes with calcium and magnesium and increasing the oxalate absorption and formation of renal stones [12, 17].

A moderate intake of soluble fibre may be included in the diet of patients with SBS to slow gastric emptying and improve osmotic diarrhoea [17]. For example, fibre supplements of pectin had no effect on energy or macronutrient absorption; therefore, patients may not benefit from pectin supplements to increase overall intestinal absorption. Some patients with end-ostomy with soluble fibre supplements included in the diet report a decrease in stool loss or ostomy effluent [12, 17]. Depending on patient tolerance, the recommended amount of fibre intake is 10–15 g/day [4].

The first choice in patients with chronic intestinal failure treated with enteral nutrition (EN) is polymeric isotonic enteral diets [12].

12.2.2 Phases of Diet Management in SBS

The diet management in SBS comprises three phases:

12.2.2.1 The Acute Phase (Immediate Post-operative Phase)

The acute period, which occurs immediately post-operative and lasts 3–4 weeks, is characterized by significant malabsorption, diarrhoea and dehydration, secondary to the loss of intestinal absorptive capacity [22, 23]. In this phase it is important to prevent complications, like dehydration and malnutrition.

The main recommendations consist of initiating parenteral nutrition (PN), in order to bypass the gastrointestinal tract and to supply adequate macronutrients, electrolytes, trace elements and vitamins to prevent malnutrition and managing fluid and electrolyte imbalances, as major complications can occur, such as dehydration and acute renal failure [15, 24].

EN must be started as soon as possible, given the fact that enteral feeding has a role in stimulating intestinal adaptation and decreasing the risk of bacterial translocation and liver dysfunction associated with prolonged parenteral nutrition. EN should begin with low-fat isotonic formulas, in order to decrease osmotic diarrhoea and steatorrhoea [13].

Initiation of oral nutrition should begin when the number and volume of stools decrease and the patient starts to gain weight, and it can be recommended to provide 5% of the total calories intake and increase this ratio every 3–7 days, concomitant with the reduction of PN to 10–15 hours, according to patient tolerance [4].

In case of high-output diarrhoea, especially in patients with jejunostomas, the management of dehydration consists of oral rehydration solutions that contain appropriate amounts of glucose, sodium and water [17].

12.2.2.2 The Adaptation Phase (3–24 Months Post-operative)

In this phase, the intestinal absorptive capacity improves secondary to structural and functional changes that depend on the residual bowel length and presence of a colon in continuity. The remaining bowel presents hyperplasia, an increase in the villous height and crypt depth and overall absorptive surface area [24].

It is important to taper gradually PN as oral or enteral intake improves, with regular monitoring of weight, serum electrolytes and vitamin levels [25].

The principal recommendations in this phase include encouraging patients to consume small, frequent meals in order to optimize nutrient absorption [26], with diets consisting of high-protein, moderate fat intake, complex carbohydrates and oxalate restriction.

A high-protein intake is optimal in tissue repair and supports immune function and overall recovery [13]. Regarding fats, as mentioned above, LCTs are poorly absorbed in patients with SBS; therefore, MCT can be included in their diet, as they are absorbed directly into the portal circulation and require less enzymatic breakdown [15]. Complex carbohydrates, such as oats, whole grains and starchy vegetables are recommended in this phase over simple sugars that can increase diarrhoea [12].

12.2.2.3 Maintenance Phase (Beyond 24 Months Post-operative)

This phase is representative of the long-term management of SBS, as it is necessary to obtain enteral autonomy, maintain a nutritional balance and reduce the risk of complications, such as diarrhoea, dehydration and deficiencies.

Based on the residual bowel, absorptive capacity and symptoms, every patient with SBS needs an individualized diet plan [13].

In the maintenance phase, the recommendations include supplements of fat-soluble vitamins (A, D, E and K), vitamin B12 intramuscular injections in patients with ileal resections and essential minerals (calcium, magnesium and zinc supplementation) [12, 24]. Also, soluble fibre can be included in the diet, in order to improve stool consistency and slow intestinal transit [17].

Oral rehydration solutions can be continued for managing chronic fluid and electrolyte loss, especially in cases with high-output stomas [17].

12.2.3 Dietary Advices According to Phenotypes of Bowel Resection (Recommendations of American Society for Parenteral and Enteral Nutrition [ASPEN])

12.2.3.1 Type 1: End-Jejunostomy

This phenotype is known as the most severe, because patients without a colon and less than 100 cm of the jejunum are predisposed to complications, such as dehydration, electrolyte imbalances, renal failure and require long-term PN. These patients should reduce hypotonic fluids to 500 ml/day, refrain from using hypertonic solutions and decrease sugar intake, as it can increase the fluid loss through the stoma. Oral rehydration solutions (ORS) are indicated, given their composition in water and sodium. The energy requirements are 35–45 kcal/kg/day and may increase up to 60 kcal/kg/day, with a diet consisting of 20–40% carbohydrates, 20–30% proteins and 40–60% fats, without oxalate restrictions [4].

12.2.3.2 Type 2: Jejunocolic

The energy intake required for these patients consist of 35–45 kcal/kg/day and can be increased up to 60 kcal/kg/day if needed, with a diet with 50–60% carbohydrates, 20–30% proteins and 20–30% fats and low in oxalate and isotonic or hypotonic fluids. Patients in this phenotype are also at risk of long-term PN, the main symptoms being diarrhoea secondary to severe malabsorption and deficiencies in vitamins and mineral, with malnutrition [4].

12.2.3.3 Type 3: Jejunoileocolic

Patients in this phenotype, having the colon with the ileocecal valve and a portion of the terminal ileum and jejunum, generally do not present malnutrition or dehydration [4].

12.2.4 Conclusion

Diet management is crucial in patients with SBS, in order to improve outcomes and long-term quality of life, with a need for individualized approaches, nutritional supplements and appropriate hydration.

References

1. Roberts K, Shah ND, Parrish CR, Wall E. Navigating nutrition and hydration care in the adult patient with short bowel syndrome. Nutr Clin Pract. 2023;38(Suppl 1):S59–75. https://doi.org/10.1002/ncp.10951. PMID: 37115029
2. Skallerup A, Nygaard L, Olesen SS, Køhler M, Vinter-Jensen L, Rasmussen HH. The prevalence of sarcopenia is markedly increased in patients with intestinal failure and associates with several risk factors. Clin Nutr. 2018;37(6 Pt A):2029–35.

3. Graungaard S, Geisler L, Andersen JR, et al. Prevalence of sarcopenia in patients with chronic intestinal failure-how are SARC-F and the EWGSOP algorithm associated before and after a physical exercise intervention. JPEN J Parenter Enteral Nutr. 2022;47(2):246–52.
4. Utrilla Fornals A, Costas-Batlle C, Medlin S, Menjón-Lajusticia E, Cisneros-González J, Saura-Carmona P, Montoro-Huguet MA. Metabolic and nutritional issues after lower digestive tract surgery: the important role of the dietitian in a multidisciplinary setting. Nutrients. 2024;16(2):246. https://doi.org/10.3390/nu16020246. PMID: 38257141; PMCID: PMC10820062
5. Oke SM, Rye B, Malietzis G, Baldwin-Cleland R, Bottle A, Gabe SM, Lung PFC. Survival and CT defined sarcopenia in patients with intestinal failure on home parenteral support. Clin Nutr. 2020;39:829–36.
6. Køhler M, Olesen SS, Rasmussen HH. Body composition predicts clinical outcome in patients with intestinal failure on long-term home parenteral nutrition. Clin Nutr ESPEN. 2018;28:193–200. https://doi.org/10.1016/j.clnesp.2018.08.004. Epub 2018 Aug 31
7. Cruz-Jentoft AJ, Baeyens JP, Bauer JM, Boirie Y, Cederholm T, Landi F, Martin FC, Michel JP, Rolland Y, Schneider SM, Topinková E, Vandewoude M, Zamboni M; European Working Group on Sarcopenia in Older People. Sarcopenia: European consensus on definition and diagnosis: report of the European Working Group on sarcopenia in older people. Age Ageing. 2010;39(4):412–23. https://doi.org/10.1093/ageing/afq034. Epub 2010 Apr 13. PMID: 20392703; PMCID: PMC2886201
8. Kawakami R, Tanisawa K, Ito T, Usui C, Miyachi M, Torii S, Midorikawa T, Ishii K, Muraoka I, Suzuki K, Sakamoto S, Higuchi M, Oka K. Fat-free mass index as a surrogate marker of appendicular skeletal muscle mass index for low muscle mass screening in sarcopenia. J Am Med Dir Assoc. 2022;23(12):1955–1961.e3. https://doi.org/10.1016/j.jamda.2022.08.016. Epub 2022 Sep 28. PMID: 36179769
9. Korzilius JW, van Asseldonk MJMD, Wanten GJA, Zweers-van Essen HEE. Body composition of adults with chronic intestinal failure receiving home parenteral nutrition: a descriptive cohort study. JPEN J Parenter Enteral Nutr. 2024;48(6):718–25. https://doi.org/10.1002/jpen.2658. Epub 2024 Jun 8
10. Fassini PG, Nicoletti CF, Pfrimer K, Nonino CB, Marchini JS, Ferriolli E. Bioelectrical impedance vector analysis as a useful predictor of nutritional status in patients with short bowel syndrome. Clin Nutr. 2017;36(4):1117–21. https://doi.org/10.1016/j.clnu.2016.07.011. Epub 2016 Jul 27. PMID: 27491548
11. Jones DJ, Lal S, Gittins M, Strauss BJG, Burden ST. Practical measurement of body composition using bioelectrical impedance, air displacement plethysmography and ultrasound in stable outpatients with short bowel syndrome receiving home parenteral nutrition: comparison of agreement between the methods. J Hum Nutr Diet. 2019;32(3):288–94. https://doi.org/10.1111/jhn.12613. Epub 2018 Nov 22. PMID: 30467908; PMCID: PMC6587511
12. Pironi L, Cuerda C, Jeppesen PB, Joly F, Jonkers C, Krznarić Ž, Lal S, Lamprecht G, Lichota M, Mundi MS, Schneider SM, Szczepanek K, Van Gossum A, Wanten G, Wheatley C, Weimann A. ESPEN guideline on chronic intestinal failure in adults—update 2023. Clin Nutr. 2023;42(10):1940–2021. https://doi.org/10.1016/j.clnu.2023.07.019. Epub 2023 Jul 29
13. Jeppesen PB. Spectrum of short bowel syndrome in adults: intestinal insufficiency to intestinal failure. JPEN J Parenter Enteral Nutr. 2014;38(1 Suppl):8S–13S. https://doi.org/10.1177/0148607114520994.
14. Iyer K, DiBaise JK, Rubio-Tapia A. AGA clinical practice update on Manag Short Bowel Syndrome: expert review. Clin Gastroenterol Hepatol: Official Clin Pract J Am Gastroenterolog Assoc. 2022;20(10):2185–2194.e2. https://doi.org/10.1016/j.cgh.2022.05.032.
15. Pironi L, Arends J, Bozzetti F, Cuerda C, Gillanders L, Jeppesen PB, Joly F, Kelly D, Lal S, Staun M, Szczepanek K, Van Gossum A, Wanten G, Schneider SM, Home Artificial Nutrition & Chronic Intestinal Failure Special Interest Group of ESPEN. ESPEN guidelines on chronic intestinal failure in adults. Clin Nutr (Edinburgh, Scotland). 2016;35(2):247–307. https://doi.org/10.1016/j.clnu.2016.01.020.

16. O'Keefe SJ, Buchman AL, Fishbein TM, Jeejeebhoy KN, Jeppesen PB, Shaffer J. Short bowel syndrome and intestinal failure: consensus definitions and overview. Clin Gastroenterol Hepatol: Off Clin Pract J Am Gastroenterolog Assoc. 2006;4(1):6–10. https://doi.org/10.1016/j.cgh.2005.10.002.
17. Parrish CR, DiBaise JK. Managing the adult patient with short bowel syndrome. Gastroenterol Hepatol. 2017;13(10):600–8. PMCID: PMC5718176 PMID: 29230136
18. Matarese LE, O'Keefe SJ, Kandil HM, Bond G, Costa G, Abu-Elmagd K. Short bowel syndrome: clinical guidelines for nutrition management. Nutr Clin Pract: Off Publ Am Soc Parent Enteral Nutr. 2005;20(5):493–502. https://doi.org/10.1177/0115426505020005493.
19. McIntyre PB, Fitchew M, Lennard-Jones JE. Patients with a high jejunostomy do not need a special diet. Gastroenterology. 1986;91:25–33.
20. Cosnes J, Evard D, Beaugerie L, Gendre JP, Le Quintrec Y. Improvement in protein absorption with a small peptide-base diet in patients with high jejunostomy. Nutrition. 1992;8:406–11.
21. Byrne TA, Wilmore DW, Iyer K, Dibaise J, Clancy K, Robinson MK, Chang P, Gertner JM, Lautz D. Growth hormone, glutamine, and an optimal diet reduces parenteral nutrition in patients with short bowel syndrome: a prospective, randomized, placebo-controlled, double-blind clinical trial. Ann Surg. 2005;242(5):655–61. https://doi.org/10.1097/01.sla.0000186479.53295.14.
22. Guillen B, Atherton NS. Short Bowel Syndrome. [Updated 2023 Jul 17]. In: StatPearls [Internet]. Treasure Island: StatPearls Publishing; 2025. Available from: https://www.ncbi.nlm.nih.gov/books/NBK536935/.
23. Tappenden KA. Pathophysiology of short bowel syndrome: considerations of resected and residual anatomy. JPEN J Parenter Enteral Nutr. 2014;38(1 Suppl):14S–22S. https://doi.org/10.1177/0148607113520005.
24. Pironi L, Sasdelli AS, Pazzeschi C, Chapter 2—Short Bowel Syndrome (SBS): classification, underlying causes, and global footprint. In: Corrigan ML, Roberts K, Steiger E, editors. Adult Short Bowel Syndrome. Academic Press; 2019. p. 17–25., ISBN 9780128143308. https://doi.org/10.1016/B978-0-12-814330-8.00002-0.
25. Matarese LE. Nutrition and fluid optimization for patients with short bowel syndrome. JPEN. 2013;37(2):161–70.
26. Wall EA. An overview of short bowel syndrome management: adherence, adaptation, and practical recommendations. J Acad Nutr Diet. 2013;113(9):1200–8.

13 Home Parenteral Nutrition in Long-Term Intestinal Failure

Liliana Mirea, Raluca Ungureanu, and Dragoş Ene

13.1 Introduction

The European Society for Clinical Nutrition and Metabolism (ESPEN) defines intestinal failure (IF) as "The reduction of gut function below the minimum necessary for the absorption of macronutrients and/or water and electrolytes, such that intravenous supplementation is required to maintain health and/or growth" [1].

Functional classification categorizes IF into three subtypes based on its onset, metabolic profile, and expected outcome. This chapter focuses on long-term intestinal failure or type III IF, which is a permanent or long-term condition. It may be either irreversible or reversible, but is usually seen in patients with irreversible bowel damage. The most common cause results from a massive surgical resection leading to short bowel syndrome (SBS). The length and functionality of the remaining small bowel determine nutritional independence or parenteral nutrition (PN) dependence.

Home parenteral nutrition (HPN) administration is the main medical treatment for management of SBS, a type III chronic intestinal failure (CIF), promoting quality of life with a structured and specialized multidisciplinary team following discharge from acute hospital settings. Alongside medical treatment, intestinal rehabilitation, and, in some cases, intestinal transplantation might be required.

L. Mirea · R. Ungureanu (✉)
Faculty of Medicine, Carol Davila University of Medicine and Pharmacy, Bucharest, Romania

Anesthesiology and Intensive Care Clinic, Clinical Emergency Hospital, Bucharest, Romania

D. Ene
Faculty of Medicine, Carol Davila University of Medicine and Pharmacy, Bucharest, Romania

General Surgery Department, Clinical Emergency Hospital, Bucharest, Romania

A. Trifan et al. (eds.), *Short Bowel Syndrome in Adults*,
https://doi.org/10.1007/978-3-031-95848-9_13

13.2 Epidemiology of Long-Term Intestinal Failure Requiring HPN

The prevalence and incidence of long-term IF vary across different countries and healthcare systems due to variations in disease etiology, access to specialized care, and the availability of HPN programs. The estimated prevalence of CIF ranges from 5 to 80 cases per million population, with the highest reported rates in countries with well-established HPN programs [2, 3].

The incidence of long-term IF is also variable, depending on factors such as the prevalence of short bowel syndrome (SBS), intestinal dysmotility disorders, and postsurgical complications. A large European multicenter survey analyzing chronic IF due to short bowel syndrome (SBS-IF) reported that around 60% of CIF cases were attributed to SBS, making it the leading cause of long-term IF requiring HPN [4–6].

With advances in surgical intestinal-sparing techniques, intestinal rehabilitation strategies, and the use of pharmacological therapies like glucagon-like peptide-2 (GLP-2) analogs (e.g., teduglutide), the incidence of permanent CIF has seen some reductions. However, due to improved survival rates and better access to HPN, the overall prevalence of CIF is increasing in many developed countries. While the prevalence of long-term IF remains low compared to other chronic conditions, the growing number of survivors with complex intestinal disorders has led to an increased need for structured HPN programs.

13.3 Role of Home Parenteral Nutrition

The medical management of PN in home care settings differs from that in hospitalized patients as it involves a transfer of main responsibility from healthcare personnel to patients and caregivers. To be eligible for HPN, patients must be clinically and metabolically stable and well trained for self-managing PN outside the hospital setting, either at home or in ambulatory care facilities [4, 7]. The decision to initiate HPN requires a thorough clinical, nutritional, and psychosocial evaluation to ensure its appropriateness, safety, and long-term feasibility.

HPN plays a vital role in the long-term management of CIF by providing essential nutrients, fluids, and electrolytes intravenously to patients who are unable to meet their nutritional needs by other routes and who can be safely managed outside of the hospital [8]. Without adequate nutritional support, patients with CIF face severe malnutrition, dehydration, and life-threatening metabolic imbalances. HPN is the standard of care, allowing patients to maintain an acceptable quality of life. Moreover, HPN facilitates intestinal rehabilitation, as some patients with reversible CIF may experience adaptation of the remaining bowel over time, reducing their dependence on PN.

Studies have shown that patients managed with structured HPN programs, under the supervision of a multidisciplinary nutrition support team (NST), achieve better outcomes, including reduced hospital admissions and improved overall well-being.

These teams typically include physicians, dietitians, nurses, and pharmacists who oversee nutritional monitoring, catheter care, infection prevention, and patient education to ensure safe and effective home management.

In certain cases, CIF due to SBS may be reversible due to intestinal adaptation and/or rehabilitation programs. Thus, patients should be promptly sent to IF centers competent in both medical and surgical management in order to increase the likelihood of discontinuing HPN, avoiding HPN failure, and providing timely evaluation for further intestinal transplantation (ITx) eligibility [9].

13.4 Indications of Home Parenteral Nutrition

The objectives and attributes of the HPN program, together with the distinct requirements of the patient, may vary throughout different clinical situations.

The degree of PN dependence varies among patients, from total (or exclusive), when the patient's nutritional needs are covered by parenteral route, to supplemental (partial or complementary), when the patient tolerates some oral or enteral route. HPN should be administered as the principal treatment for patients with transient-reversible or permanent-irreversible CIF [1]. However, whereas all patients with CIF require HPN, not all patients receiving HPN have CIF, and these terms shall not be considered equivalent [8, 9].

Consequently, according to ESPEN guidelines, four clinical situations for the use of HPN may be distinguished depending on gastrointestinal function and causative illness, alongside patient characteristics [8, 10]:

1. HPN as the primary life-saving intervention for a patient with CIF resulting from a benign condition.
2. HPN for CIF resulting from malignant disorders, often transiently occurring during curative treatments.
3. HPN incorporated into a palliative care regimen for terminal malignant conditions to prevent mortality due to malnutrition. However, exclusion of HPN from patients with a poor prognosis and no prospect for treatment should occur only after consultation with the patients and/or their designated family members.
4. HPN is used to avoid or address malnutrition in individuals with an operational intestine who refuse alternative forms of medicinal nutrition ("no-CIF situation").

Additionally, the indications and prognosis of individuals requiring HPN for CIF vary based on the underlying etiology. Based on pathophysiological classification, IF can be categorized into five primary conditions, which could be the consequence of a variety of abdominal or systemic conditions [1, 5, 11–13]:

- **SBS,** which is the most common cause of chronic IF, resulting from extensive surgical resection of the small intestine with a remnant small bowel fragment of less than 200 cm.

- **Intestinal dysmotility disorders**, secondary to conditions impairing peristalsis of gut content in the absence of fixed occluding lesions, such as chronic intestinal pseudo-obstruction (CIPO), severe diabetes-induced dysmotility, or systemic sclerosis leading to ineffective nutrient absorption. These patients often have a functioning but uncoordinated gut, leading to intestinal stasis, malnutrition, and bacterial overgrowth.
- **Intestinal fistulas** are abnormal connections between the bowel and other organs or skin, leading to loss of nutrients and fluids.
- **Extensive mucosal disease** like radiation enteritis or severe Crohn's disease, where the intestinal lining is damaged, resulting in protein-losing enteropathy and nutrient deficiencies.
- **Mechanical obstruction**, secondary to structural abnormalities, such as strictures or tumors that block the passage of food and fluids.

Additionally, there are no absolute contraindications to the use of PN. Nevertheless, the presence of specific metabolic diseases and organ failures may be associated with reduced tolerance to PN and may necessitate adaptation of the HPN program to meet the patient's specific clinical requirements.

13.5 Patients' Assessment and Selection for Home Parenteral Nutrition Application

All patients eligible for admission into an HPN program must have proven prolonged CIF that, if left untreated, will result in worsening nutritional and/or fluid status, and must have completed a sufficient trial of enteral nutrition (EN). ESPEN has established guidelines for determining HPN eligibility, which include medical, metabolic stability, functional ability, psychosocial aspects of the patient, and family suitability [14].

However, before initiating HPN, a comprehensive risk assessment must be conducted to identify potential complications and ensure that the patient is suitable for long-term intravenous (IV) therapy.

HPN requires active patient and caregiver participation and a stable home environment to ensure adherence and prevent complications. Patients with severe depression, anxiety, or cognitive impairment may have difficulty managing HPN. Additionally, lack of caregiver support can increase nonadherence and complication rates. Patients must be psychologically prepared for long-term intravenous therapy; thus, psychological screening is recommended to assess compliance risk, depression, and quality-of-life concerns.

The patient and/or caregiver must be capable of learning sterile techniques for catheter care and infusion management. Careful assessment should be performed in patients who refuse or are unable to comply with treatment protocols. Higher risk of complications is also seen in patients who live in an environment that cannot support safe home infusion therapy. A clean, sanitary, and stable home setting with reliable electricity and refrigeration for HPN storage is needed.

For a safe HPN program, the patient shall be sufficiently metabolically stable and emotionally able to cope with HPN therapy outside the acute hospital setting.

Patients on HPN require significant lifestyle adaptations, including managing daily intravenous infusions and preventing complications. Additionally, candidates for HPN or their family caregivers must get training and supervision from an HPN specialist to guarantee familiarity with HPN techniques and complications related to catheter care, preparation of PN admixtures, infusion techniques, and storage methods. They must also be instructed on what to avoid and the appropriate actions to take in the event of any complications.

13.6 Central Venous Access Device Selection and Care for Long-Term HPN

The selection of the central venous access devices (CVADs) and the positioning of the exit site must be determined by a proficient HPN NST in conjunction with the patient [15]. The exit site of the CVAD must be readily visible and accessible for patients managing their own care. Tunneled CVADs, such as Hickman, Broviac, or Groshong, as well as totally implantable devices (ports), are typically selected for long-term HPN exceeding 6 months. Conversely, peripherally inserted central catheters (PICCs) may be utilized if HPN is anticipated to last less than 6 months. The preferred site for CVAD placement is the upper vena cava, accessed via the internal jugular vein or subclavian vein. Regardless of the catheter type or insertion site, positioning the CVAD tip at the junction of the superior vena cava and right atrium minimizes the risk of complications [8].

While implantable ports or central venous catheters (CVCs) are the norm for long-term parenteral nutrition administration, a surgically created arteriovenous fistula (AVF) may be a viable alternative in certain circumstances such as preventing CVAD-related infections. Therefore, AVFs may be a valuable alternative to other methods of providing HPN.

For a more in-depth discussion on the detailed aspects of CVADs, Chap. 14 provides an extensive analysis and suggestions.

13.7 Components of Parenteral Nutrition Formulations

For CIF patients, the protein and energy requirements should be tailored to each patient's individual characteristics, nutritional needs, disease state, metabolic status, and hydration balance.

The HPN admixture must fulfill the patient's requirements [8]. A PN regimen generally has 40–50 components, including macronutrients (carbohydrates, lipids, and amino acids), water, electrolytes, and micronutrients (vitamins and trace elements). PN may be administered from distinct containers or as an admixture, ideally in a single-container unit of PN commonly referred to as two-in-one (containing carbohydrates and amino acids, with lipids infused separately) or all-in-one or "3 in

1" bags (all-in-one [AIO] that contains all macronutrients in a single bag). Additionally, those within a singular container unit may be tailored as customized admixtures or presented as ready-to-use formulations. These customized compounding units provide the advantage of adapting the formulations to the individual requirements of patients, particularly those necessitating long-term PN therapy, with rapidly fluctuating metabolic demands or in cases with specific disease-related metabolic derangements [8].

The admixture should be administered cyclically or constantly, depending on the circumstances. High nutritional contents in these formulations frequently result in elevated osmolality, hence often prohibiting peripheral venous delivery. Consequently, central venous access is frequently essential, with pump-assisted delivery recommended to increase tolerance.

Energy requirement The argument over the optimal energy source has ended. Glucose, lipids, and amino acids are widely acknowledged as vital energy substrates, although they may assume different roles in certain therapeutic scenarios. However, limited data is available to clarify energy prescription for HPN patients. Establishing energy requirements cannot be accomplished by a single-set formula, but it must rely on nutritional evaluation that includes disease-specific considerations. A research showed that the energy needs of HPN patients may be fulfilled by providing 1.4 times the resting energy expenditure (REE), or around 30 kcal/kg/d. No substantial difference was seen between predicted REE by using the Harris-Benedict equations and that measured with indirect calorimetry [16]. However, most stable individuals on HPN are effectively maintained on 20 to 35 kilocalories of total energy per kilogram per day [7, 16]. The objectives of therapy and periodic reassessment should clarify the energy requirements in an HPN prescription. Nevertheless, the replenishment of body cell mass will be different from those for maintenance needs. Certain patients have a considerable oral intake, which may be partially digested and absorbed. The colon has been shown to function as an energy-recovering organ [17]. Consequently, HPN energy needs may be adjusted based on residual gastrointestinal function. A cross-sectional investigation indicated that the maintenance of partial bowel function led to a decrease in HPN energy requirements [18].

Carbohydrates The sources of energy for HPN prescriptions originate from glucose and fat emulsions (1,7). Glucose constitutes 50–60% of total caloric intake. HPN solutions include dextrose with concentrations ranging from 5% to 35%, which can be modified according to glycemic balance. Potential consequences include hyperglycemia requiring glucose monitoring and insulin treatment, as well as increased CO_2 generation, which is especially significant in individuals with chronic hypercapnia. Optimal blood glucose regulation, defined as values below 180 mg/dL (10.0 mmol/L) during HPN infusion and stable hemoglobin A1c (HbA1c) levels under 7% in diabetic individuals, may be accomplished with constant surveillance [1]. Additionally, delivery of glucose dictates the maximum permissible rate of PN infusion: a maximum of 5–7 mg glucose/kg/min, equating to about 350 g of glucose over 12 h for a 70-kg adult, or 3–6 g glucose/kg per day [4].

Protein Requirements (Amino Acids) Protein in HPN admixtures is provided as L-amino acids. Actual commercially available formulations for PN contain the nine essential amino acids (histidine, isoleucine, leucine, lysine, methionine, phenylalanine, threonine, tryptophan, and valine) in proportions ranging from 38% to 57%, while nonessential amino acids constitute 43–62% of the total amino acids [19]. Amino acid solutions are available in concentrations between 5% and 15%, with or without electrolytes. High-strength solutions with nitrogen levels of up to 30 g/L facilitate the manufacturing of more concentrated mixtures when the volume to be infused daily should be reduced due to other causes.

Amino acid requirements vary depending on patient disease status, with some experiencing significant stoma losses or protein-losing enteropathy, while others have needs more comparable to those of healthy individuals. The intestine's protein-sparing properties, which enable the progressive release of nutrients following bolus feeding, are lacking in HPN; hence, continuous infusions have an advantage over bolus amino acid infusions [20]. Currently, the predominant way for assessing the effectiveness of PN is by the measurement of nitrogen balance. However, a research indicated that amino acid solutions deliver 17% less protein precursor than the combined amount of their individual amino acids [21]. Thereby, protein prescriptions must take into consideration the nonequivalence of amino acids to dietary protein intake.

Nonetheless, the incorporation of certain amino acids (glutamine, cysteine, and taurine) into the parenteral formula to reduce complications is not advised [14].

International guidelines recommend that healthy individuals require 0.8–1 g/kg/d of protein, associated with sufficient energy for optimal nitrogen utilization. Most stable patients on HPN are effectively sustained on regimens delivering 0.8–1.4 g of protein (0.13–0.24 g of nitrogen) per kilogram per day [7, 22].

Lipids (Intravenous Lipid Emulsions [ILE]) Lipids provide nonprotein energy and are a source of essential fatty acids (EFAs), reducing glucose dependency in long-term HPN patients. Furthermore, clinical experiences with the latest generation of intravenous lipid emulsions indicate that the function of lipids exceeds the role as conventional energy substrates, and they may serve as an immunomodulatory element (Table 13.1).

The guidelines stipulate that intravenous energy sources should consist of lipids comprising 15–30% of total caloric intake and 30–50% of nonprotein calories. The ideal dosage of lipids for individuals on HPN is not definitively determined. Lipid emulsions are especially important for individuals entirely reliant on HPN, since a minimum of 1 g/kg/week is required to prevent EFA deficiency (EFAD). Patients on long-term PN with lipid-free or less lipid-containing high-glucose solutions may

Table 13.1 Comparison of different intravenous lipid emulsion products used in PN

Lipid source	Composition	Clinical benefits	Potential risks
Soybean oil-based (standard ILE, 100% LCTs)	High in omega-6 PUFAs	Cost-effective, widely used	Pro-inflammatory, associated with IFALD risk
MCT/LCT-based	Mix of MCTs (50%) and LCTs (50%)	Better tolerance, rapid oxidation	Moderate IFALD risk
Olive oil-based (80% olive oil, 20% soybean oil)	Lower omega-6 content, high in MUFAs	Less pro-inflammatory, hepatic protection	Higher cost
Fish oil-based (omega-3-rich, 100% or blended)	High in EPA/DHA omega-3 FA	Anti-inflammatory, hepatoprotective, reduces IFALD risk	Higher cost, limited availability

Abbreviations: *FA* fatty acid, *MCT* medium-chain triglyceride, *LCT* long-chain triglyceride, *MUFA* monounsaturated fatty acid, *PUFA* polyunsaturated fatty acid, *EPA* eicosapentaenoic acid, *DHA* docosahexaenoic acid, *IFALD* intestinal failure-associated liver disease

develop hyperinsulinemia, which inhibits the mobilization of EFAs from adipose tissue. EFAs such as linoleic acid and alpha-linolenic acid are fractions of lipids that cannot be generated in vivo [7, 23]. Modifying a soybean oil-based lipid emulsion to a fish oil- or olive oil-based lipid emulsion may be safe in terms of supplying enough EFA.

When administering a soybean-based lipid emulsion, the dosage should not exceed 1 g/kg/d. Administration of soybean oil lipid emulsion in higher doses was associated with significantly increased risk of development of intestinal failure-associated liver disease (IFALD). Preliminary data indicates that lipid emulsions alternative to soybean oil-based lipid emulsions might reduce the likelihood of hepatic damage associated with PN in patients susceptible to hepatic dysfunction [1, 24, 25]. Alternative lipid sources such as olive oil, medium-chain triglycerides (MCT), and fish oil should be used to decrease soybean oil concentration.

Triglycerides should be checked monthly, and if there is an increase over 400 mg/dl, it should be withheld or the dosage should be reduced. However, withholding ILE infusion longer than 2 weeks may induce EFAD.

Fluid and Electrolytes Maintaining hydration and electrolyte balance is important in HPN, particularly in patients with high-output fistula, SBS, or chronic diarrhea. These patients require regular monitoring of dehydration signs and symptoms, fluid balance, laboratory testing, and 24-hour urine output, together with prompt fluid adjustments and supplementation, because they often experience significant fluid and electrolyte losses. Precise intravenous supplementation to prevent dehydration and electrolyte imbalances is essential to avoid chronic renal failure and other complications.

The dose recommendations for PN fluid and electrolytes are derived from clinical experience due to the absence of randomized research. Fluid requirements vary based on patient physiology, underlying disease, and ongoing losses. The volume of total parenteral nutrition (TPN) in average adult needs is about 25–35 mL/kg/day, or approximately 1500–2500 mL/day of fluid. The PN formula will be modified in order to normalize laboratory tests regarding electrolytes and mineral balance.

Electrolytes are critical for many cellular functions. They must be carefully monitored and replaced based on the patient's ongoing losses and metabolic state. Recommended electrolyte doses are: 1–1.5 mmol/kg/day for sodium, potassium, and chloride; 0.3–0.5 mmol/kg/kg/day for phosphate; and 0.1–1.15 mmol/kg/day for calcium and magnesium. Furthermore, consistent assessment of acid–base status (serum levels of chloride and bicarbonate) is necessary, since metabolic acidosis or metabolic alkalosis may arise.

Micronutrients Micronutrients include vitamins and trace elements employed for metabolic processes, immunological function, and the prevention of deficits.

Vitamins Patients on long-term HPN are susceptible to deficiencies; thus, clinical manifestations and biochemical indicators of vitamin insufficiency or toxicity should be routinely assessed. Water-soluble vitamins (B complex and vitamin C) are not stored in significant amounts in the body and need regular supplementation. Additionally, those vitamins are absorbed actively from the upper intestine, except for vitamin B12, which is selectively absorbed from the distal 60 cm of the ileum [26]. Fat-soluble vitamins (A, D, E, and K) are stored in the body's adipose tissues and liver; however, absorption is compromised in individuals with intestinal failure. Baseline blood vitamin concentrations should be assessed at the initiation of HPN and thereafter at least annually. Furthermore, the significance of baseline vitamin levels prior to initiating HPN is important, as this allows for the administration of replacement doses of vitamins until resolution occurs. Consequently, vitamin dosages in HPN may be modified as required. The method of vitamin supplementation may be tailored to certain characteristics of the particular patient. Vitamins are administered as a multivitamin formulation, including both water-soluble and fat-soluble vitamins [1].

Trace elements Trace elements are inorganic nutrients required in minute amounts. More than dozen trace elements are considered vital for biological activities (for enzymatic reactions, cellular function, and immunity); however, only nine are often included in PN regimens. Deficiencies or toxicities can cause severe metabolic disturbances. Patients with increased losses, malnutrition, or depletion prior to initiating PN may have heightened needs. The guidelines for vitamins may be extended to trace elements regarding monitoring and dosing. Standard PN solutions lack trace components due to chemical stability concerns and must be included into the PN solution just before to patient administration [1, 27].

Additives and special considerations It is generally advised that medications should not be added to PN admixtures unless they are absolutely essential. The choice to include drug additives must be justified by evidence about the physicochemical compatibility and stability of both the medicine and the final admixture. Although no recommendations can currently be made on the ideal strategy for establishing glycemic control in HPN patients, the incorporation of insulin into HPN admixtures has been shown as safe in several case series for managing hyperglycemia in diabetic or glucose-intolerant individuals.

Methods of delivering PN admixtures HPN must be delivered via an infusion pump to ensure safety and efficacy. The utilization of an electronic (ambulatory) infusion pump with suitable delivery settings is regarded as best practice. A portable pump enhances the quality of life compared to stationary pumps, as it allows those patients to achieve greater independence. The advantages encompassed sustaining optimal flow, minimal disturbance, extended battery longevity, and enhanced likelihood of social and occupational recovery. The widely recognized maximum hanging time for a ready-to-use admixture is 24 h. At the completion of a cyclic PN infusion, the infusion rate must be decreased in order to minimize insulin requirements and prevent rebound hypoglycemia [8, 14]. Continuous infusion (24-h) is often used in unstable patients or those with high fluid needs; however, cyclic infusion (12–16 h overnight) is preferred for long-term HPN patients, allowing for increased mobility and better quality of life, and also reducing the risk of hepatic complications (IFALD).

13.8 Monitoring and Management of HPN Patients

The objective of monitoring is to ensure and enhance the quality of life by evaluating the nutritional effectiveness and PN regimen tolerance, to prevent and detect nutritional deficits or toxicities, and to avoid or promptly identify and treat HPN-related complications [8]. Those measures are taken in order to optimize PN formulations in accordance with evolving requirements.

All patients must undergo frequent reassessment of their metabolic, nutritional, and overall health status. Although evidence-based guidelines for monitoring are lacking due to insufficient published data, the interval between reviews should be tailored to the patient, care environment, and duration of nutritional support. Intervals may be extended as the patient stabilizes on nutritional support. Following hospital release, the HPN NST maintains regular contact with patients and caregivers, first every few days, transitioning to weekly, and ultimately monthly, as the patient gains competence. Additionally, patients and caregivers must be educated in self-monitoring their state of nutrition, fluid balance, and infusion catheter, as well as in identifying early signs and symptoms of complications. The clinician in touch must be ready to elucidate any uncertainties and monitor clinical parameters and overall health status.

Furthermore, the quality of life of patients should be assessed using validated instruments as an integral component of routine clinical practice. The home parenteral nutrition–quality of life (HPN-QoL®) is a treatment-specific questionnaire designed for patients with CIF due to benign underlying diseases. The questionnaire comprises 48 items and concentrates on symptomatic, emotional, and physical concerns. In practice, the quality of care can be evaluated by examining a variety of factors, including the number of catheter-related events, the patient's incidence of hospital readmission, the quality of life, weight change, and the incidence of dehydration [28].

In clinically stable patients, body weight, body composition, hydration status, energy and fluid balance (urine output and stoma output), and biochemical parameters (hemoglobin, ferritin, albumin, C-reactive protein, electrolytes, venous blood gas analysis, kidney function, liver function, and glucose) should be assessed at all scheduled intervals (every 3–6 months).

Deficiencies in vitamins and trace elements may require an extended period in order to manifest clinical signs and symptoms, so a 6–12-month evaluation interval is suitable. Monitoring micronutrients is important, particularly for those patients undergoing intestinal rehabilitation and an ongoing weaning protocol from HPN. Therefore, clinical manifestations and biochemical indicators of vitamin and trace metal deficiency or toxicity should be assessed at least annually. Additionally, bone metabolism and bone mineral density should be assessed yearly or according to established guidelines [8].

Optimizing the formulation of PN is crucial to address the evolving requirements of these patients and to prevent metabolic disorders. Dextrose concentration must be raised in patients undergoing weight loss to guarantee sufficient calorie intake, while it should be decreased in instances of hyperglycemia to avoid insulin resistance and metabolic stress. Protein consumption must be increased in hypercatabolic conditions, such as infections, to facilitate tissue regeneration and improve immunological activity. In hypertriglyceridemia, lipid content should be reduced (and changed with fish oil-based emulsions), especially in intestinal failure-associated liver disease (IFALD). Fluid management requires supervision; as adequate administration is essential for patients susceptible to dehydration, such as those with SBS or with high-output stomas, whereas restriction is required in certain cases of heart failure or renal illnesses to reduce the risk of fluid overload. Electrolytes must be modified according to serum levels and continuous losses.

13.9 Complications Associated with Long-Term HPN

In spite of its advantages, HPN is linked to potential complications, such as central venous catheter-related complications (such as catheter-related bloodstream infections [CRBSIs], thrombosis, obstruction/migration, or loss of vascular access), as well as metabolic imbalances, nutritional deficiencies or toxicities, HPN-associated liver disease, or metabolic bone diseases. The consequences on quality of life, such as the development of psychological and sleeping disorders that impede socioprofessional rehabilitation, should not be neglected.

13.9.1 CVAD-Related Complications

Complications associated with CVADs are a significant concern for patients who are receiving HPN.

The risk of mechanical, infectious, and thrombotic complications is elevated by the prolonged use of catheters. Nutrient delivery can be disrupted and catheter replacement may be necessary due to mechanical complications, including catheter occlusion, dislodgment, and fracture. CRBSIs are among the most severe complications, frequently requiring catheter removal and antibiotic therapy, often requiring hospitalization due to sepsis. Thrombosis, which is induced by the formation of a thrombus around the catheter, can lead to venous obstruction, edema, and an elevated risk of pulmonary embolism. This may necessitate the use of anticoagulation therapy or the replacement of the catheter. In order to reduce CVAD complications and guarantee the long-term safety and efficacy of HPN therapy, it is imperative to implement preventive measures, such as meticulous aseptic technique, routine catheter care, regular purging of catheter lumen, and patient education. Prompt intervention and early detection are essential for the management of these complications in order to prevent significant outcomes and ensure continuous nutrition support.

13.9.2 Disease-Related Complications Associated with HPN

Renal Failure and Stones Chronic fluid and electrolyte losses, especially in patients with high-output fistula, can lead to dehydration and kidney dysfunction. Another proposed mechanism for renal injury is recurrent CRBSI; however, this has not been conclusively shown by the data. The administration of nephrotoxic drugs and preexisting renal conditions may also contribute significantly. Renal calculi and nephrocalcinosis are associated with heightened oxalate absorption, hypovolemia, and dehydration. Hypomagnesemia and metabolic acidosis may elevate the risk of renal precipitates, particularly uric acid calculi. In those who suffer from SBS, increased absorption of oxalate may occur due to fatty acids sequestering calcium and inhibiting the complexation of oxalate. Absorbed oxalate can precipitate in the renal tubules, causing tubular injury, necrosis, and atrophy. Prevention has to focus on adequate parenteral administration, optimal hydration, and high urine output. Preventive strategies involving decreased oxalate consumption and cholestyramine administration have been documented, although their efficacy is not consistently found. A low-fat diet or the substitution of MCT and oral calcium supplements during meals may also be investigated. It is advisable to manage renal failure and renal stones in patients with CIF in accordance with established criteria for these disorders.

Metabolic Bone Disease The risk of bone loss is further raised by long-term HPN, which is in addition to the risk factors of the individual (e.g., postmenopausal, lack of exercise). There are numerous factors that are associated with HPN and intestinal failure, such as suboptimal vitamin D levels, low calcium absorption or ingestion, high amino acid load, electrolyte imbalance, aluminum contamination, and cyclic infusion [29, 30].

Despite the fact that patients receive additional oral and IV supplementation, the prevalence of vitamin D insufficiency and deficiency is well documented [31]. Therefore, it is recommended that those patients should be routinely monitored for metabolic bone disease by serum and urinary biochemistry alongside annual bone mineral density testing (dual-energy X-ray absorptiometry [DEXA] scanning). Additionally, PN regimen modification with high-dose vitamin D, calcium and phosphate supplementation, and other management strategies should be implemented accordingly. Supplementary preventive measures that apply to the general population should also be recognized for patients on HPN [14].

Hepatic Complications Intestinal failure-associated liver disease (IFALD) is a significant consequence of sustained HPN, marked by hepatic impairment. It presents as hepatic steatosis, cholestasis, fibrosis, or cirrhosis and is frequently associated with excessive dextrose and lipid infusion, recurrent infections, and poor enteral stimulation. Risk factors involve extended utilization of soybean oil-derived lipid emulsions, overfeeding, and bacterial translocation from the gastrointestinal tract. Strategies for prevention and management emphasize changing parenteral nutrition composition, which includes minimizing carbohydrate overload, limiting the dose of soybean oil-based lipid emulsion to less than 1 g/kg/day or utilizing fish oil-based lipid emulsions, implementing cycling mode of infusion in order to provide fasting intervals, and encouraging minimal enteral intake wherever feasible. Consistent monitoring of liver function (aspartate aminotransferase [AST], alanine aminotransferase [ALT], alkaline phosphatase [ALP], gamma-glutamyl transferase [GGT], and bilirubin levels) is essential for prompt identification and management. In advanced instances, hepatic fibrosis and liver failure may occur, potentially requiring intestine and liver transplantation. Enhancing PN formulations and preserving gut integrity via enteral nutrition can markedly diminish the risk and advancement of IFALD.

More details linked with each of these complications are extensively discussed in dedicated chapters.

13.10 Operational and Healthcare System Considerations

13.10.1 Structure of HPN Programs

The structure of HPN programs is designed to provide comprehensive, multidisciplinary care to patients with CIF, ensuring safe and effective long-term nutrition support.

ESPEN guidelines emphasize the need for structured patient selection, informed consent, and comprehensive training for both patients and caregivers to minimize complications and improve adherence to treatment. A well-organized HPN program needs a well-coordinated operational framework that integrates healthcare providers, patients, and supporting institutions to ensure safe and effective care. Also, ensuring seamless collaboration between hospital-based nutrition support teams (NSTs), home care providers, and general practitioners is important for ongoing patient monitoring, emergency management, and overall quality of care. Also, coordination between healthcare providers, home care services, and suppliers is needed for timely delivery of nutritional solutions, equipment, and medical supplies [32].

A key operational consideration is the standardization of clinical protocols, ensuring that patients receive appropriate, high-quality treatment regardless of geographic location. These programs include patient education on catheter care, infection prevention, and troubleshooting complications, along with regular clinical and laboratory monitoring to assess metabolic status, nutritional adequacy, and organ function. Additionally, structured programs emphasize psychosocial support, helping patients adapt to the demands of HPN while maintaining quality of life.

By integrating standardized protocols, telemedicine support, and emergency response plans, well-structured HPN programs enhance patient safety, minimize complications, and improve long-term outcomes for individuals requiring lifelong parenteral nutrition.

13.10.2 Cost and Economic Burden of Long-Term HPN

The cost and economic burden are significant, affecting healthcare systems, insurers, and patients. HPN involves high costs starting with the specialized nutrient formulations, central venous catheter maintenance, infusion pumps, sterile supplies, and home healthcare services. Additionally, expenses arise from regular laboratory monitoring, medical consultations, hospitalizations, and the need for multidisciplinary care. The average annual cost per patient varies by country, with estimates ranging from 60.000 to 85.000 € per year, depending on the complexity of care and healthcare system coverage [33].

Insurance reimbursement and national healthcare policies play a crucial role in determining accessibility, with disparities in coverage leading to financial strain for patients and families in certain regions. While HPN allows patients to live outside the hospital and maintain a better quality of life, it poses challenges in terms of long-term affordability, cost-effectiveness, and equitable access to care. Strategies to optimize HPN efficiency, prevent complications, and explore alternative therapies like intestinal rehabilitation and transplantation can help reduce costs and improve healthcare sustainability [34].

13.11 Conclusion

HPN is a life-saving therapy for patients with CIF due to SBS, enabling them to maintain adequate nutrition outside the hospital setting. However, it requires careful monitoring, individualized management, and a multidisciplinary approach to ensure long-term safety and effectiveness.

Moving forward, advancements in HPN formulations, lipid emulsions, and remote patient monitoring will continue to enhance patient outcomes. Standardized HPN protocols, patient education, and multidisciplinary team collaboration are key to minimizing complications and improving the quality of life for individuals on long-term HPN. As research progresses, efforts to optimize intestinal adaptation, reduce metabolic complications, and explore innovative therapies will further refine HPN management, ensuring better long-term survival and functional independence for patients with CIF.

References

1. Pironi L, Cuerda C, Jeppesen PB, Joly F, Jonkers C, Krznari Z, et al. ESPEN guideline on chronic intestinal failure in adults—update 2023. Clin Nutr. 2023;42(10):1940–2021.
2. Pironi L, Goulet O, Buchman A, Messing B, Gabe S, Candusso M, et al. Outcome on home parenteral nutrition for benign intestinal failure: a review of the literature and benchmarking with the European prospective survey of ESPEN. Clin Nutr. 2012;31(6):831–45.
3. Brandt CF, Hvistendahl M, Naimi RM, Tribler S, Staun M, Brøbech P, et al. Home parenteral nutrition in adult patients with chronic intestinal failure: the evolution over 4 decades in a tertiary referral center. J Parenter Enter Nutr. 2017;41(7):1178–87.
4. Pironi L, Boeykens K, Bozzetti F, Joly F, Klek S, Lal S, et al. ESPEN guideline on home parenteral nutrition. Clin Nutr. 2020;39(6):1645–66.
5. Pironi L, Konrad D, Brandt C, Joly F, Wanten G, Agostini F, et al. Clinical classification of adult patients with chronic intestinal failure due to benign disease: an international multicenter cross-sectional survey. Clin Nutr. 2018;37(2):728–38.
6. Lezo A, Diamanti A, Marinier EM, Tabbers M, Guz-Mark A, Gandullia P, et al. Chronic intestinal failure in children: an international multicenter cross-sectional survey. Nutrients. 2022;14(9)
7. Staun M, Pironi L, Bozzetti F, Baxter J, Forbes A, Joly F, Jeppesen P, Moreno J, et al. ESPEN guidelines on parenteral nutrition: Home Parenteral Nutrition (HPN) in adult patients. Clin Nutr. 2009;28(4):467–79.
8. Pironi L, Boeykens K, Bozzetti F, Joly F, Klek S, Lal S, et al. ESPEN practical guideline: home parenteral nutrition. Clin Nutr. 2023;42(3):411–30.
9. Joly F, Baxter J, Staun M, Kelly DG, Hwa YL, Corcos O, et al. Five-year survival and causes of death in patients on home parenteral nutrition for severe chronic and benign intestinal failure. Clin Nutr. 2018;37(4):1415–22.
10. Cederholm T, Barazzoni R, Austin P, Ballmer P, Biolo G, Bischoff SC, et al. ESPEN guidelines on definitions and terminology of clinical nutrition. Clin Nutr. 2017;36(1):49–64.
11. Pironi L, Arends J, Baxter J, Bozzetti F, Pelaez RB, Cuerda C, et al. ESPEN endorsed recommendations: definition and classification of intestinal failure in adults. Clin Nutr. 2015;34(2):171–80.
12. Klek S, Forbes A, Gabe S, Holst M, Wanten G, Irtun O, et al. Management of acute intestinal failure: a position paper from the European Society for Clinical Nutrition and Metabolism (ESPEN) Special Interest Group. Pain Anesth Intens Care. 2017;0(2(79)):72–87
13. Quigley EMM. Enteric dysmotility: validating the Wingate/Bangkok classification. Gastroenterology. 2010;139(1):346–8.
14. Cuerda C, Pironi L, Arends J, Bozzetti F, Gillanders L, Jeppesen PB, et al. ESPEN practical guideline: clinical nutrition in chronic intestinal failure. Clin Nutr. 2021;40(9):5196–220.
15. Schneider PJ. Nutrition support teams: an evidence-based practice. Nutr Clin Pract. 2006;21(1):62–7.

16. Koea JB, Wolfe RRSJ. Total energy expenditure during total parenteral nutrition: ambulatory patients at home versus patients with sepsis in surgical intensive care. Surgery. 1995;118(1):54–62.
17. Carbonnel F, Cosnes J, Chevret S, Beaugerie L, Ng Y, Malafosse M, et al. The role of anatomic factors in nutritional autonomy after extensive small bowel resection. J Parenter Enter Nutr. 1996;20(4):275–80.
18. Bekker Jeppesen P, Staun M, Mortensen PB. Adult patients receiving home parenteral nutrition in Denmark from 1991 to 1996: who will benefit from intestinal transplantation? Scand J Gastroenterol. 1998;33(8):839–46.
19. Yarandi SS, Zhao VM, Hebbar G, Ziegler TR. Amino acid composition in parenteral nutrition: what is the evidence? Curr Opin Clin Nutr Metab Care. 2011;14(1):75–82.
20. Soeters PB, Van De Poll MCG. Amino acids, protein and the intestine. Home Parenter Nutr. 2006:234–58.
21. Hoffer LJ. How much protein do parenteral amino acid mixtures provide? Am J Clin Nutr. 2011;94(6):1396–8.
22. Hoffer LJ, Bistrian BR. Appropriate protein provision in critical illness: a systematic and narrative review. Am J Clin Nutr. 2012;96(3):591–600.
23. Jeppesen PB, Hoy CE, Mortensen PB. Essential fatty acid deficiency in patients receiving home parenteral nutrition. Am J Clin Nutr. 1998;68(1):126–33.
24. Mundi MS, Klek S, Martindale RG. Use of lipids in adult patients requiring parenteral nutrition in the home setting. J Parenter Enter Nutr. 2020;44(S1):S39–44.
25. Martindale RG, Berlana D, Boullata JI, Cai W, Calder PC, Deshpande GH, et al. Summary of proceedings and expert consensus statements from the international summit "Lipids in Parenteral Nutrition.". J Parenter Enter Nutr. 2020;44(S1):S7–20.
26. Thompson WG, Wrathell E. The relation between ileal resection and vitamin B12 absorption. Can J Surg. 1977;20(5):461–4.
27. Hardy G, Reilly C. Technical aspects of trace element supplementation. Curr Opin Clin Nutr Metab Care. 1999;2(4):277–85.
28. Baxter JP, Fayers PM, McKinlay AW. The clinical and psychometric validation of a questionnaire to assess the quality of life of adult patients treated with long-term parenteral nutrition. J Parenter Enter Nutr. 2010;34(2):131–42.
29. Buchman AL, Moukarzel A. Metabolic bone disease associated with total parenteral nutrition. Clin Nutr. 2000;19(4):217–31.
30. Seidner DL. Parenteral nutrition-associated metabolic bone disease. J Parenter Enter Nutr. 2002;26(5 SUPPL):S37.
31. Bharadwaj S, Gohel TD, Deen OJ, Coughlin KL, Corrigan ML, Fisher J, et al. Prevalence and predictors of vitamin D deficiency and response to oral supplementation in patients receiving long-term home parenteral nutrition. Nutr Clin Pract. 2014;29(5):681–5.
32. Pironi L, Cuerda C, Jeppesen PB, Joly F, Lal S, Lamprecht G, et al. Operational recommendations for the implementation of home parenteral nutrition program of care according to the guidelines of the European society for clinical nutrition and metabolism. Clin Nutr ESPEN. 2024;63:668–75.
33. Canovai E, Ceulemans LJ, Peers G, De Pourcq L, Pijpops M, Hoffman I, et al. Cost-effectiveness of intestinal transplantation compared to parenteral nutrition in adults. Transplantation. 2021;105(4):897–904.
34. Canovai E, Ceulemans LJ, Peers G, De Pourcq L, Pijpops M, De Hertogh G, et al. Cost analysis of chronic intestinal failure. Clin Nutr. 2019;38(4):1729–36.

Long-Term Venous Access for HPN: Types, Devices, and Complications

14

Liliana Mirea, Raluca Ungureanu, and Dragoş Ene

14.1 Introduction

For patients unable to meet the nutritional needs by oral or enteral route due to persistent gastrointestinal failure, like short bowel syndrome, home parenteral nutrition (HPN) is the only way to deliver essential nutrients to sustain the energy demands of the organism. Effective and safe venous access is an important part of any program of home parenteral nutrition. Optimal positioning of central vascular access device (CVAD) will help to minimize complications associated with its use. Prompt recognition and treatment of venous catheter malfunction and associated complications due to prolonged use warrants a decrease in associated morbidity and mortality. For optimal HPN program and CVAD outcomes, these patients should be managed at intestinal failure centers by multidisciplinary teams that include interventional radiologists and use evidence-based protocols implemented by trained staff.

L. Mirea · R. Ungureanu (✉)
Faculty of Medicine, Carol Davila University of Medicine and Pharmacy, Bucharest, Romania

Anesthesiology and Intensive Care Clinic, Clinical Emergency Hospital, Bucharest, Romania

D. Ene
Faculty of Medicine, Carol Davila University of Medicine and Pharmacy, Bucharest, Romania

General Surgery Department, Clinical Emergency Hospital, Bucharest, Romania

A. Trifan et al. (eds.), *Short Bowel Syndrome in Adults*,
https://doi.org/10.1007/978-3-031-95848-9_14

14.1.1 Challenges and Goals of Vascular Access Selection in Delivering HPN

Long-term parenteral nutrition (PN) patients face additional challenges compared to acute care, such as maintaining venous access due to vein exhaustion or stenosis, as well as the logistical complexities of managing PN at home, which demand patient education and support. Also, patients with conditions such as very long-term HPN or recurrent infections often experience venous depletion due to scarring, thrombosis, or vein exhaustion. Similarly, individuals with prior vascular surgeries may have compromised venous anatomy, making it difficult to establish or maintain reliable vascular access.

Establishing adequate vascular access necessitates careful planning, proficient insertion, and continuous maintenance. Vascular access management involves more than catheter placement; it includes strategic device selection, compliance with evidence-based insertion and care guidelines, meticulous monitoring, and a proactive strategy for complication avoidance. By emphasizing these characteristics, healthcare practitioners may guarantee that PN stays a secure, efficacious, and sustainable intervention, eventually enhancing outcomes while balancing comfort and quality of life for patients dependent on nutritional support. These efforts frequently need a multidisciplinary team approach, including clinical knowledge, patient education, while also acknowledging the financial ramifications connected with PN therapy [1].

14.2 Vascular Access Devices for Home Parenteral Nutrition

14.2.1 Central Venous Access Device Characteristics

Central venous access is essential for HPN delivery, especially for prolonged treatment or when high-osmolarity solutions are necessary without inducing venous irritation.

The optimal catheter material is typically flexible, robust, chemically inert, nonthrombogenic, radiopaque, and resistant to kinking. It needs to have a measuring scale on its side. Flexible catheters with a small diameter that efficiently float in the bloodstream are less prone to causing injuries. Contemporary CVADs are often composed of polyurethane or silicone rubber. Some are coated with antiseptics or antibiotics, or these agents are included into the catheter polymer to minimize infectious complications arising from bacterial proliferation and migration within the catheter [2, 3].

CVADs can be categorized based on the distance between the intravenous (IV) entrance point and the cutaneous exit point into nontunneled or tunneled catheters. In catheter selection, the clinician must evaluate the necessity for multiple lumens (one, two, or three), acknowledging that multilumen catheters are to be utilized exclusively in scenarios requiring the simultaneous infusion of incompatible solutions, such as for patients receiving concurrent chemotherapy [4]. Another aspect is the type of external catheter terminus—external hub vs. totally implanted device (TID) [2, 4, 5]. Also, CVADs may possess either an open-end tip or a valve-ended tip. Numerous devices possess supplementary orifices on their lateral walls, situated only proximal to the tip, which may affect flow dynamics and flushing requirements.

Certain catheters have an antibacterial agent, such as minocycline, integrated into the material [6]. Some catheters have an additional cuff composed of collagen impregnated with silver ions; the collagen cuff expands to 2–3 times its initial size, while the silver serves as an antibacterial agent [7]. Antimicrobial catheters are not commonly employed in contemporary practice because of little differences in outcomes and higher costs [8, 9].

All of these factors—material, design, number of lumens, and catheter configuration—play an essential role in optimizing patient safety, comfort, and outcomes when using CVADs for long-term HPN.

14.2.2 Types of Central Venous Access Devices

Short-term CVADs These types of CVADs are not suitable for HPN due to elevated risk of complications, especially infections. They are commonly employed in acute care environments, such as ICUs or hospitals, for patients necessitating prompt vascular access for short-term treatment spanning days to a few weeks.

Peripherally Inserted Central Catheters (PICC Lines) PICC lines are central venous catheters measuring 50–60 cm in length and of small diameter (20–22 gauge), typically made from silicone or polyurethane. They are inserted via a peripheral vein, commonly located in the antecubital fossa (basilic, brachial, or cephalic), and advanced into the central veins with assistance of an electrocardiogram (ECG) electrode or fluoroscopy. PICC lines represent a flexible alternative due to their ease of insertion and might be particularly advantageous in patients with acute intestinal failure, as an initial approach for intermediate duration PN (no longer than 6 months), which can be converted to a tunneled catheter if long-term home parenteral nutrition is needed. However, they have a significantly elevated risk of thrombosis and occlusion owing to their small diameters and reduced flow rates. Furthermore, the likelihood of dislodgement is heightened due to the absence of a cuff to secure the catheter to soft tissues. The location of the exit site on the arm limits normal arm mobility, rendering everyday tasks challenging and nearly unfeasible for patients carrying out the treatments by themselves. Movement of the arm may result in catheter migration of up to 9 cm, which might lead to endothelial injury, deep vein thrombosis (DVT), or serious adverse events such as heart perforation or arrhythmias. PICCs need to be secured and covered with a sterile dressing. Phlebitis and the associated infection risks, although often less than those observed with short-term CVADs, continue to be a concern, especially when catheters are inadequately managed [10–17]. Several centers employ tunneling techniques for the PICC to reduce the risk of infection and thrombosis Their study demonstrated the effectiveness of the tunneling approach; nonetheless, they concluded that the degree to which tunneling a PICC diminishes problems requires more investigation [18].

Tunneled Catheters Tunneled catheters are intended for prolonged PN, frequently utilized in patients with chronic intestinal failure (CIF). Typically, these catheters are surgically implanted, with a segment of the catheter tunneled subcutaneously prior to emerging from the skin. The subcutaneous tunnel acts as a barrier to diminish infection risk, rendering these devices more appropriate for extended usage in comparison to nontunneled CVADs. Usually, these CVADs have a strengthened outer section, including a thicker-walled sheath and a Dacron cuff, which becomes infiltrated with fibrous tissue over time, thereby securing the catheter and acting as a physical barrier against infection. Some of them also have a secondary cuff composed of collagen impregnated with silver ions, which serves as a chemical barrier against bacteria and infection [7, 19]. Tunneled catheters provide durability and offer frequent access without jeopardizing safety, rendering them optimal for HPN environments. The surgical insertion procedure is more intrusive; however, it is often well tolerated.

- The Broviac catheter possesses a narrow internal diameter, enabling reduced flow rates ranging from 25 to 65 ml/min. Initially developed for children, it is often utilized by adults [20]. The reduced dimensions are thought to diminish the risk and occurrence of thrombosis due to an improved catheter-to-vessel ratio, as the smaller device occupies less vascular space than the Hickman catheter [21, 22].
- The Hickman catheter possesses a larger internal diameter, facilitating increased flow rates. Further developed devices are also available with double or triple lumens [23]. Hickman catheters must be secured until the cuff is embedded. This is accomplished by either suturing along the line or employing a detachable stitch fixation device, which can be either sutured in position or mounted with an adhesive securing mechanism.
- Valved catheters have a valve located at either the distal or proximal extremity of the catheter. The Groshong catheter operates similarly to Broviac and Hickman catheters; however, it is distinct due to its slit-like opening located toward the distal end, which serves as a valve. The valve withstands negative intrathoracic pressure, preventing possible air embolism. The valve needs a positive pressure for activation. The valve's closure, when positive pressure decreases, restricts the retrograde flow of venous blood into the catheter. The valve necessitates the utilization of a pressurized system for infusion delivery and may modify the rate of continuous infusion medication [24].

Implanted Ports Implanted ports, or port-a-caths, are entirely internal devices situated beneath the skin, typically in the chest area. A small reservoir, or port, is linked to a catheter that is located in a central vein, enabling recurrent vascular access devoid of an external apparatus. Ports are especially beneficial for intermittent long-term utilization, as shown in cancer patients undergoing chemotherapy or patients on prolonged PN. They are aesthetically discreet and present a reduced risk of infection relative to external catheters, as they stay encapsulated beneath the skin when not in use. Ports are accessed using a non-coring Huber needle, enhancing comfort and reducing the risk of contamination during inactive periods. Nonetheless, the surgical insertion and extraction necessitate operating room resources. Notwithstanding these disadvantages, implanted ports provide a dependable and patient-centered solution for prolonged venous access. They employ the skin as a natural barrier against infection, allowing patients to swim and wash without complications. They have the lowest infection rates among all long-term CVADs, need minimal ongoing maintenance, allow for extended flush intervals (3–4 weeks), and are characterized by durability. Additionally, the advantages of TID over external catheters include the absence of dressing requirements while not in use, the ability given to patients to swim and bathe without issue, and also less body distortion for the patient. Fortunately, if patients have daily infusion requirements, the benefit of a hidden lumen diminishes when the Huber needle is in situ for 5 to 7 days per week. Frequent puncturing of the skin above the port may result in ulceration and inflammation of the skin over time. However, the management of infections using antibiotic-lock treatment is more complex in TIDs, and localized infections frequently need device removal [3]. Each port membrane is rated for survival between 1000 and 2000 punctures before the chance of failure increases, related to needle size and operator proficiency. The needle may be accidentally removed, disrupting infusions and posing a danger of extravasation. Various sizes and lengths of needles are available to accommodate varied skin fat thicknesses over the port. In an emergency, a normal needle (orange, blue, or green) may be utilized.

14.3 The Choice of CVAD and Exit Site

The process of selection of a CVAD for HPN requires the involvement of a multidisciplinary nutrition support team (NST), including the patient, an anesthetist, a radiologist, or a surgeon assigned for insertion.

The patient's participation is essential in identifying the position of the cutaneous exit, in order to assure optimal self-care and accessibility. Placement should avoid proximity to wounds, previous exit sites, tracheostomies, stomas, or fistulas to reduce complications. Tunneled catheters, as well as TIDs, are generally recommended for long-term HPN beyond 6 months because of their decreased risk of complications. A single-lumen CVAD is preferred over multiple-lumen devices due to the increased risk of infection associated with the latter. The internal jugular vein or subclavian vein is the preferable access site, with right-sided insertion decreasing the risk of venous thrombosis relative to the left side. Irrespective of the catheter type, the tip must be placed near the intersection of the superior vena cava and right atrium, since this positioning minimizes the risk of thrombosis. The selection of single-lumen vs. multiple-lumen catheters is dependent upon the etiology of intestinal failure, anticipated duration of PN support, infusion frequency and composition, and additionally drugs used concomitantly. The use of the femoral vein for HPN is often discouraged due to the susceptibility of the groin exit point to contamination and an increased risk of venous thrombosis. However, if the femoral vein is utilized due to limited access to the upper superior vena cava, tunneling is essential to enhance the management of the catheter exit site and secure attachment for prolonged use, despite the fact that access via the femoral veins is not advisable [27]. In acute intestinal failure, multiple-lumen catheters may be required to support simultaneous treatments. As intestinal failure advances, the requirements for intravenous support may alter, necessitating modifications in the kind and placement of CVADs. Even PICCs can be utilized for intermediate periods, especially during the transition to outpatient treatment. However, PICC lines are not recommended if the expected duration of PN is prolonged over 6 months. In a domestic environment, devices should be easy to use for patients or caregivers to operate with limited professional oversight. This encompasses simplified flushing methods, secure dressings, and instruction on sterile techniques to avoid infections. Implanted ports are especially appropriate for outpatient care because of reduced susceptibility to contamination and the enhanced freedom and comfort they provide to patients. These devices enhance quality of life, allowing patients to perform everyday activities while undergoing long-term PN [4, 16, 17, 25–27].

14.4 Insertion Techniques for Vascular Access Devices

14.4.1 Pre-insertion Assessment and Planning

Thorough pre-insertion evaluation and strategizing are essential for the secure and effective placement of a vascular access device for HPN. These procedures reduce complications and enhance device functionality by customizing the approach to the patient's clinical requirements and anatomical factors. Significant elements refer to assessing the patient's coagulation status and performing imaging studies to evaluate venous anatomy.

The chosen vein for vascular access must be based on patient's wishes, venipuncture technique, potential complications, catheter site maintenance, and the risks. Traditional landmark-based treatments are less accurate and entail more risks, leaving image-guided techniques, such as ultrasonography and fluoroscopy, the favored options in contemporary practice.

14.4.2 Infection Prevention Measures during Insertion

Preventing infections during the placement of CVADs is important in order to diminish the likelihood of catheter-related bloodstream infections (CRBSIs). It is recommended to conduct central venous catheterization in a setting that facilitates aseptic procedures. All healthcare practitioners participating in the process must execute thorough hand hygiene utilizing an alcohol-based hand rub or soap and water, and don personal protective equipment, including sterile gowns, sterile gloves, hats, and masks that cover both the mouth and nose. The patient must be completely covered with a sterile barrier to reduce exposure to contaminants. This entails employing extensive sterile drapes to shield nonsterile regions, and exclusively sterile equipment, catheters, and devices must be utilized. All materials must undergo inspection to confirm sterility prior to commencing the operation. The insertion site must be sanitized with a suitable antiseptic solution, such as a 2% chlorhexidine solution, for a minimum of 30 seconds. The area must be allowed to dry thoroughly prior to continuation [4, 27]. In the presence of a contraindication to chlorhexidine, povidone–iodine or 70% alcohol may be utilized.

Contamination of any component utilized in the catheter insertion process might result in the dissemination of microorganisms into the catheter's lumen and subsequently into the bloodstream. Clinicians should evaluate the need for utilization of antibiotic-coated catheters for certain patients, considering their infection risk. Nonetheless, these antimicrobial-coated devices should not be considered a replacement for conventional infection control protocols, and comprehensive preventative methods must be maintained [27]. After insertion, the site must be covered with a sterile dressing. When utilizing a chlorhexidine-impregnated dressing, the insertion site must be inspected regularly for indications of irritation, allergic reactions, or necrosis.

14.4.3 Documentation and Confirmation

Proper records ensure traceability, adherence to clinical standards, and provide a reference for managing complications. Verification of catheter placement is mandatory to ascertain that the device is accurately situated inside the central venous system. Confirmation methods encompass imaging techniques, notably chest X-ray, which is the common technique for verifying placement. Furthermore, ultrasonography guidance during insertion can verify venous access; nevertheless, it does not guarantee the correct positioning of the CVAD's tip. Fluoroscopy may be employed during the insertion. Electrocardiography (ECG) guidance is a method that utilizes alterations in ECG waves to verify the accurate positioning of catheter tips, frequently employed as a supplementary tool to imaging.

14.5 Maintenance of Vascular Access Devices

Adhering to proper catheter care methods is vital for preserving the performance and durability of vascular access devices utilized for PN. Consistent daily care reduces the likelihood of complications.

14.5.1 Flushing Protocols

Regular flushing of the catheter is essential to prevent obstruction due to fibrin, blood clots, or residual PN solution, and to confirm the catheter's integrity and performance before to and during PN delivery. ESPEN guidelines advise against the use of a heparin lock because it promotes intraluminal biofilm formation, increasing the likelihood of CRBSIs [16, 28, 29] Additionally, NaCl 0.9% flushing appears not to be inferior to heparin flushing regarding CVAD occlusion. However, in some instances, such as central lines with elevated thrombosis risks, heparinized saline may be employed to avoid clot formation, particularly in central catheters and ports that are not in continuous use. The dosage (e.g., 10–100 units/mL) and frequency are dependent upon the device type and institutional guidelines. For individuals with a history of recurrent infections, specific solutions containing antiseptics (ethanol, citrate) or antibiotics may be utilized to prevent or cure infections.

Flushing is commonly conducted prior to and subsequent to the administration of PN solution, drugs, or other fluids. Valved catheters (e.g., Groshong catheters) are designed with an internal valve that inhibits blood reflux and often need just saline flushes, typically eliminating the need for heparin locks. Flush at regular intervals (e.g., every 12–24 h) if the catheter is not in continuous use; for dormant catheters (e.g., implanted ports), flushing may be planned every 7–30 days, depending upon the device type. Flushing must consistently be conducted using aseptic technique and following the disinfection of the catheter hub or injection port with a suitable antiseptic. Flushing should be performed via a push-pause (pulsatile) technique to generate turbulence within the catheter, dislodging debris and preventing accumulation along the catheter walls. Refrain from applying excessive force during flushing to prevent catheter rupture. If resistance is met, refrain from flushing; evaluate for potential occlusion or catheter impairment. Generally, employ a flush volume that is no less than double the internal capacity of the catheter and any supplementary devices (often 5–10 mL of saline). Secure the catheter while administering the final 0.5 mL of solution or immediately before to detaching the syringe to reduce blood reflux into the catheter.

14.5.2 Catheter Inspection, Dressing Changes, and Maintenance

Regular examination of the catheter site is essential to detect early indications of problems. Erythema, edema, sensitivity, exudate, or warmth at the insertion site may signify infection or discomfort. During this operation, the integrity of the catheter should be assessed by inspecting it for leaks, kinks, or damage and confirming that all connections are secure and caps are clean. Catheters must be expeditiously removed when they are no longer needed. Ensuring a clean and sterile dressing over the catheter insertion site diminishes the likelihood of infections. Transparent dressings are generally replaced every 7 days, whereas gauze, utilized for individuals with exudate or adhesive allergies, may be changed every 48 h or sooner if they become dirty, moist, or loose. The dressing must be meticulously removed, followed by a thorough evaluation of the insertion site. It is essential to disinfect the region using an antiseptic solution, such as chlorhexidine. The next step is to apply a sterile transparent or gauze dressing, ensuring it is secure yet not too tight, so preserving patient comfort and skin integrity. The area must be allowed to air-dry thoroughly prior to the application of a new sterile dressing.

14.5.3 Patient and Caregiver Education

Education for patients and caregivers maintaining vascular access at home emphasizes practical instruction in catheter maintenance, including dressing changes, flushing procedures, and the identification of infection or device failure indicators. Visual aids, checklists, and written directives can enhance learning and increase confidence. In outpatient or HPN settings, equipping patients with knowledge regarding sterile handling and emergency care is important for minimizing problems.

14.6 Complications Related to Vascular Access in Home Parenteral Nutrition

Recognizing and identifying possible complications of long-term CVADs is crucial for maintaining safe care. Clinicians must meticulously weigh the risks and advantages when evaluating device removal, since line extraction may be imperative in some circumstances, while reinsertion presents its own concerns. It is often wise to evaluate the feasibility of preserving an existing line and its alignment with the patient's best interests. In noncritical care environments, CVADs utilized for PN are susceptible to problems including CRBSIs, site infections, catheter dislodgement, occlusions, venous thrombosis, and device malfunction or failure [1, 30, 31].

14.6.1 Infectious Complications

CRBSI rates in experienced referral centers can be expected to range from 0.14 to 1.09 episodes per catheter year [17, 32–35]. Patients receiving PN encounter an increased risk of complications compared to those utilizing CVADs for other indications. The nutrient-dense PN solution, with high levels of glucose, amino acids, and lipids, carries an optimal environment for the proliferation of bacteria and fungi, especially staphylococci, enterococci, and *Candida* species. Thus, PN treatment is considered an independent risk factor for CRBSIs [30, 36, 37]. Additionally, other variables increase the chance of developing CRBSIs, including patient-related elements such as immunosuppression from underlying diseases, critical illness, or extended hospitalizations. Catheter colonization occurs when microbial pathogens proliferate in a specimen without exhibiting systemic or localized signs of infection. Semiquantitative (>15 colony-forming units [CFU]) or quantitative (>1000 CFU) catheter cultures may assist in differentiating substantial from nonsignificant colonization. Catheter-associated infections can be classified as local, including exit-site infections, tunnel infections, or port pocket infections, or systemic, in the form of CRBSIs. Exit-site infections often respond favorably to wound care and medication, whereas tunnel infections frequently necessitate catheter removal and IV antibiotic treatment.

CRBSIs are a major infectious complication linked with vascular access devices. CRBSIs may be classified according to the route of colonization into those arising from the catheter lumen and those originating from the external catheter surface and might originate from skin puncture sites, hub contamination, or dissemination from another septic focus [38].

14.6.1.1 Diagnosis

Diagnosing a CRBSIs necessitates clinical evaluation and laboratory analysis. Local clinical manifestations include erythema, discomfort, edema, or exudation of serous or purulent fluid at the exit site or TID pocket. Tunnel infection manifests as a painful, inflammatory pattern along the subcutaneous tunnel.

General clinical manifestations may include nonspecific symptoms such as subfebrile temperature and chills, progressing to systemic signs like hypotension or alterations in mental state indicative of sepsis or septic shock. Symptoms may manifest 1–3 h following the initiation of a new infusion or after catheter closure. Laboratory assessment is optimally conducted by quantitative or semiquantitative blood culture drawn through the catheter lumen or by obtaining paired quantitative blood cultures peripherally and from the catheter. In the latter scenario, it is important to observe the differential time-to-positivity (DTP) to determine if the infection is catheter-related, assuming the catheter remains in situ. Moreover, alternative possible sources of infection must be excluded with complete clinical evaluation and imaging investigations [39].

14.6.1.2 Management

The ESPEN recommendations advocate for the management of CRBSIs in accordance with the existing recommendations on long-term intravascular catheters.

When CRBSI is suspected, unwarranted CVAD removal puts the patient at the danger of reinsertion, as many cases are found to be noninfected.

A conservative approach may be reasonable for treating simpler infections caused by *Staphylococcus aureus*, coagulase-negative staphylococci, and gram-negative bacilli, utilizing systemic antibiotics and antibiotic-lock therapy before considering catheter removal. In cases where catheter removal is impractical, after obtaining a swab from the skin surrounding the exit site, along with a blood sample for culture, antibiotic-lock treatment should be administered for 7–10 days, up to 2 weeks, alongside standard systemic antibiotic therapy. Antibiotic treatment should be tailored based on culture results. This scenario is rational for suspected intraluminal infections in the absence of tunnel or pocket infection with the scope to preserve the device while eradicating the infection [17]. Additionally, in suspected cases of endoluminal infection, it is advised to temporarily cease infusion until laboratory findings become available, while peripheral PN is administered temporarily [40, 41]. If infection is not proven, PN therapy can be initiated on the same CVAD [40, 41].

However, catheter removal is necessary in instances of tunnel infections, port abscesses, septic shock, or major infections such as endocarditis, metastatic infections, and when paired blood cultures indicate the presence of fungi or virulent bacteremia. The reinsertion of long-term devices should be deferred until suitable systemic antibiotic therapy, guided by the susceptibilities, has commenced and subsequent blood cultures results are negative. However, the successful rescue of infected implanted ports by antibiotic therapy is uncommon, necessitating the removal of most devices.

Antibiotic coverage must be adjusted according to local antibiograms and the patient's risk factors. As important as initiating therapy, the de-escalation of treatment depending on culture results and sensitivity testing is essential. Administering antibiotics through other routes can enhance the likelihood of eliminating a catheter infection. If an indwelling port reservoir is contaminated, antibiotics must be administered through another access route. Nevertheless, attempting to preserve a catheter poses a danger of severe metastatic consequences, such as septic arthritis, osteomyelitis, spinal epidural abscess, or other septic emboli [42].

Although the majority of infections caused by coagulase-negative staphylococci heal without concerns, those caused by other microbes may result in potentially serious problems. *Staphylococcus aureus* bacteremia can lead to acute endocarditis, and all patients should be assessed preferably using transesophageal echocardiography. The treatment duration for simple bacteremia should be up to 10 days. For complex infections, a minimum treatment duration of 6 weeks is advised. In instances of fungal infections, catheter removal and systemic antifungal medication are necessary for certain individuals.

14.6.1.3 Strategies to Prevent Infections

Research indicates that several measures can reduce the incidence of catheter-associated infections [15].

- Establishment of a written policy and the education of healthcare professionals, patients, and family members is important in preventing infectious complications. Guidelines underscore the necessity of hand decontamination before and during the care of CVADs [43]. They advocate for the use of soap and water or alcohol-based gels or foams free of water. A randomized trial demonstrated that interactive video-based instruction for both staff and patients decreases catheter-related infection (CRI) in HPN patients [44].
- Site care must be performed according to an established plan, at a minimum frequency of once weekly, and whenever the dressing gets moist or soiled. Chlorhexidine 2% is suggested for antisepsis of the hands, catheter exit site, and skin prior to catheter placement. Stopcocks, catheter hubs, and other sample ports must consistently be cleaned, ideally with 2% chlorhexidine in 70% isopropyl alcohol. Intravenous administration sets must be replaced every 24 h.

- Additionally, avoiding CVADs after manipulating ostomy bags is recommended.
- Locks with taurolidine inhibits microbial adherence to catheter surfaces and biofilm. The use of taurolidine decreased CRBSIs without any side effects or the development of bacterial resistance [45, 46].
- In certain situations of repeated CRBSI, a priority in the care is the reeducation of the patient and/or caregiver. Additionally, the use of an antimicrobial catheter lock should be taken into account. While certain data indicates that antibiotic- or antimicrobial-locking solutions reduce the likelihood of CRBSI, fears over antibiotic resistance and inadequate assessment of possible adverse effects remain. Therefore, the regular application of these procedures is not widely endorsed [47].
- Additionally, in selected patients, a surgically produced arteriovenous fistula might be an option in patients with repeated CRBSIs.
- Catheter removal as soon as they are no longer needed further reduces infection risk and helps preserve long-term venous access options [48].

Current guidelines include a topic about strategies that have been demonstrated to be unsuccessful for the prevention of CRBSI, including the use of in-line filters, regular catheter replacement, antibiotic prophylaxis, and heparin administration. Furthermore, catheter locking with 70% ethanol to prevent CRBSI is not recommended because its use is associated with systemic toxicity, catheter occlusion, and catheter damage [16]. However, other studies showed that locking of CVADs with a combination of heparin and vancomycin has demonstrated efficacy in diminishing gram-positive infections. Antibiotic locks may also be beneficial in instances of recurrent line infections [2, 49]. There is no conclusive evidence that the utilization of needle-free connections diminishes the incidence of CRBSI in HPN patients. Additionally, selecting a suitable insertion site and strictly following maximal barrier measures during insertion are essential in periprocedural period.

14.6.2 Mechanical Complications

Mechanical complications frequently arise and can considerably affect therapeutic efficacy and patient safety. Complications encompass catheter kinking, malposition, vascular perforation, and other associated difficulties necessitating prompt detection and intervention to prevent severe repercussions.

14.6.2.1 Catheter Malposition and Kinking

Catheter malposition and kinking occur when the catheter tip is improperly situated in the targeted central vein, migrates after implantation, or bends or twists, therefore blocking flow and impairing functionality. It frequently arises from incorrect positioning, inadequate catheter length, or patient movement.

It is identified by difficulties with flushing or aspirating blood, infusion pump alarms signaling excessive resistance, or observable distortion in the catheter pathway. The management in this scenario involves externally repositioning the catheter if obvious kinking is observed around the insertion site; in instances of internal kinks, imaging may be required to evaluate the kink's location. The catheter tip may contact the vascular wall, which may be assessed using a chest scan. If repositioning is unsuccessful, catheter replacement may be necessary. To prevent complications, it is essential to ensure the right catheter length during implantation and to secure the device with the scope to reduce movement [50].

14.6.2.2 Catheter Occlusion

Catheter occlusion results from an obstruction in the catheter lumen due to fibrin, blood clots, or precipitates from PN formula. Today, many approaches are utilized in clinical practice to remove occlusions from a central venous catheter's internal lumen, with the selected method contingent upon resource availability and the suspected underlying cause of the obstruction [51]. The mechanical cleaning of the catheter's interior lumen using specialized brushes is a successful and generally applicable method for addressing occlusions. The initial comparison research evaluating both mechanical and pharmacological techniques revealed a superior success rate with brushes in contrast to thrombolysis [52]. Nevertheless, the mechanical restoration of catheter patency is frequently constrained by restricted access to necessary devices, hence maintaining the relevance and demand for pharmacological methods. This technique requires filling the catheter's inner lumen with a pharmacological solution designed to dissolve and eliminate the cause of the obstruction. The efficacy of the pharmacological approach depends on the selection of the suitable medication according to the precise etiology of the blockage. Intraluminal thrombosis denotes the formation of a thrombus within the catheter. It may manifest as either a partial or total blockage. Blood clots in the catheter lumen can be treated by providing thrombolytic agents, usually using a thrombolytic "lock" introduced into the catheter twice, with each application retained for 30 to 60 min. If this procedure fails, a guide wire or snare may be employed to extract a clot from the catheter's tip [53, 54]. Most medication precipitates can be effectively dissolved by using "locks" with sterile 0.1 molar hydrochloric acid solution or 4% citrate solution [55]. Occlusions resulting from fat emulsions are most effectively addressed by filling the catheter lumen with 70% ethyl alcohol for a minimum of 30 min (an "ethanol lock"). Due to blockage essentially diminishing the capacity of the catheter's internal channel, the suitable medication solution must be administered gradually and in a volume initially less than the catheter's fill capacity, permitting enough time to dissolve. Prior to each consecutive application, it is recommended to completely evacuate the contents from the catheter lumen [56]. To prevent CVAD occlusion, it is suggested to flush catheters with saline [17].

Pinch-off syndrome arises when subclavian long-term CVADs experience shear stresses between the first rib and clavicle. The risk is considered increased due to more medial vein punctures with landmark approaches, as the catheter traverses anteriorly between the clavicle and first rib before entering the subclavian vein. Frequent compression in active individuals may result in line breakage, extravasation, translocation, and embolization. Lateral punctures of the axillary vein with ultrasound guidance are believed to mitigate this risk. A postural influence on catheter functionality may be observed clinically, with enhanced aspiration and flushing when the patient is supine and elevates the ipsilateral arm, as opposed to while in an upright position. Infraclavicular discomfort, accompanied by dermal alterations and edema, may signify fluid extravasation from a damaged catheter [57, 58].

14.6.2.3 Thrombosis

Catheter-related venous thrombosis (CRVT) is a significant complication that leads to the loss of central venous access and may necessitate intestinal transplantation (ITx) if it involves two or more central venous vessels. CRVT may present clinically or remain subclinical, arising shortly after catheter placement or manifesting later in individuals with prolonged catheterization. CVRT may be asymptomatic; nevertheless, symptoms might include edema, discomfort, and erythema along the catheterized vein. Thrombosis refers to the development of a blood clot within a vein, which may arise from catheter-tip-induced endothelial damage [15]. The subclavian vein is preferred for catheterization because of its decreased incidence of thrombosis compared to other veins. Thrombosis may result in catheter obstruction or embolization. Diagnosis can be validated using ultrasound or venography.

CRVT is often managed with anticoagulant therapy. Initial anticoagulation therapy often consists of low molecular weight heparin, followed by vitamin K antagonists, except in oncologic patients and those with inadequate oral absorption, for whom low molecular weight heparin is favored. The duration of anticoagulation for a patient is based upon specific case features (risk factors, thrombus size and characteristics, and catheter extraction) but typically ranges from 3 to 6 months, and in certain instances, may be indefinite. The choice of keeping the catheter must be conditional upon individual criteria. Catheter removal is typically justified when HPN is no longer required, if it is infected or obstructed, if there are contraindications to anticoagulant therapy, or if symptoms and signs continue after anticoagulation [10, 59–62].

Thrombolytic agents are not frequently used, except in cases of massive thrombosis with clinical signs of severe form, in the absence of hemorrhagic risk, especially if thrombus formation is recent (previous 10 days). Additionally, catheter-directed thrombolysis may be used in some instances. Also, a superior vena cava filter might be inserted if the patient has contraindications for anticoagulation treatment or the thrombus increases in size under treatment [17].

In patients with persistent thrombosis and failure of anticoagulation or thrombolysis, catheter mechanical interventions (aspiration, fragmentation, thrombectomy, balloon angioplasty, or stenting) or surgical procedures (thrombectomy, venoplasty, venous bypass, or decompression at the venous thoracic outlet) might be indicated.

Diverse techniques have been employed to minimize CRVT:

- Minimizing damage to the venous wall during catheter insertion in order to prevent venous thrombosis.

- Ultrasound-guided catheterization, selecting a catheter with the lowest diameter, and optimal positioning of the catheter tip is associated with decreased risk of thrombosis.
- CVADs manufactured from silicon or polyurethane are less frequently linked to local thrombosis compared to those constructed from polyethylene.
- Catheter puncture site location with the right jugular vein being favored for its direct access to the right atrium, as left-sided catheters have been linked to an increased risk of thrombosis.

Using heparin-impregnated catheters or routine prophylaxis with low-dose warfarin or heparin is not recommended as no evidence exists to justify the regular application of these preventative treatments for all patients; however, it might be an option in high-risk patients [17].

14.6.2.4 Vessel Perforation and Extravasation

Vascular perforation and extravasation are serious complications that arise when the catheter penetrates the vascular wall during insertion or due to inappropriate catheter management. The intensity and manifestation depend on the drug, its concentration, and the volume extravasated. Alarm signals include severe discomfort in the chest, shortness of breath, edema, and low blood pressure. Imaging may reveal the extravasation of contrast or PN solution into adjacent tissues or bodily cavities. Infusion must be stopped promptly if perforation or extravasation is suspected; the catheter should be removed, and the patient should be monitored for consequences such as hematoma or pneumothorax. In severe instances, it may necessitate surgical or interventional radiology procedures for repairing the vessel. Techniques to minimize these complications are: refrain from applying excessive force during insertion, use ultrasound guidance during insertion, and verify location with imaging prior to commencing PN [63].

14.6.2.5 Catheter Fracture or Breakage

This problem frequently occurs due to the repetitive compression of the exterior segment of a line. In the event of a fracture, there exists a risk of venous air embolism; hence, the line must be promptly clamped proximal to the fracture utilizing artery forceps or an equivalent instrument. In certain instances, exterior fractures may be rectified by substituting the compromised segment of the line with a specific repair kit. Ports or cuffs that penetrate the skin often require total excision and substitution.

14.6.2.6 Venous Stenosis

Venous stenosis denotes the constriction of a vein, frequently resulting from endothelial damage or inflammation due to extended catheter utilization. The continuous presence of a catheter might irritate the venous wall, leading to fibrosis and subsequent stenosis. This is suspected when there is edema of the arm or neck on the catheter side, diminished blood return, or challenges in progressing parenteral nutrition solutions through the catheter. Severe stenosis may lead to the development of collateral veins. Management involves repositioning the catheter to an alternative location to facilitate the recovery of the damaged vein; in severe situations, interventional procedures such as angioplasty or stent implantation may be necessary. To prevent difficulties, the smallest feasible catheter size should be utilized to minimize vein irritation.

14.7 Special Considerations in Vascular Access

14.7.1 Pediatric Patients

Establishing vascular access in pediatric patients, particularly newborns and infants, poses distinct challenges due to their fragility, small vessel size, developmental factors, and the necessity for prolonged nutritional support in several instances. To address these issues, meticulous preparation is necessary, including smaller-caliber catheters particularly developed for newborns and infants. Numerous pediatric patients necessitating PN possess chronic conditions, such as short bowel syndrome or congenital gastrointestinal anomalies, which require extended vascular access; therefore, tunneled catheters (e.g., Broviac or Hickman) are favored for long-term utilization due to their resilience and reduced infection risks. This group is at an elevated risk for CRBSIs due to underdeveloped immune systems and challenges in sustaining aseptic care standards. This group has specific developmental issues, as they are continuously developing, which may result in catheter migration or require adjustments in catheter length and positioning over time.

14.7.2 Patients with Limited Venous Access

Patients with poor venous access pose considerable problems and necessitate novel and flexible strategies to facilitate the management of vascular access. These patients, sometimes owing to chronic diseases, several previous catheterizations, or venous depletion from thrombosis or scarring, necessitate innovative methods to establish and sustain dependable venous access. When upper extremity and neck veins are unavailable, translumbar catheter insertion into the inferior vena cava (IVC) under fluoroscopic supervision is a viable alternative. A surgical method to expose and directly cannulate a vein may be used in complicated circumstances.

14.8 Advances in Vascular Access Devices

14.8.1 Antimicrobial-Coated Catheters

Antimicrobial-coated catheters signify a notable improvement in vascular access devices. These catheters are engineered to reduce the risk of CRBSIs. The coatings often incorporate antimicrobial or antiseptic solutions that prevent microbial colonization and biofilm development. Catheters coated with silver or silver sulfadiazine provide antibacterial qualities and are effective against a wide range of bacteria and some fungi. Chlorhexidine–silver sulfadiazine coatings amalgamate the antiseptic attributes of chlorhexidine with the antibacterial advantages of silver sulfadiazine, offering prolonged protection. Antibiotic coatings comprise chemicals like minocycline and rifampin, which effectively inhibit bacterial growth on the catheter surface. Biofilm inhibition coatings impede biofilm development on catheter surfaces, which can lead to chronic infections and antibiotic resistance.

Although antimicrobial-coated catheters provide particular benefits, there are limitations and concerns, including expense, the potential for abuse leading to the emergence of resistant organisms, and their cost-effectiveness and therapeutic efficacy being most reserved in high-risk patients. The preventive effect may decline over time, requiring vigilant monitoring.

14.9 Conclusion

This chapter has offered an in-depth examination of vascular access devices in patients receiving HPN therapy. It describes the essential components of vascular access management, encompassing device selection, insertion procedures, and prevention and management of complications. By implementing evidence-based methods, healthcare practitioners may guarantee the safe, effective, and sustainable administration of PN.

Continuous education, interdisciplinary collaboration, consistent monitoring, and follow-up guarantee that patients and their caregivers are adequately prepared to provide accurate HPN treatment.

References

1. Martincich I, Cini K, Lapkin S, et al. Central venous access device complications in patients receiving parenteral nutrition in general Ward settings: a retrospective analysis. J Parenter Enter Nutr. 2020;44(6):1104–11.
2. Casey AL, Mermel LA, Nightingale P, et al. Antimicrobial central venous catheters in adults: a systematic review and meta-analysis. Lancet Infect Dis. 2008;8(12):763–76.
3. Lubos S. Central parenteral nutrition. In: Basics in clinical nutrition. 5th ed. Prague: Galén; 2019. p. 328–36.
4. Pittiruti M, Hamilton H, Biffi R, et al. ESPEN guidelines on parenteral nutrition: central venous catheters (access, care, diagnosis and therapy of complications). Clin Nutr. 2009;28(4):365–77.
5. Ryder M. Device selection: a critical strategy in the reduction of catheter- related complications. Nutrition. 1996;12(2):143–5.
6. Darouiche RO, Raad II, Heard SO, et al. A comparison of two antimicrobial-impregnated central venous catheters. N Engl J Med. 1999;340(1):1–8.
7. Denny DF. Placement and management of long-term central venous access catheters and ports. Am J Roentgenol. 1993;161(2):385–93.
8. Gilbert R, Brown M, Rainford N, et al. Antimicrobial-impregnated central venous catheters for prevention of neonatal bloodstream infection (PREVAIL): an open-label, parallel-group, pragmatic, randomised controlled trial. Lancet Child Adolesc Heal. 2019;3(6):381–90.

9. Loveday HP, Wilson JA, Pratt RJ, et al. Epic3: national evidence-based guidelines for preventing healthcare-associated infections in NHS hospitals in England. J Hosp Infect. 2014:86(S1).
10. Baskin JL, Pui CH, Reiss U, et al. Management of occlusion and thrombosis associated with long-term indwelling central venous catheters. Lancet. 2009;374(9684):159–69.
11. Nadroo AM, Glass RB, Lin J, et al. Changes in upper extremity position cause migration of peripherally inserted central catheters in neonates. Pediatrics. 2002;110(1 I):131–6.
12. Puel V, Caudry M, Le Métayer P, et al. Superior vena cava thrombosis related to catheter malposition in cancer chemotherapy given through implanted ports. Cancer. 1993;72(7):2248–52.
13. Hacking MB, Brown J, Chisholm DG. Position dependent ventricular tachycardia in two children with peripherally inserted central catheters (PICCs). Paediatr Anaesth. 2003;13(6):527–9.
14. Verdino RJ, Pacifico DS, Tracy CM. Supraventricular tachycardia precipitated by a peripherally inserted central catheter. J Electrocardiol. 1996;29(1):69–72.
15. Pironi L, Boeykens K, Bozzetti F, et al. ESPEN guideline on home parenteral nutrition. Clin Nutr. 2020;39(6):1645–66.
16. Pironi L, Boeykens K, Bozzetti F, et al. ESPEN practical guideline: Home parenteral nutrition. Clin Nutr. 2023;42(3):411–30.
17. Cuerda C, Pironi L, Arends J, et al. ESPEN practical guideline: clinical nutrition in chronic intestinal failure. Clin Nutr. 2021;40(9):5196–220.
18. Giustivi D, Gidaro A, Baroni M, et al. Tunneling technique of PICCs and midline catheters. J Vasc Access. 2022;23(4):610–4.
19. Sands MJ. Vascular access in the adult home infusion patient. J Parenter Enter Nutr. 2006;30(SUPPL. 1)
20. Leibundgut K, Müller C, Müller K, et al. Tunneled, double lumen Broviac catheters are useful, efficient and safe in children undergoing peripheral blood progenitor cell harvesting and transplantation. Bone Marrow Transplant. 1996;17(4):663–7.
21. Nifong TP, McDevitt TJ. The effect of catheter to vein ratio on blood flow rates in a simulated model of peripherally inserted central venous catheters. Chest. 2011;140(1):48–53.
22. Spencer TR, Mahoney KJ. Reducing catheter-related thrombosis using a risk reduction tool centered on catheter to vessel ratio. J Thromb Thrombolysis. 2017;44(4):427–34.
23. Bjeletich J, Hickman RO. The Hickman indwelling catheter. Am J Nurs. 1980;80(1):62.
24. Goossens GA. Flushing and locking of venous catheters: available evidence and evidence deficit. Nurs Res Pract. 2015;2015:1–12.
25. Moir D, Bodenham A. A narrative review of long-term central venous access devices for the intensivist. J Intens Care Soc. 2018;19(3):236–46.
26. Pironi L, Cuerda C, Jeppesen PB, et al. ESPEN guideline on chronic intestinal failure in adults—update 2023. Clin Nutr. 2023;42(10):1940–2021.
27. Practice guidelines for central venous access 2020. Anesthesiology. 2020;132(1):8–43.
28. Pironi L, Arends J, Bozzetti F, et al. ESPEN guidelines on chronic intestinal failure in adults. Clin Nutr. 2016;35(2):247–307.
29. Brito AR d O, Nishinari K, Saad PF, et al. Comparison between saline solution containing heparin versus saline solution in the lock of totally implantable catheters. Ann Vasc Surg. 2018;47:85–9.
30. Chopra V, O'Horo JC, Rogers MAM, et al. The risk of bloodstream infection associated with peripherally inserted central catheters compared with central venous catheters in adults: a systematic review and meta-analysis. Infect Control Hosp Epidemiol. 2013;34(9):908–18.
31. Dougherty L. Frequency, diagnosis, and management of occlusive and mechanical PICC complications. Peripher Inser Cent Venous Catheter. 2014:85–94.
32. Bozzetti F, Mariani L, Boggio Bertinet D, et al. Central venous catheter complications in 447 patients on home parenteral nutrition: an analysis of over 100.000 catheter days. Clin Nutr. 2002;21(6):475–85.
33. Clare A, Teubner A, Shaffer JL. What information should lead to a suspicion of catheter sepsis in HPN? Clin Nutr. 2008;27(4):552–6.

34. Dibb M, Carlson G, Abraham A, et al. Salvage of central venous catheters in HPN catheter-related blood stream infections is safe and effective: 18 years experience from a national centre. Gut. 2012;61:A14–5.
35. Dibb M, Teubner A, Theis V, et al. Review article: the management of long-term parenteral nutrition. Aliment Pharmacol Ther. 2013;37(6):587–603.
36. Fonseca AG, Burgermaster M, Larson E, et al. The relationship between Total parenteral nutrition and central line-associated blood stream infections. FASEB J. 2016;30(S1)
37. Marra AR, Opilla M, Edmond MB, et al. Epidemiology of bloodstream infections in patients receiving long-term total parenteral nutrition. J Clin Gastroenterol. 2007;41(1):19–28.
38. Sitges-Serra A, Girvent M. Catheter-related blood-stream infections. World J Surg. 1999;23:365–77.
39. Vashi PG, Virginkar N, Popiel B, et al. Incidence of and factors associated with catheter-related bloodstream infection in patients with advanced solid tumors on home parenteral nutrition managed using a standardized catheter care protocol. BMC Infect Dis. 2017;17(1):372.
40. Oncu S, Oncu S, Ozturk B, et al. Elimination of intraluminal colonization by antibiotic lock in catheters. Tohoku J Exp Med. 2004;203(1):1–8.
41. Messing B, Man F, Colimon R, et al. Antibiotic-lock technique is an effective treatment of bacterial catheter-related sepsis during parenteral nutrition. Clin Nutr. 1990;9(4):220–5.
42. Ho A, Bravery K. Central venous access devices (long term). Clin Guidel Gt Orm Str Hosp Child. 2009; 2:Appendix 1.
43. O'Grady N, Alexander M, Burns L, et al. Background information: strategies for prevention of catheter-related infections in adult and pediatric patients. Centres Dis Control Prev. 2015;
44. Smith CE, Curtas S, Kleinbeck SVM, et al. Clinical trial of interactive and videotaped educational interventions reduce infection, reactive depression, and rehospitalizations for sepsis in patients on home parenteral nutrition. J Parenter Enter Nutr. 2003;27(2):137–45.
45. Liu Y, Zhang AQ, Cao L, et al. Taurolidine lock solutions for the prevention of catheter-related bloodstream infections: a systematic review and meta-analysis of randomized controlled trials. PLoS One. 2013;8(11)
46. Wouters Y, Causevic E, Klek S, et al. Use of catheter lock solutions in patients receiving home parenteral nutrition: a systematic review and individual-patient data meta-analysis. J Parenter Enter Nutr. 2020;44(7):1198–209.
47. Zacharioudakis IM, Zervou FN, Arvanitis M, et al. Antimicrobial lock solutions as a method to prevent central line-associated bloodstream infections: a meta-analysis of randomized controlled trials. Clin Infect Dis. 2014;59(12):1741–9.
48. Elliott TSJ, Tebbs SE. Prevention of central venous catheter-related infection. J Hosp Infect. 1998;40(3):193–201.
49. Niël-Weise BS, Stijnen T, van den Broek PJ. Anti-infective-treated central venous catheters for total parenteral nutrition or chemotherapy: a systematic review. J Hosp Infect. 2008;69(2):114–23.
50. Hartnell GG, Wilde PH. Nonsurgical repositioning of central venous catheters. Radiology. 1988;168(2):581.
51. Dibb M, Lal S. Home parenteral nutrition: vascular access and related complications. Nutr Clin Pract. 2017;32(6):769–76.
52. Allan PJ, McMahon M, Abraham A, et al. Reduced need for replacement of long term parenteral nutrition catheters following endoluminal brushing. Clin Nutr. 2015;34(1):146–50.
53. Walker TG. Prevention of dialysis catheter malfunction with recombinant tissue plasminogen activator. Yearb Diagnostic Radiol. 2011;2011:260–5.
54. Rosovsky RP, Kuter DJ. Catheter-related thrombosis in cancer patients: pathophysiology, diagnosis, and management. Hematol Oncol Clin North Am. 2005;1:183–202.
55. Shulman RJ, Reed T, Pitre D, et al. Use of hydrochloric acid to clear obstructed central venous catheters. J Parenter Enter Nutr. 1988;12(5):509–10.
56. Gundogan K, Dave NJ, Griffith DP, et al. Ethanol lock therapy markedly reduces catheter-related blood stream infections in adults requiring home parenteral nutrition: a retrospective study from a Tertiary Medical Center. J Parenter Enter Nutr. 2020;44(4):661–7.

57. Aitken Delmar R, Minton JP. The "pinch-off sign": a warning of impending problems with permanent subclavian catheters. Am J Surg. 1984;148(5):633–6.
58. Andris DA, Krzywda EA, Scht-Lte W, et al. Pinch-off syndrome: a rare etiology for central venous catheter occlusion. J Parenter Enter Nutr. 1994;18(6):531–3.
59. Malhotra S, Punia VPS. Upper extremity deep vein thrombosis. J Assoc Physicians India. 2004;52(MAR):237–41.
60. Liem TK, Yanit KE, Moseley SE, et al. Peripherally inserted central catheter usage patterns and associated symptomatic upper extremity venous thrombosis. J Vasc Surg. 2012;55(3):761–7.
61. Dumantepe M, Tarhan A, Ozler A. Successful treatment of central venous catheter induced superior vena cava syndrome with ultrasound accelerated catheter-directed thrombolysis. Catheter Cardiovasc Interv. 2013;81(7):E269.
62. Van RCJ, Tesselaar MET, Osanto S, et al. Deep vein thrombosis associated with central venous catheters—a review. J Thromb Haemost. 2005;3(11):2409–19.
63. Doellman D, Hadaway L, Bowe-Geddes LA, et al. Infiltration and extravasation: update on prevention and management. J Infus Nurs. 2009;32(4):203–11.

Monitoring and Management of Trace Elements in Short Bowel Syndrome

15

Anca Trifan, Laura Huiban, Georgiana-Emmanuela Gîlcă-Blanariu, and Ștefan Andrei Chiriac

15.1 Introduction

Prognosis and survival of short bowel syndrome (SBS) patients rely on how well the remaining bowel adapts, along with targeted nutritional therapies in combination with a personalized pharmacological management. Individual care plans are tailored based on several patient-related factors, such as the length of the remaining bowel, the bowel sections in place, the degree of intestinal adaptation, and the patient's adherence to all dietary recommendations, nutrient supplementation, and medication [1].

Beyond the challenge of optimal utilization of macronutrients and vitamins, an essential role is attributed to trace elements, which are involved in a wide range of physiological processes, from immune defense and hematopoiesis to antioxidant response, metabolic bone disease, neurocognitive function, and many others [2]. Moreover, trace elements, together with vitamins, are critical for the proper utilization of macronutrients, and optimizing the micronutrient status involves fine-tuning between nutritional intervention, pharmacotherapy, and personalized supplementation. Especially after transitioning to enteral autonomy, various micronutrients, including trace elements, can become deficient [3].

In SBS, trace element deficiencies are often associated with malabsorption and nutritional changes and pose significant concerns due to their participation in vital processes. In many cases of SBS, trace element deficiencies are addressed by oral supplementation, as the patients are usually reaching Emergency Care Units with various forms of dehydration and anemia [4]. Partial or total parenteral or enteral

A. Trifan · L. Huiban · G.-E.Gîlcă-Blanariu (✉) · Ș. A. Chiriac
Faculty of Medicine, Gastroenterology Department,
Grigore T. Popa University of Medicine and Pharmacy, Iași, Romania

Institute of Gastroenterology and Hepatology, St. Spiridon Emergency Hospital,
Iași, Romania

A. Trifan et al. (eds.), *Short Bowel Syndrome in Adults*,
https://doi.org/10.1007/978-3-031-95848-9_15

nutrition is also contributing to trace element deficiencies (i.e., zinc and copper) due to insufficient or imbalanced microelement formulation [5–7].

There are several trace elements to be evaluated when monitoring the nutritional status of SBS patients, and considering the complex pathomechanisms involved in these deficiencies, careful consideration should be offered to their monitoring and management. Current recommendations endorse evaluation of trace element levels at baseline and tailored monitoring thereafter, with adjustments made based on individual patient needs and clinical circumstances, in order to avoid both deficiencies and toxicities [8].

15.2 Mechanisms of Trace Element Deficiencies in Short Bowel Syndrome

The pathomechanisms contributing to trace element deficiency in SBS are associated with the consequences of anatomical and physiological changes that result from surgical shortening of the small intestine. In patients suffering from diseases affecting the small intestine (such as Crohn's disease), significant portions of the duodenum, ileum, or jejunum are surgically removed for therapeutic purposes [9–11]. In this context, the size of the small intestine loss could be proportional to the nutritional deficiencies, as the surface area and the distribution of functional structures available for nutrient absorption decrease [10]. The most common trace element deficiencies associated with malabsorptive syndrome in SBS patients are iron, zinc, copper, selenium, and magnesium deficiencies. Consequently, due to the portions that were surgically removed, the ability of the body to absorb specific nutrients is affected (e.g., the loss of significant portions of the duodenum could lead to iron or copper malabsorption, while a shorter ileum leads to zinc and copper loss) [12–14].

The changes occurring in the small intestine as a result of anatomical alterations lead to impaired hormonal-modulated digestive functions, such as increased intestinal motility and gastric emptying [15, 16]. In these cases, while the transit time increases, the contact between food bolus and gastric epithelia, as well as between luminal content and small intestine epithelia, decreases, promoting trace element loss through feces [17]. The normal mechanism of intestinal motility and synchronization of digestion steps could be altered by ileal resection, leading to more rapid transit of the chyme from the duodenum to the colon [18, 19].

The insufficient contact between the intestinal content and lumen prevents the efficient absorption of trace elements and other nutrients, the digestion of which is vitally provided by the small intestine. Irregular digestive patterns as well as chronic diarrhea could also contribute to trace element malabsorption. In SBS cases that result from extensive small intestine resection, chronic diarrhea affects electrolyte, water, and trace element homeostasis and could be the main cause of severe dehydration [4, 17, 20].

Many reports acknowledged the predominance of dysbiosis in SBS patients [21–23]. Alongside the significant contribution of gut microbiota to digestion, its quantitative and qualitative traits are important to the symbiotic relationship between the microbiota and host. Several reports showed that digestive alterations in SBS could also be sustained by significant bacterial overgrowth (such as in small intestine bacterial overgrowth syndrome [SIBO]) that leads to nutrient competition and trace element absorption inhibition mediated by bacterial metabolic products (e.g., hydrogen sulfide) [24–28]. SIBO was reported in both adult and pediatric cases of SBS with similar pathophysiological traits [25, 26].

Furthermore, the changes in gastrointestinal tract integrity and hormonal modulation could also contribute to the alteration of glandular organ function, such as bile and pancreas (i.e., bile salt loss and pancreatic enzyme deficiency). Bile salts' implication in trace element absorption is most important for selenium and copper as their transport mainly relies on lipids, being soluble in fats [29]. In some cases, bile salt-mediated luminal hyperosmolarity could inhibit trace element absorption [29, 30]. As pancreatic dysfunction is often reported in SBS patients, not only is trace element absorption impaired but the absorption of other nutrients as well [31].

There are primarily two causes of iron deficiency in SBS patients: resection of significant portions of the duodenum and proximal jejunum and reduced acid production in the stomach [32, 33]. It is currently accepted that acidic environment provided by gastric secretion contributes to the preparation of calcium and iron ions for absorption (Fe^{3+} to Fe^{2+}) [34, 35]. In this context, the loss of chyme acidity prevents this conversion and thus iron absorption within the proximal sections of the small intestine. A recent study reported that necrotizing enterocolitis could be a major cause of SBS and iron deficiency in pediatric cases [36]. Another important process that contributes to the efficiency of iron absorption is the bile acid-mediated breakdown of dietary lipids that increases the bolus residency in the stomach [37, 38]. Increased levels of dietary iron could also be lost due to chronic diarrhea [39].

Magnesium is another vital trace element, the absorption of which is often affected by SBS, primarily due to malabsorptive syndrome and chronic diarrhea [31, 40]. Similar to other trace elements, the resection of significant segments of the ileum contributes to decreased magnesium absorption area. Lipid digestion is also important in magnesium absorption; thus, impaired bile salt secretion indirectly contributes to magnesium loss [41, 42].

Selenium, similar to magnesium, is implicated in neuromuscular mediation. Frequent reports have shown that SBS patients are often affected by muscle weakness and impaired cognitive functions as a result of selenium and magnesium deficiencies [20, 43]. Surgical removal of duodenum and jejunum could contribute to selenium deficiency due to loss of absorption areas [44]. Alterations in pancreatic digestive activity as a result of impaired gastrointestinal tract could play an important role in defective transport of selenium [45]. Gut microbiota was also reported as significant contributors to selenium absorption; therefore, dysbiosis could be a cause of compromised selenium metabolism [46].

Another trace element that was recently reported as a significant modulator of the immune system and pancreatic activity is zinc. It was shown that decreased zinc levels are associated with poor alkaline phosphatase activity, leading to altered thyroid functions and autoimmune anemia [47, 48]. In turn, poor pancreatic activity impairs zinc- and fat-mediated absorption of other trace elements [49]. Other mechanisms through which zinc is lost during digestion include loss of absorption areas due to jejunal resection and increased fecal excretion due to chronic diarrhea [50, 51].

Impaired intestinal transport due to increased luminal permeability, altered metabolism, and diarrhea was previously associated with copper deficiencies in SBS [52]. In contrast to other trace elements, copper absorption is modulated by several transport proteins within duodenum and proximal jejunum. Also, copper homeostasis could be altered by hepatic function impairment due to long-term parenteral nutrition [53].

Other trace elements that are deficient in SBS are manganese, iodine, chromium (Cr), molybdenum, and fluoride [54]. Also, different from iron, magnesium, and copper, the luminal absorption of manganese could be performed by all the segments of small intestine [55, 56], while bile acids only contribute to manganese uptake [57]. Little is known about the mechanisms of manganese deficiency in SBS patients; however, mechanisms similar to those of other trace elements (including parenteral nutrition) were reported as potential contributors [58]. Despite these limitations, the importance of manganese deficiency in SBS is highly under observation due to its severe effects. Manganese deficiency might not be as aggressive but is associated with oxidative stress, in contrast to major trace element deficiencies that were previously described [56]. As a functional component of metalloenzymes, manganese deficiency could lead to liver failure and cholestasis associated with oxidative stress, while the excess could determine Parkinson's-like neurological manifestations due to basal ganglia accumulation [59]. By contrast, iodine deficiency in SBS was often associated with reduced transit time and insufficient intake due to dietary changes in SBS [60].

Loss of ileum and parenteral nutrition are primarily predisposing to chromium deficiency in SBS [61, 62]. Chromium deficiency causes chromodulin complex impairment that leads to glucose intolerance, insulin resistance, altered tissular use of insulin, and lipid metabolism impairment [62, 63]. Parenteral nutrition that provides iron in excess could determine chromium deficiency due to unbalanced competition for transferrin-modulated transport [59]. The occurrence of Cr(IV), Cr(V), and Cr(VI) is carcinogenic, while excessive apport of Cr(III) and Cr(VI) could lead to oxidative stress [64]. Similar to magnesium, selenium, and manganese, chromium deficits were associated with neuropathies [65].

Besides zinc, selenium, and iron, thyroid function is also modulated by iodide. In SBS, iodine deficiency could occur due to impaired gastric digestion and duodenal resection [60]. Molybdenum deficiency was reported in SBS patients relying on parenteral nutrition; however, it is hard to diagnose due to extremely low plasmatic levels, but oxidative stress and impaired sulfite and purines catabolism are suggestive [66]. Cobalt deficiency in SBS was associated with defective vitamin B12 absorption, which is associated with previously described mechanisms (intestinal dysmotility, dysbiosis, and bacterial overgrowth) [67].

15.3 Diagnosis and Monitoring of Trace Element Deficiencies: Clinical and Biological Aspects

15.3.1 Clinical Assessment

The diagnosis of trace element deficiencies begins with a detailed clinical examination. A thorough medical history should be obtained, with emphasis on obtaining information regarding the underlying medical conditions that could lead to deficiencies of trace elements such as previous extensive intestinal resections, intestinal ischemia, and Crohn's disease. Diet-related risk factors should also be excluded, such as reduced nutrient intake due to other causes.

Several signs and symptoms can be noted in relation to specific deficiencies [8]. Key clinical aspects include the following:

- Zinc deficiency [68]:
  - Loss of appetite, irritability, altered smell and taste, photophobia
  - Cutaneous disturbances: squamous plaques, periorificial localization (angular cheilitis), paronychia, thinning of hair
  - Delayed wound healing
  - Predisposition to infections
- Copper deficiency [4]:
  - Clinical manifestations of anemia (pallor, asthenia, dyspnea)
  - Predisposition to infections due to neutropenia
  - Paresthesia and ataxia, often the consequence of neuropathy
  - Osteoporosis and predisposition to bone fractures
- Selenium deficiency [69]:
  - Unremarkable clinical examination in marginal selenium deficiency
  - Muscular weakness and myalgia
  - Heart failure-related symptoms in case of severe deficiency
  - Immune dysfunction leading to a higher risk of viral infections
  - Clinical manifestations linked to hypothyroidism
- Iron deficiency [8]:
  - Clinical manifestations of anemia (pallor, asthenia, dyspnea)
  - Hair loss
  - Brittle nails
- Magnesium deficiency [4]:
  - Muscle cramps
  - Tremor
  - Cardiac arrhythmias
  - Neuromuscular irritability

15.3.2 Biological Assessment

In order to early identify deficiencies in trace elements, a routine biological monitoring of these is recommended, even in the absence of typical clinical manifestations. The recommended surveillance interval is variable, depending on the nutritional status as well as on the risk level of the patient. In case of total parenteral nutrition, trace elements should be monitored on a monthly basis, while in those that require oral or enteral nutrition, an interval of 3–6 months is considered sufficient. However, in patients with high ostomy output or in cases presenting with chronic diarrhea, a monthly evaluation of trace elements should be performed [8, 64].

The most frequently used and readily available method for evaluation in the clinical practice is the plasma or serum level of the trace elements. During the parenteral nutrition phase, measuring the serum or plasma levels of trace elements is very reliable, since changes in level can be abrupt and serum monitoring can facilitate optimum follow-up. However, after weaning off parenteral nutrition, low-grade chronic deficits could arise and as studies have shown both in SBS [70, 71]and in other types of chronic diseases with malabsorption—such as inflammatory bowel disease [72]—hair evaluation could be a reliable option to monitor this type of low-grade chronic deficiency.

The main drawback of this approach is the potentially higher associated costs and lower accessibility of the method, compared to serum evaluation. Therefore, the currently validated method for implementation in clinical practice references the plasma or serum level of trace elements.

The following trace elements should be evaluated:

- *Zinc:* Either plasma or serum zinc levels can be evaluated. However, plasma levels are not sensitive to the dietary zinc intake. Thus, serum levels are preferred. Serum zinc levels are considered normal between 70 and 250 μg/dl in adults; levels lower than 60 μg/dL are indicative of deficiency. Zinc levels should be measured using special metal-free tubes in order to reduce the risk of errors. Lower zinc levels can be found in cases of myocardial infarction, estrogen therapy, fever, and sepsis. Also, albumin levels can influence the results; thus, zinc levels should be correlated with serum albumin and C-reactive protein (CRP). Ancillary tests such as alkaline phosphatase, a zinc-dependent enzyme that can show low levels in case of zinc deficiency, or urinary zinc, which is also potentially low in case of zinc deficiency, can be used but are not diagnostic. As zinc levels can frequently oscillate, often a therapeutic trial followed by clinical improvement of symptoms is suggestive of deficiency [1, 2, 6].
- *Copper:* The assessment of copper deficiency should include both serum copper as well as ceruloplasmin levels. The normal range of plasma copper is between 70 and 140 μg/dL. Levels lower than 70 μg/dL are found in deficiency; however, if ceruloplasmin levels are also decreased, a differential diagnosis with Wilson disease should be considered. Ancillary tests include a complete blood count (CBC) that can show anemia and neutropenia, and rarely thrombocytopenia [4, 8, 64].

- *Selenium:* Normal plasma selenium concentrations vary between 60 and 150 ng/mL. However, in cases of clinically relevant deficiency, the levels are usually lower than 40 ng/mL. Ancillary tests include plasma glutathione peroxidase (GPx) and urinary selenium levels that can show low levels, further supporting the diagnostic [8, 64, 69].
- *Iron*: Iron deficiency assessment should include serum iron levels, ferritin, transferrin saturation, and total iron-binding capacity (TIBC). In the case of iron deficiency, the levels of all of these biological markers are usually decreased, with the exception of TIBC, which is high. However, one of the most common indicators of iron deficiency is the presence of anemia, as shown by low hemoglobin levels in the CBC. The profile of iron-deficient anemia is microcytic, hypochromic with a low reticulocyte count [8, 64].
- Magnesium: Serum magnesium under 1.5 mg/dL indicates deficiency. However, as 99% of magnesium is stored intracellularly and only 1% is circulating in the plasma, a normal result is not entirely indicative of adequate levels. A better assessment can be obtained when using urinary magnesium. Associated electrolyte imbalances are frequently found, notably hypokalemia, hypocalcemia, hyponatremia, and hypophosphatemia; thus, these should also be actively assessed in cases of magnesium deficiency [4, 8, 64].

15.4 Management of Trace Element Deficiencies

A comprehensive nutritional evaluation should be performed in all SBS patients, addressing both macro- and micronutrient deficiencies. The evaluation of trace elements uses mainly serum levels and optimally involves the support of a dietician with expertise in SBS. The long-term monitoring involves—beyond measuring the serum levels of trace elements—regular assessment of fluid balance, weight fluctuations, bone density, liver and kidney function, and electrolyte balance [8].

Most frequently, the monitored trace elements are iron, calcium, magnesium, and phosphorus, since they are parameters at-hand in the everyday clinical practice, and their deficiencies have an easily noticeable clinical impact. Other trace elements useful to be monitored in SBS patients are zinc, selenium, chromium, and copper, which can be deficient in this patient category with sometimes a less obvious clinical impact [73] (Table 15.1).

Since currently available parenteral nutrition formulas include trace elements to maintain a proper balance of micronutrients [74], the risk of developing trace element deficiencies emerges especially at the phase of weaning parenteral nutrition, as several studies report significant deficiencies both at this point [75–77] and also after successfully discontinuing parenteral nutrition [54].

The preferred route of administration for managing trace element deficiencies is the oral route, especially after discontinuation of parenteral nutrition, which should be possible in more than half of the SBS patients after 2–5 years [78].

The SBS patients have variable needs of some micronutrients, depending on the moment of evaluation. Therefore, patients with increased gastrointestinal losses

Table 15.1 Disorders associated with trace element deficiencies in SBS

Type of element	Consequence of deficit
Iron	Anemia, glossitis
Calcium	Osteoporosis
Magnesium	Anxiety, impaired sleep, tetany, arrhythmia
Zinc	Stomatitis, alopecia, immune dysfunction
Selenium	Thyroid dysfunction, infertility
Copper	Ataxia, cytopenia
Chromium	Neuropathy
Phosphorus	Ataxia, paresthesia

might require higher amounts of zinc and selenium, while those with cholestasis should receive lower levels of copper and manganese. Additionally, long-term PN often leads to elevated levels of manganese and chromium [64].

One important factor impacting micronutrient deficiency is small bowel length, since this aspect is a key contributor to reaching enteral autonomy [79], especially at the time of weaning off parenteral nutrition. However, the residual bowel has the capacity to adapt within a certain degree [80], which can explain the variable reports of trace element deficiencies during total enteral nutrition ranging from 25% [3] to 83.9% [75]. Other factors which should be considered when managing trace elements after weaning off parenteral nutrition, beyond the remaining small bowel length, are: the presence of small bowel bacterial overgrowth, altered transit time, the presence or absence of remaining colon, and the presence of chronic changes of the intestinal mucosa [81].

In patients with SBS, the deficiency of divalent cations—including calcium, zinc, and magnesium—can result from various factors, such as a diminished absorptive surface area, an accelerated transit time, and the binding of these cations to unabsorbed fats present in the intestinal lumen [1].

In the subgroup of SBS patients with colon in continuity, dietary adjustments can improve several mineral statuses. For example, the adoption of a low-fat diet is important to minimize loss of magnesium, calcium, zinc, and copper [82], while a low-oxalate intake is useful to decrease the risk of oxalate nephrolithiasis, in addition to optimum calcium intake, considering that calcium binds oxalate in the gut. Calcium supplementation is also essential in preventing loss of bone mineral density, with special consideration to be exerted in patients with SBS following bile acid sequestrant treatment, since their use can impair both calcium and iron absorption and maintain suboptimal levels of these micronutrients [83].

As far as magnesium supplementation is concerned, there is a wide range of magnesium salts available for oral administration: magnesium sulfate, hydroxide, chloride, acetate, carbonate, gluconate, lactate, citrate, aspartate, pyroglutamate, oxide, and diglycinate. However, many of these compounds are not well absorbed and can worsen diarrhea or increase stoma output. For instance, studies indicate that magnesium acetate tends to produce less diarrhea than magnesium gluconate.

Magnesium oxide is a popular choice because it offers a higher amount of elemental magnesium compared to the other salts, with typical administration at night, when the slower intestinal transit allows for better absorption. Additionally, magnesium diglycinate (a chelated form) is absorbed as efficiently as magnesium oxide in the proximal jejunum and after an ileal resection, generating fewer bowel movements than magnesium oxide [84].

Zinc is a trace element that could be deficient in SBS patients, especially in patients with large-volume gastrointestinal output. In these cases, often high doses of oral zinc supplements are needed. Additionally, low serum zinc levels may occur as a result of reduced serum albumin—the primary protein responsible for binding zinc—which does not always indicate a true zinc deficiency. Consequently, falsely decreased zinc levels can be identified in the context of inflammation; that is why zinc measurement should be accompanied by evaluation of both albumin and CRP [5, 85]. However, the zinc supplementation should be carefully monitored, since it can lead to negative clinical effects even at moderate doses. Moreover, high levels of zinc can lead to reduced copper levels, since copper binds most strongly to metallothionein [86].

A summary of the current standard recommendations for trace element supplementation can be found in Table 15.2. One should consider that doses for each trace

Table 15.2 Usual supplementation requirements in SBS patients [8, 87]

Trace element	Recommended supplementation	Typical dose
Iron	Oral or intravenous (IV)*	100–200 mg per day or every other day
Calcium		1000–3000 mg per day (careful consideration of dose, due to risk of calcium oxalate nephrolithiasis in SBS patients with extensive ileal resection and intact colon)
Magnesium	Oral or IV*	50–500 mg elemental magnesium (lactate or gluconate) Additional IV may be required (2 g magnesium sulfate biweekly)
Zinc	Oral	220 mg tablet (equivalent of 50 mg elemental zinc) (zinc sulfate tablet up to 220 mg three times daily)
Selenium	Oral	100–200 μg daily
Chromium	Oral	100–200 μg, 1–3 daily
Copper	Oral or IV*	From 2 mg elemental copper daily
Phosphate (as sodium and potassium salts)	Oral	250–2000 mg per day
Manganese	For patients requiring parenteral nutrition	

* depending on degree of deficit

element need to be personalized, with tailored doses based on the level of deficit, but also considering several patient-related factors, from diet and underlying associated chronic diseases to concomitant pharmacotherapy and patient's adherence to medical interventions.

15.5 Conclusions

Trace element deficiencies are frequent among SBS patients, especially during the process of intestinal rehabilitation. The levels of trace elements need to be monitored regularly in order to promptly identify deficiency and guide supplementation. The most common trace element deficiencies are iron, zinc, copper, selenium, and magnesium deficiencies, although other deficiencies such as phosphate, chromium, and manganese can arise in this patient category.

Individualized trace element supplementation together with close follow-up and nutritional monitoring are essential to ensure optimum evolution of patients with SBS and to avoid both deficiencies and potential toxicities.

References

1. Wall EA. An overview of short bowel syndrome management: adherence, adaptation, and practical recommendations. J Acad Nutr Diet. 2013;113(9):1200–8. https://doi.org/10.1016/j.jand.2013.05.001.
2. Bailey RL, West KP Jr, Black RE. The epidemiology of global micronutrient deficiencies. Ann Nutr Metab. 2015;66(suppl 2):S22–33.
3. Ubesie AC, Kocoshis SA, Mezoff AG, Henderson CJ, Helmrath MA, Cole CR. Multiple micronutrient deficiencies among patients with intestinal failure during and after transition to enteral nutrition. J Pediatr. 2013;163(6):1692e6
4. Braga CB, Ferreira IM, Marchini JS, Cunha SF. Copper and magnesium deficiencies in patients with short bowel syndrome receiving parenteral nutrition or oral feeding. Arq Gastroenterol. 2015;52(2):94–9.
5. Sundaram A, Koutkia P, Apovian CM. Nutritional management of short bowel syndrome in adults. J Clin Gastroenterol. 2002;34(3):207–20.
6. Sriram K, Lonchyna VA. Micronutrient supplementation in adult nutrition therapy: practical considerations. JPEN J Parenter Enteral Nutr. 2009;33(5):548–62.
7. Jin J, Mulesa L, Carrilero RM. Trace Elements in Parenteral Nutrition: Considerations for the Prescribing Clinician. Nutrients. 2017;9(5):440.
8. Iyer K, DiBaise JK, Rubio-Tapia A. AGA clinical practice update on management of short bowel syndrome: expert review. Clin Gastroenterol Hepatol. 2022;20(10):2185–2194.e2.
9. Robinson MK, Wilmore DW. Short bowel syndrome. In: Holzheimer RG, Mannick JA, editors. Surgical treatment: evidence-based and problem-oriented. Munich: Zuckschwerdt; 2001. Available from: https://www.ncbi.nlm.nih.gov/books/NBK6974/.
10. Jang KU, Yu CS, Lim SB, Park IJ, Yoon YS, Kim CW, Lee JL, Yang SK, Ye BD, Kim JC. Factors affecting poor nutritional status after small bowel resection in patients with Crohn disease. Medicine (Baltimore). 2016;95(30):e4285.
11. Tappenden KA. Anatomical and physiological considerations in short bowel syndrome: emphasis on intestinal adaptation and the role of enterohormones. Nutr Clin Pract. 2023;38:S27–34.

12. Engels LG, van den Hamer CJ, van Tongeren JH. Iron, zinc, and copper balance in short bowel patients on oral nutrition. Am J Clin Nutrition. 1984;40(5):1038–41.
13. Saboor M, Zehra A, Qamar K, Moinuddin. Disorders associated with malabsorption of iron: a critical review. Pak J Med Sci. 2015;31(6):1549–53.
14. Moon N, Aryan M, Westerveld D, Nathoo S, Glover S, Kamel AY. Clinical manifestations of copper deficiency: a case report and review of the literature. Nutr Clin Pract. 2021 Oct;36(5):1080–5.
15. Besterman HS, Adrian TE, Mallinson CN, Christofides ND, Sarson DL, Pera A, Lombardo L, Modigliani R, Bloom SR. Gut hormone release after intestinal resection. Gut. 1982;23(10):854–61.
16. Ahmed M, Ahmed S. Functional, diagnostic and therapeutic aspects of gastrointestinal hormones. Gastroenterol Res. 2019;12(5):233–44.
17. Torres C, Vanderhoof JA. Chronic complications of short bowel syndrome. Curr Paediatr. 2006;16(5):291–7.
18. Garcia-Casado J, Martinez-de-Juan JL, Ponce JL. Intestinal motility. In: Akay M, editor. Wiley encyclopedia of biomedical engineering; 2006. https://doi.org/10.1002/9780471740360.ebs0649.
19. Schmidt T, Pfeiffer A, Hackelsberger N, Widmer R, Meisel C, Kaess H. Effect of intestinal resection on human small bowel motility. Gut. 1996 Jun;38(6):859–63.
20. Utrilla Fornals A, Costas-Batlle C, Medlin S, Menjón-Lajusticia E, Cisneros-González J, Saura-Carmona P, Montoro-Huguet MA. Metabolic and nutritional issues after lower digestive tract surgery: the important role of the dietitian in a multidisciplinary setting. Nutrients. 2024;16(2):246.
21. Engstrand Lilja H, Wefer H, Nyström N, Finkel Y, Engstrand L. Intestinal dysbiosis in children with short bowel syndrome is associated with impaired outcome. Microbiome. 2015 May;4(3):18.
22. Piper HG, Fan D, Coughlin LA, Ho EX, McDaniel MM, Channabasappa N, Kim J, Kim M, Zhan X, Xie Y, Koh AY. Severe gut microbiota dysbiosis is associated with poor growth in patients with short bowel syndrome. J Parenteral Enteral Nutrit. 2017;41:1202–12.
23. Carter J, Bettag J, Morfin S, Manithody C, Nagarapu A, Jain A, Nazzal H, Prem S, Unes M, McHale M, et al. Gut microbiota modulation of short bowel syndrome and the gut–brain axis. Nutrients. 2023;15(11):2581.
24. Dibaise JK, Young RJ, Vanderhoof JA. Enteric microbial flora, bacterial overgrowth, and short-bowel syndrome. Clin Gastroenterol Hepatol. 2006 Jan;4(1):11–20.
25. Joly J, Mayeur C, Bruneau A, Noordine ML, Meylheuc T, Langella P, Messing B, Duée PH, Cherbuy C, Thomas M. Drastic changes in fecal and mucosa-associated microbiota in adult patients with short bowel syndrome. Biochimie. 2010;92(7):753–61.
26. McGrath KH, Pitt J, Bines JE. Small intestinal bacterial overgrowth in children with intestinal failure on home parenteral nutrition. JGH Open. 2019;3(5):394–9.
27. Goulet O, Joly F. Intestinal microbiota in short bowel syndrome Microbiote intestinal dans le syndrome du grêle court. Gastroenterol Clin Biol. 2010;34(S1):37–43.
28. Mareş CR, Săsăran MO, Mărginean CO. Small intestinal bacterial overgrowth and childhood malnutrition: a comprehensive review of available evidence. Nutrients. 2024;16(24):4319.
29. Boyer JL. Bile formation and secretion. Compr Physiol. 2013 Jul;3(3):1035–78.
30. Harries JT, Sladen GE. The effects of different bile salts on the absorption of fluid, electrolytes, and monosaccharides in the small intestine of the rat in vivo. Gut. 1972 Aug;13(8):596–603.
31. Parrish CR, DiBaise JK. Managing the adult patient with short bowel syndrome. Gastroenterol Hepatol (N Y). 2017;13(10):600–8.
32. Duro D, Jaksic T, Duggan C. Multiple micronutrient deficiencies in a child with short bowel syndrome and normal somatic growth. J Pediatr Gastroenterol Nutr. 2008 Apr;46(4):461–4.
33. Lin B, Wang Y, Zheng J, Zhu C. A case report of anemia associated with short bowel syndrome corrected by EPO during nutrition therapy. J Clin Images Med Case Rep. 2024;5(2):2872.
34. Shkembi B, Huppertz T. Calcium absorption from food products: food matrix effects. Nutrients. 2022;14:180.

35. Ems T, St Lucia K, Huecker MR. Biochemistry, iron absorption. [Updated 2023 Apr 17]. In: StatPearls [Internet]. Treasure Island: StatPearls Publishing; 2025. Available from: https://www.ncbi.nlm.nih.gov/books/NBK448204/.
36. Fawole R. Iron deficiency anemia in children with short bowel syndrome. Grad Med Edu Res J. 2024;6(1)
37. DeWayne Ashmead H. The absorption and metabolism 01 iron amino acid chelate. Arch Latinoam Nutr. 2001;51(1, Supl. 1):13–21.
38. Arnaud M, Diego M, Christophe Z, Andreas S, Zimmermann MB. The effect of lipids, a lipid-rich ready-to-use therapeutic food, or a phytase on iron absorption from maize-based meals fortified with micronutrient powders. Am J Clin Nutr. 2017;105(6):1521–7.
39. Jeejeebhoy KN. Short bowel syndrome: a nutritional and medical approach. CMAJ. 2002;166(10):1297–302.
40. Parish CR, DiBaise JK. Short bowel syndrome in adults—Part 3. Hydrating the adult patient with short bowel syndrome. In: Nutrition issues in gastroenterology, Series #138. Practical gastroenterology; 2015.
41. Schuchardt JP, Hahn A. Intestinal absorption and factors influencing bioavailability of magnesium-an update. Curr Nutr Food Sci. 2017;13(4):260–78.
42. Zuvarox T, Belletieri C. Malabsorption syndromes. [Updated 2023 Jul 24]. In: StatPearls [Internet]. Treasure Island: StatPearls Publishing; 2025. Available from: https://www.ncbi.nlm.nih.gov/books/NBK553106/.
43. Burns DP, Drummond SE, Wölfel S, Murphy KH, Szpunar J, O'Halloran KD, Mackrill JJ. Impaired upper airway muscle function with excessive or deficient dietary intake of selenium in rats. Antioxidants (Basel). 2024;13(9):1080.
44. Montoro-Huguet MA, Belloc B, Domínguez-Cajal M. Small and large intestine (I): malabsorption of nutrients. Nutrients. 2021;13(4):1254.
45. Saito Y. Selenium transport mechanism via selenoprotein P—its physiological role and related diseases. Front Nutr. 2021;8:685517.
46. Cai J, Su W, Chen X, Zheng H. Advances in the study of selenium and human intestinal bacteria. Front Nutr. 2022;9:1059358.
47. Cho YE, Lomeda RA, Ryu SH, Sohn HY, Shin HI, Beattie JH, Kwun IS. Zinc deficiency negatively affects alkaline phosphatase and the concentration of Ca, Mg and P in rats. Nutr Res Pract. 2007 Summer;1(2):113–9.
48. Kido T, Hachisuka E, Suka M, et al. Interleukin-4 administration or zinc supplementation is effective in preventing zinc deficiency–induced hemolytic anemia and splenomegaly. Biol Trace Elem Res. 2021;199:668–81.
49. Easley D, Krebs N, Jefferson M, Miller L, Erskine J, Accurso F, Hambidge KM. Effect of pancreatic enzymes on zinc absorption in cystic fibrosis. J Pediatr Gastroenterol Nutr. 1998;26(2):136–9.
50. DiBaise JK. Management of short bowel syndrome in adults. In: Connor RF, editor. UpToDate. Wolters Kluwer. Last updated: Feb 06, 2023. [Accessed on February 20, 2025].
51. Kumpf VJ. Pharmacologic management of diarrhea in patients with short bowel syndrome. J Parenter Enter Nutr. 2014;38:38S–44S.
52. Bender MT, Frye JW, Parrish C, Copland AP. Less copper than a modern penny: a case of insidious copper deficiency and short bowel syndrome? Am J Gastroenterol. 2018;113:S1383–4.
53. Prohaska JR. Role of copper transporters in copper homeostasis. Am J Clin Nutr. 2008 Sep;88(3):826S–9S.
54. Tuokkola J, Olkkonen E, Gunnar R, Pakarinen M, Merras-Salmio L. Vitamin and trace element status and growth in children with short bowel syndrome being weaned off parenteral nutrition. J Pediatr Gastroenterol Nutr. 2025 Feb;80(2):318–25. https://doi.org/10.1002/jpn3.12427.
55. Lutz TA, Schroff A, Scharrer E. Effects of calcium and sugars on intestinal manganese absorption. Biol Trace Elem Res. 1993;39:221–7.
56. Li L, Yang X. The essential element manganese, oxidative stress, and metabolic diseases: links and interactions. Oxidative Med Cell Longev. 2018, 2018:7580707.

57. Ahmad TR, Higuchi S, Bertaggia E, Hung A, Shanmugarajah N, Guilz NC, Gamarra JR, Haeusler RA. Bile acid composition regulates the manganese transporter Slc30a10 in intestine. J Biol Chem. 2020;295(35):12545–58.
58. Stehle P, Stoffel-Wagner B, Kuhn K. Parenteral trace element provision: recent clinical research and practical conclusions. Eur J Clin Nutr. 2016;70:886–93.
59. Pogatschnik Cassandra. Trace Element Supplementation and Monitoring in the Adult Patient on Parenteral Nutrition. Practical Gastroenterology, Nutrition Issues In Gastroenterology, Series #129, 2014.
60. Passos ACV, Barros F, Damiani D, Semer B, Cespedes WCJ, Sannicola B, Tannuri ACA, Tannuri U. Hypothyroidism associated with short bowel syndrome in children: a report of six cases. Arch Endocrinol Metab. 2018;62(6):655–60.
61. Brown RO, Forloines-Lynn S, Cross RE, Heizer WD. Chromium deficiency after long-term total parenteral nutrition. Dig Dis Sci. 1986 Jun;31(6):661–4.
62. Afzal S, Ocasio Quinones GA. Chromium deficiency. [Updated 2024 Jun 7]. In: StatPearls [Internet]. Treasure Island, StatPearls Publishing; 2025. Available from: https://www.ncbi.nlm.nih.gov/books/NBK582150/.
63. Lewicki S, Zdanowski R, Krzyżowska M, Lewicka A, Dębski B, Niemcewicz M, Goniewicz M. The role of Chromium III in the organism and its possible use in diabetes and obesity treatment. Ann Agric Environ Med. 2014;21(2):331–5.
64. Berger MM, Shenkin A, Dizdar OS, Amrein K, Augsburger M, Biesalski HK, Bischoff SC, Casaer MP, Gundogan K, Lepp HL, de Man AME, Muscogiuri G, Pietka M, Pironi L, Rezzi S, Schweinlin A, Cuerda C. ESPEN practical short micronutrient guideline. Clin Nutr. 2024 Mar;43(3):825–57.
65. Moukarzel A. Chromium in parenteral nutrition: too little or too much? Gastroenterology. 2009;137(5 Suppl):S18–28.
66. Shenkin A, Talwar D, Ben-Hamouda N, Amrein K, Casaer MP, de Man A, Dizdar OS, Gundogan K, Lepp HL, Rezzi S, van Zanten AR, Berger MM, ESPEN Micronutrient Special Interest Group (SIG-MN). LLL 44-1 Micronutrients in clinical nutrition: trace elements. Clin Nutr ESPEN. 2024;61:369–76.
67. Morotti F, Terruzzi J, Cavalleri L, Betalli P, D'Antiga L, Norsa L. Vitamin B12 deficiency presenting as intestinal pseudo-obstruction in short bowel syndrome: a case report. Nutrition. 2023 Feb;106:111895.
68. Sanna A, Firinu D, Zavattari P, Valera P. Zinc status and autoimmunity: a systematic review and meta-analysis. Nutrients. 2018;10(1):68. https://doi.org/10.3390/nu10010068.
69. Rayman MP. Selenium and human health. Lancet. 2012;379(9822):1256–68. https://doi.org/10.1016/S0140-6736(11)61452-9.
70. Hambidge KM. Zinc deficiency in man: its origins and effects. Phil Trans R Soc Lond B. 1981;294:129–44.
71. Jeejeebhoy K. Zinc: an essential trace element for parenteral nutrition. Gastroenterology. 2009;137(5 Suppl):S7–12. https://doi.org/10.1053/j.gastro.2009.08.014.
72. Gîlcă-Blanariu GE, Coroabă A, Ciocoiu M, et al. Hair EDX analysis-a promising tool for micronutrient status evaluation of patients with IBD? Nutrients. 2021;13(8):2572. https://doi.org/10.3390/nu13082572.
73. Livingstone C. Zinc: physiology, deficiency, and parenteral nutrition. Nutr Clin Pract. 2015;30:371e82.
74. Domellof M, Szitanyi P, Simchowitz V, et al. ESPGHAN/ESPEN/ESPR guidelines on pediatric parenteral nutrition: iron and trace minerals. Clin Nutr Edinb Scotl. 2018;37:2354.
75. Feng H, Zhang T, Yan W, et al. Micronutrient deficiencies in pediatric short bowel syndrome: a 10-year review from an intestinal rehabilitation center in China. Pediatr Surg Int. 2020;36:1481–7. https://doi.org/10.1007/s00383-020-04764-3.
76. Ubesie AC, Cole CR, Nathan JD, et al. Micronutrient deficiencies in pediatric and young adult intestinal transplant patients. Pediatr Transplant. 2013;17:638–45. https://doi.org/10.1111/petr.12132.

77. Yang CF, Duro D, Zurakowski D, Lee M, Jaksic T, Duggan C. High prevalence of multiple micronutrient deficiencies in children with intestinal failure: a longitudinal study. J Pediatr. 2011;159(1):39–44.e1.
78. Amiot A, Messing B, Corcos O, et al. Determinants of home parenteral nutrition dependence and survival of 268 patients with non-malignant short bowel syndrome. Clin Nutr. 2013;32:368–74.
79. Chatzidaki V, Wood R, Alegakis A, Lawson M, Fagbemi A. Parenteral support and micronutrient deficiencies in children with short bowel syndrome: a comprehensive retrospective study. Clin Nutr ESPEN. 2023;58:270–6. https://doi.org/10.1016/j.clnesp.2023.10.008.
80. Billiauws L, Thomas M, Bihan J, Joly F. Intestinal adaptation in short bowel syndrome. What is new? Nutr Hosp. 2018;35(3):731–7.
81. Beattie LM, Barclay AR, Wilson DC. Short bowel syndrome and intestinal failure in infants and children. Pediatric Child Health. 2010;20(10):485e91.
82. Ovesen L, Chu R, Howard L. The influence of dietary fat on jejunostomy output in patients with severe short bowel syndrome. Am J Clin Nutr. 1983;38:270–7.
83. Berger MM, Shenkin A, Schweinlin A, Amrein K, Augsburger M, Biesalski HK, Bischoff SC, Casaer MP, Gundogan K, Lepp HL, de Man AME, Muscogiuri G, Pietka M, Pironi L, Rezzi S, Cuerda C. ESPEN micronutrient guideline. Clin Nutr. 2022;41(6):1357–424. https://doi.org/10.1016/j.clnu.2022.02.015.
84. Nightingale JMD. Management of patients with a short bowel. World J Gastroenterol. 2001;7(6):741–51.
85. Salota R, Omar S, Sherwood RA, Raja K, Vincent RP. Clinical relevance of trace element measurement in patients on initiation of parenteral nutrition. Ann Clin Biochem. 2016;53:680e5.
86. Hordyjewska A, Popiolek L, Kocot J. The many "faces" of copper in medicine and treatment. Biometals: Int J Role Metal Ions Biol Biochem Med. 2014;27:611e21.
87. Matarese LE, Steiger E. Dietary and medical management of short bowel syndrome in adult patients. J Clin Gastroenterol. 2006;40(Suppl 2):S85–93. https://doi.org/10.1097/01.mcg.0000212678.14172.7a.

Enteral Feeding and Parenteral Nutrition in Short Bowel Syndrome: Current Recommendations and Unmet Needs

16

Catalina Mihai, Cristina Cijevschi, Robert Nastasa, Razvan Igna, and Anca Trifan

16.1 Introduction

Short bowel syndrome (SBS) is characterized by malnutrition and growth retardation resulting in the most frequent cases from substantial surgical resection of the small intestine. Intestinal failure (IF), a clinical manifestation of SBS, exhibits significant variability in severity based on the type and length of the remaining small intestine [1].

Three types of SBS are identified according to the anatomy of the remaining bowel: end-jejunostomy, jejunocolic anastomosis, and jejunoileal anastomosis, with the entire colon and ileocecal valve remaining intact [2]. SBS is characterized by several clinical features, such as malabsorption, electrolyte imbalances, dehydration, and starvation. It is the leading cause of chronic IF, which is defined as a reduction in gut function below the minimum threshold necessary for the absorption of water, electrolytes, and/or macronutrients. Patients with SBS often require long-term nutritional support, with parenteral nutrition (PN) being a cornerstone therapy. While PN can be lifesaving, it also presents unique challenges, such as the risk of complications and the need for ongoing monitoring [3]. Recent advancements in management have significantly reduced the morbidity and mortality associated with SBS–IF, largely due to an improved understanding of physiological changes and strategies to enhance them to achieve enteral autonomy [4].

C. Mihai · C. Cijevschi · R. Nastasa (✉) · A. Trifan
Grigore T. Popa University of Medicine and Pharmacy, Iaşi, Romania

Institute of Gastroenterology and Hepatology, St. Spiridon Emergency Hospital, Iaşi, Romania

R. Igna
Grigore T. Popa University of Medicine and Pharmacy, Iaşi, Romania

Intensive Care Department, St. Spiridon Emergency Hospital, Iaşi, Romania

A. Trifan et al. (eds.), *Short Bowel Syndrome in Adults*,
https://doi.org/10.1007/978-3-031-95848-9_16

Effective management of SBS–IF requires a multidisciplinary team approach, involving specialized physicians such as surgeons, gastroenterologists, and registered dietitians. Long-term parenteral support, which includes parenteral nutrition and/or intravenous fluids (PN/IV), is necessary for patients who are unable to meet their nutritional and hydration needs through oral intake. However, PN/IV has drawbacks. Besides being expensive, it is associated with several problems, some of which are potentially fatal [5]. Beyond nutritional support and therapies aimed at malabsorption symptoms and problems, there have historically been limited choices for managing SBS–IF, with surgery and transplantation being reserved for extreme cases.

However, novel targeted therapeutic approaches have recently been proposed to improve gut function and lessen dependency on PN/IV [6]. The costs associated with long-term home parenteral nutrition (HPN) are substantial and typically increase with prolonged patient longevity. The life-sustaining benefits of HPN are counterbalanced by its economic impact on the healthcare system, which includes direct costs related to PN, medical consultations, laboratory monitoring, home support, and hospitalizations resulting from treatment-related complications. Furthermore, non-healthcare expenses and indirect costs resulting from productivity loss contribute to the total economic burden. Despite all its disadvantages, PN in patients with SBS and IF remains the most important therapeutic method [7].

16.2 The Rationale for Parenteral/Enteral Nutrition Use

SBS–IF is characterized by diarrhea, steatorrhea, stomach discomfort, electrolyte imbalances, dehydration, and malnutrition, although the exact symptoms vary from patient to patient, depending on the extent of resection and the adaptation of the remaining bowel. Because management is complicated, a customized and all-encompassing strategy is needed. To improve fluid and nutrient absorption, the primary objectives of therapy are intestinal rehabilitation and symptom control. The ability of the remnant gut to adapt after surgical resection depends on several parameters, including age, concomitant diseases, remaining bowel length and structure, and oral food intake [8]. An end jejunostomy with less than 115 cm of small intestine left, a jejunocolic or ileocolic anastomosis with less than 60 cm of small intestine left, or a duodenostomy or jejunoileal anastomosis with less than 35 cm of small intestine left are the usual procedures performed on patients deemed to be at the highest nutritional risk [9]. Weight loss and specific clinical syndromes associated with deficiencies in a variety of micronutrients and macronutrients (calcium, magnesium, potassium, selenium, zinc, iron, vitamin B12, vitamins A, D, and K, carbohydrates, lactose, protein, and fat, among others) are among the consequences of malnutrition from SBS–IF. Each of the body's systems is affected by malnutrition, which lowers overall health and quality of life [10]. Also, mortality rates persist at elevated levels in patients with SBS–IF, varying between 25% and 32% over 5 years globally [11].

The primary objectives of SBS–IF therapy include enhanced intestinal absorption, reduced diarrhea, and prevention of dehydration. Intestinal rehabilitation is the ultimate goal to reduce and, ideally, eliminate PN/IV dependence. The cornerstone of treatment remains nutritional support. Patients require parenteral nutrition (PN)/ intravenous (IV) therapy in addition to a hypercaloric diet, enteral nutrition, proper oral rehydration, vitamin and mineral supplements, and medication to manage symptoms and consequences of SBS–IF [12].

16.3 Enteral Nutrition

Enteral nutrition (EN), although rarely used, has proven its effectiveness during the adaptation period. The presence of nutrients in the intestinal lumen stimulates the intestinal adaptation process, which occurs through mucosal hyperplasia and the trophic secretion of digestive hormones and biliopancreatic enzymes [13]. The use of EN, alone or in combination with an oral diet, has been shown to increase protein, lipid absorption, and energy intake in patients with SBS [14].

A complex composition of EN formulas containing whole proteins, complex carbohydrates, and long-chain triglycerides is recommended. Isotonic polymeric formulas are preferred over elemental ones, as they are well tolerated, less hyperosmotic, more cost-effective, and have an increased potential to enhance intestinal adaptation. The addition of fiber is beneficial only in cases of SBS when the large bowel is present [3, 15].

EN can be administered through a nasogastric tube (for short-term administration) or via endoscopic, percutaneous gastrostomy, taking into account the technical difficulties related to anatomical changes and adhesion syndrome. Slow administration of the solution into the stomach is recommended to increase intestinal transit time and improve absorption [16].

EN should be started as soon as the patient has digestive tolerance. Both the European Society for Clinical Nutrition and Metabolism (ESPEN) and the American Gastroenterological Association (AGA) recommend the use of EN in combination with or without an oral diet in stable patients with SBS–IF (normal electrolyte levels, adequate hydration, stool excretion <2 L/day), with insufficient oral intake. The adjunctive use of EN could help patients discontinue PN [3, 10].

16.4 Role of Parenteral Nutrition in Short Bowel Syndrome

PN is a life-sustaining therapy for patients with SBS who are unable to meet their nutritional needs through enteral feeding alone. PN delivers essential nutrients, including carbohydrates, proteins, fats, electrolytes, vitamins, and trace elements directly into the bloodstream, bypassing the gastrointestinal tract.

For long-term PN administration, tunneled, single-lumen central catheters (with a lower risk of infection and thrombosis) or totally implantable devices (port) are preferred [17].

16.4.1 Goals of Parenteral Nutrition

The primary goals of PN in SBS management include the following:

- Maintaining nutritional status and preventing malnutrition
- Ensuring adequate hydration and correcting electrolyte imbalances
- Supporting metabolic demands during periods of bowel adaptation and recovery
- Promoting growth and development in pediatric patients
- Reducing the risk of long-term complications associated with malnutrition

16.4.2 Prescribing Parenteral Nutrition: Process and Formulation

Prescribing PN requires a detailed and individualized approach. It involves calculating the patient's daily requirements for macronutrients, fluids, electrolytes, vitamins, and trace elements, while regularly monitoring for complications. The steps involved in prescribing PN include the following:

16.4.2.1 Initial Assessment

A thorough clinical evaluation includes assessing body weight, height, and body composition, as well as recent weight trends; evaluating laboratory parameters to assess liver function, kidney function, electrolytes, and glucose levels; and evaluating fluid balance, urine output, and signs of dehydration.

16.4.2.2 Calculation of Energy Requirements

Energy requirements depend on the patient's age, weight, clinical condition, and metabolic demands. General guidelines: adults, 25–35 kcal/kg/day; children, vary based on age and growth needs, typically higher than for adults.

Energy requirements are adjusted for stress factors, such as infections and surgeries.

16.4.2.3 Macronutrient Composition

Macronutrient delivery in PN includes carbohydrates, proteins, and fats, each tailored to meet the patient's specific needs.

- Carbohydrates: provided as glucose (dextrose). It typically contributes 50–60% of total caloric intake; infusion rates should not exceed 4–5 mg/kg/min to avoid hyperglycemia.
- Proteins: delivered as amino acids. Requirements: adults, 1–2 g/kg/day; pediatric patients, up to 3 g/kg/day to support growth and development.
- Fats: lipid emulsions provide essential fatty acids and account for 20–30% of total caloric intake. Newer emulsions containing fish oil have been shown to reduce the risk of liver toxicity compared to soybean-based emulsions.

16.4.2.4 Electrolytes, Vitamins, and Trace Elements

Electrolytes are adjusted daily based on laboratory results to maintain normal physiological levels.

- Sodium, potassium, calcium, magnesium, and phosphate are monitored and supplemented as needed.
- Vitamins: multivitamin preparations ensure adequate intake of both fat-soluble and water-soluble vitamins.
- Trace elements, including zinc, selenium, copper, manganese, and chromium, are included in PN formulations according to the recommended daily allowances.

16.4.2.5 Fluid Requirements

Fluid needs depend on the patient's clinical condition, typically 30–35 mL/kg/day. Additional fluids may be required for patients with high-output stomas or diarrhea, as well as during hot weather [18].

16.4.3 Monitoring Parenteral Nutrition

Monitoring PN is essential to ensure efficacy, prevent complications, and make necessary adjustments. Effective monitoring includes clinical assessments, laboratory tests, and imaging studies when needed.

16.4.3.1 Clinical Monitoring

- Daily weight and fluid balance: regular monitoring of body weight and fluid input/output helps detect fluid imbalances
- Vital signs: monitoring for signs of infection, particularly catheter-related infections
- Nutritional status: regular assessment of muscle mass, fat stores, and overall clinical condition

16.4.3.2 Laboratory Monitoring

- Blood glucose: checked daily initially, then adjusted based on stability to prevent hyperglycemia or hypoglycemia
- Electrolytes (sodium, potassium, magnesium, phosphate): monitored daily initially, then weekly or as clinically indicated
- Liver function tests (ALT, AST, alkaline phosphatase, bilirubin): monitored weekly to detect early signs of cholestasis or liver injury
- Triglycerides: assessed weekly to prevent hypertriglyceridemia from lipid emulsions
- Micronutrient levels: checked periodically to ensure adequate vitamin and trace element status
- Bone health markers: regular assessment of calcium, vitamin D, and bone density for patients receiving long-term PN

16.4.3.3 Imaging Studies

- Ultrasound: used to assess liver size and detect hepatobiliary complications, such as gallstones or hepatic steatosis
- DEXA scan: performed periodically for bone mineral density assessment in long-term PN patients [17]

16.4.4 Advancements in Parenteral Nutrition Formulations

Recent advancements in PN formulations have improved outcomes for patients with SBS. Notable developments include the following:

- *Lipid Emulsions*. Traditional soybean oil-based lipid emulsions have been associated with hepatotoxicity. Newer emulsions containing fish oil or mixed-oil formulations (such as soybean, olive, and fish oils) have demonstrated improved safety profiles.
- *Customized PN Solutions*. Tailored PN solutions offer individualized nutrient delivery, enabling precise control of macronutrient and micronutrient intake tailored to the patient's clinical status.
- *Amino Acid Formulations*. Improved amino acid formulations now include essential and conditionally essential amino acids, enhancing nitrogen balance and reducing the risk of catabolism.

Glucagon-like peptide-2 (GLP-2) analog therapies, such as teduglutide, promote intestinal adaptation, improve nutrient absorption, and reduce dependence on PN [19].

16.4.5 Parenteral Nutrition-Associated Complications

Complications of long-term PN are presented in Table 16.1 [20].

Table 16.1 Long-term parenteral nutrition complications

Catheter-related complications	Obstruction, thrombosis, infection
PN-associated liver disease	Cholestasis, steatosis, fibrosis, unclassified End-stage liver disease
Metabolic complications	Metabolic bone disease Iron deficiency anemia Manganese toxicity
Others	Blood clots Gallbladder disease Kidney disease Anxiety Depression

PN parenteral nutrition

Catheter-Related Complications The primary complications associated with central venous catheters are mechanical and infectious. Mechanical complications (occlusion, thrombosis) can lead to loss of venous access, representing an indication for intestinal transplantation. Thrombosis is treated with anticoagulants, although these are not recommended in primary prevention [3]. Infectious complications have a highly variable reported incidence, ranging from 0.199 to 11.5 episodes per 1000 catheter days, with *Staphylococcus* spp. being the most frequently involved. They can be prevented by observing the rules of asepsis and antisepsis, providing adequate education to the patient and the care team, and using antimicrobial locks (e.g., taurolidine) [21]. Treatment involves the administration of antimicrobial agents both locally and systemically. In severe cases, such as tunnel infections, port abscesses, severe sepsis, endocarditis, suppurative thrombophlebitis, or a positive blood culture for fungi, catheter replacement may be necessary [3].

Liver Disease PN-associated liver disease requires vigilant monitoring and the use of newer lipid formulations. ESPEN recommends the use of the term "Intestinal failure-associated liver disease (IFALD)," emphasizing that the disease's pathogenesis is multifactorial, with parenteral nutrition (PN) being only one of the etiopathogenic factors [22]. The primary mechanisms involved are increased intestinal permeability, alterations in the enterohepatic circulation of bile acids, and disruption of the intestinal microbiota and the liver–intestinal axis.

It is more common in children compared to adults and can progress to end-stage liver disease, which requires combined intestinal and liver transplantation. It is diagnosed based on modified liver tests (in the absence of pre-existing liver diseases) and can be monitored in its evolution by transient elastography [20]. Preventive measures include combating infectious or inflammatory factors (catheter infections, intestinal bacterial overgrowth), maintaining the colon and as much length of the small intestine as possible during surgical procedures, use of enteral or oral nutrition, discontinuous use of PN, avoiding overfeeding, and limiting the use of soybean-based intravenous fat emulsions [22].

16.4.6 Weaning of Parenteral Nutrition

Virtually all patients with SBS will follow parenteral nutrition (PN) in the initial period until the adaptation process reaches its maximum (usually after 1 year); over 50% of them will be able to resume oral nutrition, most of whom will do so within the first 2 years post-resection [16]. Predictive factors for PN weaning include the length and integrity of the remaining intestine, the presence of the colon and ileocecal valve, age, duration of PN, nutritional status, and gastrointestinal motility. Fasting plasma citrulline has been shown to have prognostic value in IF, with values below 20 μmol/L correlating with PN elimination [23].

The reduction and eventual elimination of PN is a progressive process, with careful monitoring of symptoms, stool and urine excretion, body weight, hydration status (daily urine volume over 1 liter, urinary Na > 20 mEq/L), electrolytes, and micronutrients. The reduction of PN is achieved either by decreasing the number of weekly administrations or by reducing the daily administered volume. The introduction of enteral nutrition as soon as the patient has oral tolerance helps the intestinal adaptation process and the abandonment of PN [24].

PN will be resumed if there are abnormalities in laboratory parameters, a weight loss of more than 1 kg/week occurs, or the volume of fecal matter exceeds 600 g/day. In patients with irreversible IF, with suboptimal remaining intestine, PN is a necessity throughout life (home PN). It is estimated that patients with residual small bowel measuring less than 100–140 cm without a colon or those with an ileo-jejunal length of 40–60 cm and colonic anastomosis will require long-term PN [13].

16.4.7 Challenges in the Long-Term Management of Parenteral Nutrition

Despite advancements, long-term PN management remains challenging. Key issues include cost and resource utilization (PN therapy is expensive and requires a multidisciplinary approach for optimal management) and patient education (ensuring adherence and understanding of catheter care is vital for preventing complications).

Managing patients with SBS on long-term PN requires a team approach comprising gastroenterologists and nutrition specialists (to oversee the patient's nutritional management and adjust PN regimens), pharmacists (to assist in the preparation and monitoring of customized PN solutions), nurses (to provide catheter care and patient education), and dietitians (to facilitate the transition to enteral feeding and support long-term dietary planning) [25].

16.5 Unmet Needs and Future Directions

Short bowel syndrome and IF are rare conditions in the general population, requiring an individualized, multidisciplinary approach with high costs to the health system. Ideally, any patient with IF should be referred to a specialized center with expertise in nutritional, medical, and surgical management to maximize the chances of long-term PN discontinuation, avoid HPN failure, and determine the optimal timing for intestinal transplantation. Despite the availability of a multidisciplinary approach, disparities in care persist [26]. Additionally, although numerous published guidelines exist for the diagnosis and management of SBS–IF, the treatment algorithms and care pathways are often inadequately defined, even within specialized SBS–IF clinics [27].

From the multidisciplinary team to the existence of dedicated national programs, from access to innovative medical therapies to intestinal transplant centers, specialized medical resources are limited. Professional societies have developed a series of management guidelines and recommendations; however, their implementation is suboptimal, particularly in low- and middle-income countries. Consequently, individuals with SBS–IF frequently experience inadequate access to financial, medical, and psychosocial support throughout their journey [28].

Recent advancements in surgical and medical therapies have been implemented to expand treatment options for SBS. The uses of Teduglutide, regenerative therapies including TESI (tissue-engineered small intestine) and SIC (small intestinalized colon), and xenotransplantation are under investigation as potential treatments for patients with SBS. However, each approach presents distinct challenges that require resolution. Currently, no definitive treatment for SBS has been established; however, ongoing research in this area is expected to facilitate the development of innovative therapies and enhance patient prognosis [1]. Until then, enteral and parenteral nutrition remain the cornerstone of SBS treatment.

References

1. Endo, et al. Clinical challenges of short bowel syndrome and the path forward for organoid-based regenerative medicine. Regen Ther. 2023;24:64–73.
2. O'Keefe SJ, et al. Short bowel syndrome and intestinal failure: consensus definitions and overview. Clin Gastroenterol Hepatol. 2006;4(1):6–10.
3. Cuerda C, et al. ESPEN practical guideline: clinical nutrition in chronic intestinal failure. Clin Nutr. 2021;40(9):5196–220.
4. Pironi L. Definitions of intestinal failure and the short bowel syndrome. Best Pract Res Clin Gastroenterol. 2016;30(2):173–85.
5. Tulsky JA, et al. A research agenda for communication between health care professionals and patients living with serious illness. JAMA Intern Med. 2017;177(9):1361–6.
6. Nightingale JMD. The short bowel. In: Nightingale JMD, editor. Intestinal failure. London: Greenwich Medical Media; 2001. p. 177–98.
7. Buchman AL. Teduglutide and short bowel syndrome: every night without parenteral fluids is a good night. Gastroenterology. 2012;143(6):1416–20.
8. Brandt CF, et al. Home parenteral nutrition in adult patients with chronic intestinal failure: the evolution over 4 decades in a tertiary referral center. JPEN J Parenter Enteral Nutr. 2017;41(7):1178–87.
9. Sundaram A, et al. Nutritional management of short bowel syndrome in adults. J Clin Gastroenterol. 2002;34:207–20.
10. American Gastroenterological Association. American Gastroenterological Association medical position statement: short bowel syndrome and intestinal transplantation. Gastroenterology. 2003;124(4):1105–10.
11. Boland E, et al. A 25-year experience with postresection short-bowel syndrome secondary to radiation therapy. Am J Surg. 2010;200(6):690–3.
12. Hofstetter S, et al. Key issues in addressing the clinical and humanistic burden of short bowel syndrome in the US. Curr Med Res Opin. 2013;29(5):495–504.
13. Lakkasani S, et al. Concise review on short bowel syndrome: etiology, pathophysiology, and management. World J Clin Cases. 2022;10(31):11273–82.
14. Joly F, et al. Tube feeding improves intestinal absorption in short bowel syndrome patients. Gastroenterology. 2009;136(3):824–31.
15. Matarese LE. Nutrition and fluid optimization for patients with short bowel syndrome. J Parenter Enter Nutr. 2013;37(2):161–70.

16. Iyer K, et al. AGA clinical practice update on management of short bowel syndrome: expert review. Clin Gastroenterol Hepatol. 2022;20(10):2185–94.
17. Pironi L, et al. ESPEN practical guideline: home parenteral nutrition. Clin Nutr. 2023;42(3):411–30.
18. Nightingale J, Woodward JM. Small Bowel and Nutrition Committee of the British Society of Gastroenterology. Guidelines for management of patients with a short bowel. Gut. 2006;55 Suppl 4(Suppl 4)
19. Pironi L, et al. ESPEN guidelines on chronic intestinal failure in adults. Clin Nutr. 2017;36(2):619.
20. Massironi S, et al. Understanding short bowel syndrome: current status and future perspectives. Dig Liver Dis. 2020;52(3):253–61.
21. Deutsch L, et al. Advances in chronic intestinal failure management and therapies. Curr Opin Gastroenterol. 2020;36(3):223–9.
22. Lal S, et al. Clinical approach to the management of intestinal failure associated liver disease (IFALD) in adults: a position paper from the Home Artificial Nutrition and Chronic Intestinal Failure Special Interest Group of ESPEN. Clin Nutr. 2018;37:1794–7.
23. Bering J, DiBaise JK. Home parenteral and enteral nutrition. Nutrients. 2022;14(13):2558.
24. Parrish CR, DiBaise JK. Managing the adult patient with short bowel syndrome. Gastroenterol Hepatol (NY). 2017;13(10):600–8.
25. Matarese LE, et al. Short bowel syndrome: clinical guidelines for nutrition management. Nutr Clin Pract. 2005;20(5):493–502.
26. Misiakos EP, et al. Short bowel syndrome: current medical and surgical trends. J Clin Gastroenterol. 2007;41(1):5–18.
27. Matarese LE, et al. Short bowel syndrome in adults: the need for an interdisciplinary approach and coordinated care. JPEN J Parenter Enteral Nutr. 2014;38(1 Suppl):60S–4S.
28. Solar H, et al. Current status of chronic intestinal failure management in adults. Nutrients. 2024;16(16):2648.

17 Drug Pharmacokinetics and Pharmacodynamics in Short Bowel Syndrome: Special Considerations

Liliana Mirea, Cristian Cobilinschi, and Ioana Marina Grintescu

17.1 Introduction

Pharmacokinetics is traditionally referred to as the study of what the body does to a drug. A more scientific definition of pharmacokinetics states that it is the study of the absorption, distribution, metabolism, and, finally, excretion of drugs and their metabolites regardless of the method of administration [1]. These basic pharmacokinetic processes can be characterized using physiological principles as well as mathematical models, in order to calculate the concentration of the drug at the site of its effect [2]. Different pharmacokinetic models are developed to better predict drug effects based on varying concentrations [1]. The optimal concentration of a drug at its site of effect may be influenced by alterations in pharmacokinetic processes, such as decreased absorption, metabolic variability, liver or kidney failure, as well as interactions with co-administered drugs [3].

Pharmacodynamics describes the effects of different drugs on the body and examines the interactions of different molecules with various biological targets. Pharmacodynamic studies focus on mechanism of action, drug responses based on interactions at the target receptor site, and drug responses in relation to plasma concentrations [4].

However, pharmacokinetics and pharmacodynamics of a drug should not be considered as separate phenomena, as the latest clinical pharmacological approaches propose an integration of both pharmacokinetics and pharmacodynamics with physiological data of patients [5]. Pharmacokinetic–pharmacodynamic integration or

L. Mirea · C. Cobilinschi (✉) · I. M. Grintescu
Department of Anesthesiology and Intensive Care II, Carol Davila University of Medicine and Pharmacy, Bucharest, Romania

Department of Anesthesiology and Intensive Care I, Clinical Emergency Hospital of Bucharest, Bucharest, Romania
e-mail: cristian.cobilinschi@umfcd.ro; ioana.grintescu@rospen.ro

A. Trifan et al. (eds.), *Short Bowel Syndrome in Adults*,
https://doi.org/10.1007/978-3-031-95848-9_17

quantitative pharmacology emphasizes the importance of concentration–response and response–time relationships over the simplified approach, based solely on peak plasma drug concentration [6]. One of the key principles of this approach includes differentiating between the rate and extent of absorption, as an independent factor influencing the effect of an orally administered drug, as well as dose regimens and modes of administration [6].

In patients with short bowel syndrome resulting from extensive intestinal resection, various disturbances in the normally expected pharmacokinetics and pharmacodynamics are anticipated. However, factors such as the time elapsed since the resection, current nutritional status, remaining bowel segments, hydration status, and liver and kidney function should be considered to optimize the pharmacological profile in these patients.

In the following sections, we discuss the impact of anatomical and pathophysiological changes that occur in patients with short bowel syndrome and their significant effects on pharmacological processes.

17.2 Pharmacokinetic Considerations in Patients with Short Bowel Syndrome

Absorption represents the process through which a drug reaches the systemic circulation after oral administration. This sequence involves a more complex mechanism than the mere presence of the drug in the gastrointestinal tract and is influenced by the absorption surface, local motility, and pH, as well as by the chemical properties of the drug [7]. The extent of absorbed drugs is determined by the product of bioavailability and the drug dose. The mathematical model of the absorption rate in the case of oral administration of drugs is best described by a first-order absorption rate. This model suggests that the absorption rate is linear and proportional to the remaining amount of drug to be absorbed [8].

Normally, the small intestine and duodenum are the main sites responsible for the absorption of most drugs, a process that is also influenced by the rate at which these drugs are transported from the stomach to this area [9]. Since absorption capacity is proportional to surface area, which is increased by the presence of intestinal villi, it decreases in the latter part of the gastrointestinal tract where the surface area is reduced [10].

Since drug absorption occurs mainly in the duodenum and the initial part of the jejunum, gastrointestinal transit time—determined by the alternation between the migrating myoelectric complex (fasted state) and digestive motility patterns (fed state)—is an important factor influencing drug absorption [11].

Drug absorption and bioavailability are also influenced by the pH of the gastrointestinal lumen. The pH of the solution influences the ratio of ionized to unionized drug fractions, depending on the drug's acid-base dissociation constant (pKa). This process is crucial for drug absorption, as only the unionized form can penetrate physiological membranes [12]. An elevated gastric pH reduces the absorption of weakly basic drugs, which require low pH for dissolution and absorption [13].

Bile salts, alone or in combination with lecithin, may play a significant role in drug absorption. Depending on the drug formulation (solid, solution, or cyclodextrin complex), bile salts can enhance absorption and increase bioavailability by preventing precipitation, facilitating solubilization, or displacing drug molecules from cyclodextrin complexes [14].

Patients with short bowel syndrome due to extensive intestinal resections exhibit alterations in all the previously described physiological mechanisms involved in normal drug absorption. Although the latest European Society of Clinical Nutrition and Metabolism (ESPEN) classification does not reference the degree of malabsorption associated with short bowel syndrome, it should be assessed individually, as it depends not only on the extent of resection but also on the anatomy of the remnant intestine and mucosal integrity [15].

As expected, a decrease in surface area impairs optimal drug absorption, with patients who have undergone extensive intestinal resection being the most affected—particularly those with short bowel syndrome type I and a jejunostomy [16].

For this reason, drugs with decreased bioavailability should be avoided in patients with short bowel syndrome and replaced with other routes of administration. Examples include bisphosphonates, pyridostigmine, levothyroxine, and cyclosporine [17, 18].

The extensive use of proton pump inhibitors and H2-receptor antagonists, commonly prescribed in patients with short bowel syndrome to reduce gastrointestinal fluid losses, may further interfere with drug absorption due to their impact on luminal pH [19]. Previous reports indicate that gastric pH may increase from 1.9 to 4.5–5 after just 5 days of omeprazole administration [20].

Boutte et al. indicated that patients with short bowel syndrome may experience increased bile acid loss, reduced enterohepatic recirculation, and a compensatory increase in hepatic bile acid synthesis [21]. All these disturbances further contribute to abnormal intestinal drug absorption.

Taking into account all these expected changes in drug absorption in patients with short bowel syndrome, drug prescriptions should always be made cautiously. The Biopharmaceutical Classification System (BCS) may be useful in selecting the most appropriate medical treatment for these patients. For example, drugs from BCS Class IV—low solubility, low permeability—such as cyclosporine, ritonavir, hydrochlorothiazide, or furosemide, should be avoided in patients with short bowel syndrome, and alternative formulations or administration routes should be considered. Nevertheless, considering the altered bile acid metabolism in patients with short bowel syndrome, drugs from BCS Class II—such as amiodarone, atorvastatin, digoxin, diclofenac, carbamazepine, and macrolides—which have low solubility and high permeability, should be replaced, especially in patients with type I short bowel syndrome [13, 22].

Very few studies have evaluated drug absorption in patients with short bowel syndrome, despite their similar pharmacological needs to other patients.

Notably, patients with short bowel syndrome often require antibiotic therapy due to catheter-related bloodstream infections (CRBSIs), which are considered the most frequent cause of hospital admission for patients with intestinal failure (IF) [23].

One of the currently established quality indicators for appropriate antimicrobial use is the early switch from intravenous to oral therapy. Therefore, pharmacological data on antimicrobial absorption are urgently needed for patients with short bowel syndrome [24].

In a study evaluating the bioavailability of different antibiotics and antifungals in short bowel syndrome patients, Korzilius et al. reported that oral clindamycin and fluconazole had a bioavailability similar to that found in healthy subjects. However, ciprofloxacin and flucloxacillin registered decreased absorption [25].

Patients with short bowel syndrome often experience psychiatric disturbances as well as reduced quality of life, making the prescription of antidepressants necessary. Faye et al. reported that expected concentration-to-dose ratios for escitalopram and citalopram were observed only in patients with at least 180 cm of remaining small bowel or those with a minimum of 80 cm of small bowel and at least 50% of their colon intact [26].

Anticoagulation and antiplatelet therapy are commonly prescribed for patients with short bowel syndrome, either due to associated cardiac conditions (such as atrial fibrillation, ischemic heart disease, or mechanical heart valves) or because bowel ischemia with superior mesenteric artery thrombosis is one of the most frequent causes of short bowel syndrome. Additionally, catheter-associated thrombosis may also necessitate prolonged anticoagulation therapy [23, 27]. In a recent systematic literature review, Mercer et al. suggested that warfarin is effective in achieving anticoagulation therapy in patients with a short bowel of less than 12 cm, with the advantage of easy monitoring through the measurement of the international normalized ratio (INR) [28]. When considering the use of direct oral anticoagulant agents (DOACs), rivaroxaban has the most available data supporting its efficacy and may be effective even in patients with a small bowel of at least 30 cm [28]. As patients with short bowel syndrome usually receive high doses of proton pump inhibitors, it was reported that rivaroxaban pharmacokinetics is not influenced by this concomitant prescription [29].

Acetylsalicylic acid absorption was evaluated in a study conducted by Faye et al., which indicated that its absorption may be effective in patients with at least 30 cm of remaining small intestine. However, the assessment technique used for platelet aggregation is not widely available in all hospitals [30]. Clopidogrel's interindividual pharmacokinetic variations make it unsuitable as an antiplatelet agent in patients with short bowel syndrome. On the other hand, ticagrelor has been reported to have rapid absorption and a safer pharmacological profile [31].

It is worth mentioning that most of the available data on orally administered drugs in patients with short bowel syndrome come from small studies, case series, and case reports, highlighting the need for more extensive research in this field. Nevertheless, the impact of increased use of glucagon-like peptide-2 analogs on drug absorption should also be investigated, alongside their effects on reducing the need for parenteral nutrition [32].

The British Intestinal Failure Alliance (BIFA), as part of the British Association for Parenteral and Enteral Nutrition (BAPEN), suggests that some drugs should be administered at higher doses than usually recommended to obtain the desired effects. However, some adverse effects should be expected in these conditions.

Patients with short bowel syndrome who have sufficient remaining colon (jejuno-ileo-colic—short bowel type 3) may soon benefit from colonic drug delivery techniques, which have recently advanced due to a better understanding of colonic physiology and promising in vitro and in vivo results [33, 34].

In this regard, given the increasing use of therapeutic drug monitoring techniques in patients with inflammatory bowel disease, it should be considered that, in the absence of solid pharmacological evidence, this type of monitoring should also be considered for patients with extensive bowel resections.

17.3 Pharmacodynamic Considerations in Patients with Short Bowel Syndrome

Patients with short bowel syndrome may not exhibit specific pharmacodynamic disturbances directly related to the disease; however, the pharmacodynamic profile of drugs may be indirectly influenced by alterations in pharmacokinetics, mainly related to the absorption process [4]. Keller et al. better describe this relationship, with pharmacokinetics being the cause (determining *drug concentration* in the compartments) and pharmacodynamics representing the effect (*the drug response*) [4].

Except during the acute phase, patients with short bowel syndrome who have achieved metabolic stability usually maintain a normal hydration status, meaning the volume of distribution for drugs is not affected. This is reflected in reported data on body composition in patients with short bowel syndrome, which shows that these patients appear thinner with decreased muscle mass, but without sarcopenia and with normal muscle function [35]. Chiplunker et al. indicated that patients with short bowel syndrome who are on long-term parenteral nutrition may develop an increased percentage of body fat compared to healthy individuals. However, it was also stated that adipose tissue is an anhydrous tissue, with no significant effects on the volume of distribution [36].

Even if patients with short bowel syndrome have an increased risk for developing Intestinal Failure-Associated Liver Disease, hepatic drug metabolism is impaired only in very late stages of the disease [37].

17.4 Conclusions

Considering the pathophysiological changes that occur secondary to the loss of extensive intestinal segments, namely decreased nutrient absorption, it is easy to appreciate that drug absorption is also affected, despite the paucity of data regarding drug pharmacokinetics in these patients. Even though there are some recommendations available, primarily based on best practices, it remains unclear how different medications should be prescribed to patients with short bowel syndrome.

To ensure the highest standard of medication safety, therapeutic drug monitoring should be available at every center dedicated to patients with short bowel syndrome. Alternatively, when possible, other formulations (such as intravenous or cutaneous) should be recommended.

References

1. Byers JP, Sarver JG. Chapter 10—Pharmacokinetic modeling. In: Hacker M, Messer W, Bachmann K, editors. Pharmacology. San Diego: Academic Press; 2009. p. 201–77.
2. Atkinson AJ. Chapter 1—Introduction to clinical pharmacology. In: Atkinson AJ, Abernethy DR, Daniels CE, Dedrick RL, Markey SP, editors. Principles of clinical pharmacology. 2nd ed. Burlington: Academic Press; 2007. p. 1–7.
3. Flood P, Rathmell JP, Urman RD. Stoelting's pharmacology & physiology in anesthetic practice, 6e. Lippincott Williams & Wilkins, a Wolters Kluwer Business; 2022. p. 12–47.
4. Keller F, Hann A. Clinical pharmacodynamics: principles of drug response and alterations in kidney disease. Clin J Am Soc Nephrol. 2018;13(9):1413–20.
5. Kumar N, Kanchan T, Unnikrishnan B, Thapar R, Mithra P, Kulkarni V, et al. Applying quantitative and systems pharmacology to drug development and beyond: an introduction to clinical pharmacologists. Indian J Pharmacol. 2018;49(5):344–7.
6. Gabrielsson J, Green AR, Van der Graaf PH. Optimising in vivo pharmacology studies-practical PKPD considerations. J Pharmacol Toxicol Methods. 2010;61(2):146–56.
7. Loftsson T. Chapter 3—Physicochemical properties and pharmacokinetics. In: Loftsson T, editor. Essential pharmacokinetics. Boston: Academic Press; 2015. p. 85–104. https://www.sciencedirect.com/science/article/pii/B9780128014110000032.
8. Rajpoot K, Tekade RK, Sharma MC, Tekade M. Chapter 2—Pharmacokinetics and biopharmaceutics: "a leader or attendant". In: Tekade RK, editor. Biopharmaceutics and pharmacokinetics considerations, Advances in Pharmaceutical Product Development and Research, vol. 1. Academic Press; 2021. p. 17–27. https://www.sciencedirect.com/science/article/pii/B9780128144251000206.
9. Severijnen R, Bayat N, Bakker H, Tolboom J, Bongaerts G. Enteral drug absorption in patients with short small bowel: a review. Clin Pharmacokinet. 2004;43(14):951–62.
10. Sardou HS, Abbaspour M, Akhgari A, Kesharwani P, Sahebkar A. Colon-targeted delivery systems of budesonide as second-line therapy in inflammatory bowel disease. J Drug Deliv Sci Technol. 2024;93
11. Deloose E, Janssen P, Depoortere I, Tack J. The migrating motor complex: control mechanisms and its role in health and disease. Nat Rev Gastroenterol Hepatol. 2012;9(5):271–85. https://doi.org/10.1038/nrgastro.2012.57.
12. Gaohua L, Miao X, Dou L. Crosstalk of physiological pH and chemical pKa under the umbrella of physiologically based pharmacokinetic modeling of drug absorption, distribution, metabolism, excretion, and toxicity. Expert Opin Drug Metab Toxicol. 2021;17(9):1103–24. https://doi.org/10.1080/17425255.2021.1951223.
13. Abuhelwa AY, Williams DB, Upton RN, Foster DJR. Food, gastrointestinal pH, and models of oral drug absorption. Eur J Pharm Biopharm. 2017;112:234–48. https://doi.org/10.1016/j.ejpb.2016.11.034.
14. Holm R, Müllertz A, Mu H. Bile salts and their importance for drug absorption. Int J Pharm. 2013;453(1):44–55. https://doi.org/10.1016/j.ijpharm.2013.04.003.
15. Billiauws L, Corcos O, Joly F. What's new in short bowel syndrome? Curr Opin Clin Nutr Metab Care. 2018;21(4):313–8.
16. Tappenden KA. Anatomical and physiological considerations in short bowel syndrome: emphasis on intestinal adaptation and the role of enterohormones. Nutr Clin Pract. 2023;38(S1):S27–34.
17. Ward N. The impact of intestinal failure on oral drug absorption: a review. J Gastrointest Surg. 2010;14(6):1045–51.
18. Patel R, Barker J, Elshaer A. Pharmaceutical excipients and drug metabolism: a mini-review. Int J Mol Sci. 2020;21(21):1–21.
19. Massironi S, Cavalcoli F, Rausa E, Invernizzi P, Braga M, Vecchi M. Understanding short bowel syndrome: current status and future perspectives. Dig Liver Dis. 2020;52(3):253–61. https://doi.org/10.1016/j.dld.2019.11.013.

20. Prichard PJ, Yeomans ND, Mihaly GW, Jones DB, Buckle PJ, Smallwood RA, et al. Omeprazole: a study of its inhibition of gastric pH and oral pharmacokinetics after morning or evening dosage. Gastroenterology. 1985;88(1 Pt 1):64–9.
21. Boutte HJ, Chen J, Wylie TN, Wylie KM, Xie Y, Geisman M, et al. Fecal microbiome and bile acid metabolome in adult short bowel syndrome. Am J Physiol Gastrointest Liver Physiol. 2022;322(1):G154–68.
22. Samineni R, Chimakurthy J, Konidala S. Emerging role of biopharmaceutical classification and biopharmaceutical drug disposition system in dosage form development: a systematic review. Turkish J Pharm Sci. 2022;19(6):706–13.
23. Jahns F, Hausen A, Keller P, Stolz V, Kalff JC, Kuetting D, et al. Life on the line—incidence and management of central venous catheter complications in intestinal failure. Clin Nutr. 2024;43(6):1627–34.
24. Kallen MC, Prins JM. A systematic review of quality indicators for appropriate antibiotic use in hospitalized adult patients. Infect Dis Rep. 2017;9(1). https://www.mdpi.com/2036-7449/9/1/6821.
25. Korzilius JW, Gompelman M, Wezendonk GTJ, Jager NGL, Rovers CP, Brüggemann RJM, et al. Oral antimicrobial agents in patients with short bowel syndrome: worth a try! J Antimicrob Chemother. 2023;78(8):2008–14. https://doi.org/10.1093/jac/dkad198.
26. Faye E, Corcos O, Lancelin F, Declèves X, Bergmann JF, Joly F, et al. Antidepressant agents in short bowel syndrome. Clin Ther. 2014;36(12):2029–33.e3.
27. Woods A, Lal S. Intestinal failure and short bowel syndrome. Med (United Kingdom). 2024;52(3):181–5. https://doi.org/10.1016/j.mpmed.2023.12.004.
28. Mercer C, Crawford A, Shapiro S, Allan PJ, Ambrose T. Anticoagulation and antiplatelet therapy in short bowel syndrome: a systematic review. Intest Fail. 2024;1:100007. https://doi.org/10.1016/j.intf.2024.100007.
29. Moore KT, Plotnikov AN, Thyssen A, Vaccaro N, Ariyawansa J, Burton PB. Effect of multiple doses of omeprazole on the pharmacokinetics, pharmacodynamics, and safety of a single dose of rivaroxaban. J Cardiovasc Pharmacol. 2011;58(6):581–8.
30. Faye E, Drouet L, De Raucourt E, Green A, Bal-dit-Sollier C, Boudaoud L, et al. Absorption and efficacy of acetylsalicylic acid in patients with short bowel syndrome. Ann Pharmacother. 2014;48(6):705–10.
31. Droppa M, Karathanos A, Gawaz M, Geisler T. Individualised dual antiplatelet therapy in a patient with short bowel syndrome after acute myocardial infarction with coronary artery stenting. BMJ Case Rep. 2015;2015:10–3.
32. Vande Casteele N, Herfarth H, Katz J, Falck-Ytter Y, Singh S. American Gastroenterological Association Institute technical review on the role of therapeutic drug monitoring in the management of inflammatory bowel diseases. Gastroenterology. 2017;153(3):835–57.e6. https://doi.org/10.1053/j.gastro.2017.07.031.
33. McCoubrey LE, Favaron A, Awad A, Orlu M, Gaisford S, Basit AW. Colonic drug delivery: formulating the next generation of colon-targeted therapeutics. J Control Release. 2023;353:1107–26. https://doi.org/10.1016/j.jconrel.2022.12.029.
34. Iyer K, DiBaise J, Rubio-Tapia A. AGA clinical practice update on management of short bowel syndrome: expert review. Clin Gastroenterol Hepatol. 2022;20:2185–94.
35. Bannert K, Karbe C, Förster RH, Sautter LF, Meyer F, Valentini L, et al. Orally compensated short bowel patients are thin, potentially malnourished but rarely sarcopenic. Clin Nutr. 2023;42(8):1480–90.
36. Chiplunker AJ, Chen L, Levin MS, Warner BW, Davidson NO, Rubin DC. Increased adiposity and reduced lean body mass in patients with short bowel syndrome. Dig Dis Sci. 2020;65(11):3271–9.
37. Lal S, Pironi L, Wanten G, Arends J, Bozzetti F, Cuerda C, et al. Clinical approach to the management of intestinal failure associated liver disease (IFALD) in adults: a position paper from the Home Artificial Nutrition and Chronic Intestinal Failure Special Interest Group of ESPEN. Clin Nutr. 2018;37(6):1794–7.

18 Management of Short Bowel Syndrome: Antisecretory, Antimotility, and Luminally Active Agents

Liana Gheorghe and Razvan Cerban

18.1 Introduction

Short bowel syndrome (SBS) is a complex, often debilitating condition that occurs following significant surgical resection of the small intestine or severe bowel disease. The limited bowel length in SBS patients leads to compromised digestion, malabsorption, and often severe diarrhea, fluid, and electrolyte imbalances [1]. Management of SBS focuses on maximizing nutrient absorption, stabilizing fluid-electrolyte balance, and improving the quality of life [2]. While parenteral nutrition (PN) and enteral feeding are commonly utilized, pharmacological interventions play a crucial role in enhancing the remaining intestinal function and minimizing fluid loss [3]. This chapter provides an overview of these agents, their mechanisms of action, clinical application, and relevant evidence supporting their use in treating SBS patients.

Pharmacologic therapy in SBS targets three main goals:

- Reducing intestinal secretion to minimize fluid loss (antisecretory agents)
- Slowing intestinal motility to enhance nutrient and fluid absorption (antimotility agents)
- Improving nutrient absorption or modifying luminal content to improve absorption (luminally active agents)

L. Gheorghe · R. Cerban (✉)
Carol Davila University of Medicine and Pharmacy, Bucharest, Romania

Center for Digestive Diseases and Liver Transplant, Fundeni Clinical Institute, Bucharest, Romania

A. Trifan et al. (eds.), *Short Bowel Syndrome in Adults*, https://doi.org/10.1007/978-3-031-95848-9_18

18.2 Antisecretory Agents

After extensive intestinal resection, gastric secretions are usually increased for the first 6–12 months after surgery. While the exact mechanism remains unclear, some researchers suggest that it may be caused by the loss of feedback mechanisms from the resected bowel segments [3].

Gastric hypersecretion is usually temporary and tends to resolve within weeks to months following resection [2]. In addition, gastric hypersecretion can cause the release of acidic content into the proximal small bowel, which will lead to altered lipid digestion due to diminished pancreatic enzyme activity and alteration of bile acids. Treating gastric hypersecretion, besides reducing the volume of secretions, can also help restore the normal intestinal pH to optimize bile salt and pancreatic enzyme activity.

18.2.1 Proton Pump Inhibitors (PPIs) and H2-Receptor Antagonists (H2RAs)

The main drugs used for gastric hypersecretion are proton pump inhibitors (PPIs) and H2-receptor antagonists (H2RAs), with PPIs having a more potent effect on acid inhibition. PPIs irreversibly inhibit the H^+/K^+ ATPase in gastric parietal cells, resulting in sustained suppression of gastric acid production. H2RAs, in contrast, block histamine receptors in gastric parietal cells, thereby reducing acid production through competitive inhibition. Studies have shown that PPIs and H2RAs can reduce gastric hypersecretion and improve clinical outcomes in SBS patients, particularly during the first 6 months following surgery [4]. In addition, patients with ileal resection, which frequently leads to loss of feedback inhibition, can also have an important benefit [5, 6]. A significant effect heterogeneity of PPIs was reported. Patients with SBS passing large amounts of wet fecal excretions (more than 2 kg/day) had better treatment results. The degree of PPIs absorption in SBS patients is difficult to estimate, so intravenous administration should always be considered in case of lack of effect of oral medication. However, despite their good tolerability, PPIs are linked to an increased risk of community-acquired pneumonia, osteoporosis, and vitamin B12 deficiency [7, 8].

18.2.2 Somatostatin Analogs

Somatostatin analogs, such as octreotide, are synthetic versions of the naturally occurring hormone somatostatin, which inhibits various gastrointestinal (GI) secretions, including gastric, pancreatic, and biliary fluids [9]. Octreotide is effective at reducing gastrointestinal secretions and can help prolong intestinal transit time. Its effectiveness is often limited by development of tachyphylaxis over time. By binding to somatostatin receptors, octreotide can reduce gastrointestinal motility and fluid secretion, which leads to a decrease in fecal output and fluid losses in patients with SBS [10].

Several studies have demonstrated that octreotide significantly reduces intestinal fluid losses in patients with SBS, although its use may be limited by side effects, such as gallstone formation and glucose and fat malabsorption [10, 11]. Additionally, somatostatin reduces splanchnic blood flow and may interfere with the use of amino acids for splanchnic protein synthesis, potentially hindering the physiological adaptation process following intestinal resection [12]. Octreotide can be given as a 72-h trial, at the dose of 300 μg/day, and if clinically effective, it can be switched to a longer-acting formulation. If there is no significant response, there is no point in continuing this drug, with as few as 5% of patients having a prolonged benefit [13]. Some patients experienced significant fluid retention associated with octreotide treatment [12].

Consequently, it is recommended to objectively monitor the effects and adjust parenteral support as needed.

18.3 Antimotility Agents

Antimotility agents reduce intestinal motility, allowing for longer contact time between nutrients and the absorptive mucosa, which enhances nutrient and water absorption in SBS patients.

18.3.1 Opioid Agonists

To decrease intestinal motility, patients should receive loperamide or diphenoxylate in conjunction with atropine as a first-line medication. Loperamide and diphenoxylate are commonly used opioid agonists in the management of SBS. These agents bind to opioid receptors in the gut, slowing intestinal motility and transit time. Loperamide and diphenoxylate act as agonists at μ-opioid receptors in the intestinal smooth muscle. This reduces peristalsis and increases the time for fluid and nutrient absorption, subsequently decreasing stool volume. Research has shown that both loperamide and diphenoxylate can effectively reduce stool output in SBS patients, especially when taken consistently before meals. In one study, patients experienced up to a 40% reduction in stool output with loperamide use [14]. Diphenoxylate is often used in conjunction with atropine to further slow transit, though side effects such as constipation may limit its use. Loperamide, typically administered at 4 mg three to four times per day, is commonly recommended. However, due to its enterohepatic circulation, higher doses of 12–24 mg at a time may be necessary for patients with terminal ileum resection. The optimal timing, dosage, and tolerability of these medications vary greatly between individuals. They are often used in combination and may be given 30–60 min before meals and at bedtime, although scientific evidence supporting this practice is limited [8].

18.3.2 Codeine and Other Narcotics

Although less commonly used due to their potential for dependency, codeine and other narcotics are occasionally considered as second-line medication in SBS management. Codeine, like loperamide, binds to μ-opioid receptors in the gut, decreasing motility and prolonging transit time.

However, because it is systemically absorbed, codeine can lead to central nervous system side effects and has a higher potential for abuse [15]. Codeine is often considered only when other antimotility agents fail, but studies have shown that it can be effective in reducing stool frequency and volume in severe cases [16, 17]. In some centers, a mixture of codeine phosphate (8 mg/mL) in doses ranging from 80 to 160 mg, or tincture of opium at 0.3–1.0 mL, is administered four times per day [12].

Loperamide and codeine can work synergistically when used together, enhancing their combined effect on slowing intestinal motility [18]. This synergy may provide greater relief from diarrhea and reduce stool output more effectively than either agent alone. However, careful monitoring is necessary to manage potential side effects and minimize the risk of dependency associated with codeine use [3].

18.3.3 Clonidine

Clonidine, available in a transdermal form, has shown some benefit in patients with high-output stool losses. Clonidine can reduce intestinal fluid secretion by binding to alpha-adrenergic receptors on enteric neurons in addition to reducing gastric and colonic motility [19, 20]. Due to its antihypertensive effect, the use of clonidine is often restricted, as patients can develop low blood pressure and a high risk of orthostatic hypotension. While antimotility agents can effectively decrease intestinal transit and reduce stool outputs, their use in patients with a dilated bowel requires caution. In such cases, antimotility drugs may even worsen diarrhea by promoting bacterial overgrowth, as slowed transit provides an ideal environment for bacterial proliferation. In order to avoid these circumstances, close monitoring and a tailored approach for each patient are essential.

18.4 Luminally Active Agents

Luminally active agents act directly in the intestinal lumen to enhance absorption, promote mucosal growth, or inhibit the breakdown of nutrients, thus helping to compensate for the reduced absorptive surface area in SBS.

18.4.1 Bile Acid Sequestrants

Bile acid sequestrants, such as cholestyramine, bind bile acids in the intestine, preventing their osmotic effects and reducing diarrhea in patients with SBS, particularly those with ileal resections.

By binding bile acids, these agents prevent their reabsorption in the colon, where bile acids can induce diarrhea through their laxative effect [15]. This is particularly relevant in SBS patients who lack a functional ileum for bile acid reabsorption. Cholestyramine can be especially useful in patients with distal ileal resection. Pancreatic enzyme replacement should be given if appropriate.

The use of bile acid sequestrants may be limited in patients with extensive resection, as these drugs can worsen steatorrhea by reducing bile acid availability for micelle formation [21].

18.4.2 Short-Chain Fatty Acid (SCFA) Supplements

Short-chain fatty acids, produced through the fermentation of non-absorbable carbohydrates, play a role in enhancing water and electrolyte absorption in the colon. SCFA supplements or prebiotics that promote SCFA production have shown potential benefits for SBS patients. SCFAs stimulate colonic absorption of sodium and water, compensating for fluid losses in the upper gastrointestinal tract. In patients with residual colon, SCFA supplements may promote mucosal adaptation and nutrient absorption. Studies on SCFAs in SBS have indicated that they can improve fluid and electrolyte balance, particularly in patients with colon-in-continuity [22, 23].

18.4.3 Oral Rehydration Solutions

Patients with SBS lacking a colon can often lose more water and sodium through their stoma than they consume orally [24]. This is particularly common in individuals with less than 100 cm of residual jejunum, where daily jejunostomy output can exceed 4 L. To maintain adequate hydration, fluids should be provided to match losses, ensuring a urine output of at least 1 L/day. In the intestinal lumen, glucose increases sodium and water absorption, using the sodium-glucose-coupled transport system [25]. Particularly in patients with high-output jejunostomies, the use of inappropriate fluids, such as hypertonic beverages (fruit juices) or low-sodium, hypotonic solutions like water, tea, and coffee, can worsen fluid losses. A common misconception among patients is that drinking large quantities of water aids hydration; however, this typically increases ostomy output, perpetuating fluid and electrolyte imbalances. Instead, glucose-electrolyte oral rehydration solutions (ORS) are preferred, as they enhance absorption and reduce secretion. ORS is particularly important in SBS patients with a high risk of dehydration. Formulas are specifically tailored to maximize sodium and water absorption and reduce losses. The ideal sodium concentration of any ORS should be between 90 and 120 mEq Na^+/L (with a carbohydrate-to-sodium ratio of 1:1) [26]. ORS has proven effective in reducing the need for parenteral hydration and is recommended as a standard intervention for managing dehydration in SBS patients [25, 27].

Most patients with SBS who still have a colon can typically stay well-hydrated by drinking hypotonic fluids. For those needing additional support, commercially prepared ORS are readily available, and there are also simple recipes for making affordable, homemade versions. Regardless of how patients hydrate themselves, it is crucial for clinicians to identify those who require parenteral fluid support based on factors such as urine output, hypotension, or the presence of acute kidney injury (Table 18.1).

Table 18.1 Comparison of pharmacologic agents for SBS management

Category	Drug class	Examples	Mechanism of action	Benefits	Potential adverse effects
Antisecretory Agents	Proton Pump Inhibitors (PPIs)	Omeprazole, Pantoprazole	Inhibit the H^+/K^+ ATPase in gastric parietal cells, reducing acid secretion	Decreases gastric hypersecretion, improves nutrient absorption	Increased risk of infections (e.g., pneumonia), osteoporosis, vitamin B12 deficiency
	H2-Receptor Antagonists (H2RAs)	Ranitidine (withdrawn), Famotidine	Block histamine receptors in parietal cells, reducing acid secretion	Alternative to PPIs, short-term relief	Less effective than PPIs, tolerance may develop over time
	Somatostatin Analogs	Octreotide	Inhibits release of GI hormones and secretions	Reduces diarrhea, decreases fluid loss	Risk of gallstones, glucose metabolism disturbances, fat malabsorption

(continued)

Table 18.1 (continued)

Category	Drug class	Examples	Mechanism of action	Benefits	Potential adverse effects
Antimotility Agents	Opioid Agonists	Loperamide, Diphenoxylate	Bind to μ-opioid receptors in intestinal smooth muscle, slowing motility	Reduces stool output, prolongs transit time	Constipation, potential bacterial overgrowth
	Codeine & Other Narcotics	Codeine, Opium tincture	Slows intestinal transit via central and peripheral opioid receptor activation	Effective in severe diarrhea cases	CNS depression, dependency risk, constipation
	Clonidine	Transdermal Clonidine	Modulates sympathetic outflow, reducing motility & secretion	Can reduce high-output stool losses	Hypotension, dry mouth, sedation
Luminally Active Agents	Bile Acid Sequestrants	Cholestyramine	Binds bile acids, preventing their diarrheogenic effect	Helps in bile acid-induced diarrhea, especially in ileal resection cases	Can worsen steatorrhea, reduces absorption of fat-soluble vitamins
	Short-Chain Fatty Acid (SCFA) Supplements	Butyrate, Acetate, Propionate	Enhance water and sodium absorption in the colon	May improve hydration, supports colonic adaptation	Limited evidence, effectiveness depends on residual colon presence
	Oral Rehydration Solutions (ORS)	WHO ORS, Custom ORS formulas	Sodium-glucose co-transport promotes water absorption	Prevents dehydration, reduces need for parenteral support	Poor compliance due to taste, not effective in all patients

18.5 Conclusion

The management of SBS with antisecretory, antimotility, and luminally active agents aims to control symptoms, reduce fluid and electrolyte loss, and improve nutrient absorption. While antisecretory agents decrease GI secretions, antimotility agents help to prolong intestinal transit, and luminally active agents directly modify intestinal content to support absorption. These therapies can be used in combination to optimize patient outcomes, but individualized treatment plans are necessary due to varying responses and potential adverse effects. Future advancements in SBS management are anticipated with the ongoing development of agents that promote intestinal adaptation, thus further reducing dependence on PN.

References

1. Massironi S, Cavalcoli F, Rausa E, Invernizzi P, Braga M, Vecchi M, et al. Understanding short bowel syndrome: current status and future perspectives. Dig Liver Dis. 2020;52(3):253–61. https://doi.org/10.1016/j.dld.2019.11.013.
2. Thompson JS, Weswman RA, Rochling FA, Mercer DF. Current management of short bowel syndrome. Curr Probl Surg. 2012;49:52–115. https://doi.org/10.1067/j.cpsurg.2011.10.002.
3. Iyer K, DiBaise JK, Rubio-Tapia A. AGA clinical practice update on management of short bowel syndrome: expert review. Clin Gastroenterol Hepatol. 2022;20(10):2185–94.e2. https://doi.org/10.1016/j.cgh.2022.05.032.
4. Jeppesen PB, Staun M, Tjellesen L, Mortensen PB. Effect of intravenous ranitidine and omeprazole on intestinal absorption of water, sodium, and macronutrients in patients with intestinal resection. Gut. 1998;43(6):763–9. https://doi.org/10.1136/gut.43.6.763.
5. Nightingale J, Woodward JM, Small Bowel and Nutrition Committee of the British Society of Gastroenterology. Guidelines for management of patients with a short bowel. Gut. 2006;55 Suppl 4(Suppl 4):iv1–12. https://doi.org/10.1136/gut.2006.091108.
6. Matarese LE, Jeppesen PB, O'Keefe SJ. Short bowel syndrome in adults: the need for an interdisciplinary approach and coordinated care. JPEN J Parenter Enteral Nutr. 2014;38(1 Suppl):60S–4S. https://doi.org/10.1177/0148607113518946.
7. Thomson AB, Sauve MD, Kassam N, Kamitakahara H. Safety of the long-term use of proton pump inhibitors. World J Gastroenterol. 2010;16(19):2323–30. https://doi.org/10.3748/wjg.v16.i19.2323.
8. Kumpf VJ. Pharmacologic management of diarrhea in patients with short bowel syndrome. JPEN J Parenter Enteral Nutr. 2014;38(1 Suppl):38S–44S. https://doi.org/10.1177/0148607113520618.
9. Lembcke B, Creutzfeldt W, Schleser S, Ebert R, Shaw C, Koop I. Effect of the somatostatin analogue sandostatin (SMS 201–995) on gastrointestinal, pancreatic and biliary function and hormone release in normal men. Digestion. 1987;36(2):108–24. https://doi.org/10.1159/000199408.
10. Nehra V, Camilleri M, Burton D, Oenning L, Kelly DG. An open trial of octreotide long-acting release in the management of short bowel syndrome. Am J Gastroenterol. 2001;96(5):1494–8. https://doi.org/10.1111/j.1572-0241.2001.03803.x.
11. Pironi L, Cuerda C, Jeppesen PB, et al. ESPEN guideline on chronic intestinal failure in adults—update 2023. Clin Nutr. 2023;42(10):1940–2021. https://doi.org/10.1016/j.clnu.2023.07.019.
12. Bass BL, Fischer BA, Richardson C, Harmon JW. Somatostatin analogue treatment inhibits post-resectional adaptation of the small bowel in rats. Am J Surg. 1991;161(1):107–12. https://doi.org/10.1016/0002-9610(91)90369-o.

13. Forbes A. Intestinal failure and short bowel syndrome. Medicine (Baltimore). 2010;39(3):178–82. https://doi.org/10.1016/j.mpmed.2010.12.010.
14. Parekh NR, Steiger E. Short bowel syndrome. Curr Treat Options Gastroenterol. 2007;10(1):10–23. https://doi.org/10.1007/s11938-007-0052-9.
15. Chan L-N. Opioid analgesics and the gastrointestinal tract. Pract Gastroenterol. 2008;32:37–50.
16. Bering J, DiBaise JK. Short bowel syndrome in adults. Am J Gastroenterol. 2022;117(6):876–83. https://doi.org/10.14309/ajg.0000000000001763.
17. Pironi L, Raschi E, Sasdelli AS. The safety of available treatment options for short bowel syndrome and unmet needs. Expert Opin Drug Saf. 2021;20(12):1501–13. https://doi.org/10.1080/14740338.2021.1940947.
18. King RF, Norton T, Hill GL. A double-blind crossover study of the effect of loperamide hydrochloride and codeine phosphate on ileostomy output. Aust N Z J Surg. 1982;52(2):121–4. https://doi.org/10.1111/j.1445-2197.1982.tb06083.x.
19. Buchman AL, Fryer J, Wallin A, Ahn CW, Polensky S, Zaremba K. Clonidine reduces diarrhea and sodium loss in patients with proximal jejunostomy: a controlled study. JPEN J Parenter Enteral Nutr. 2006;30(6):487–91. https://doi.org/10.1177/0148607106030006487.
20. McDoniel K, Taylor B, Huey W, et al. Use of clonidine to decrease intestinal fluid losses in patients with high-output short-bowel syndrome. JPEN J Parenter Enteral Nutr. 2004;28(4):265–8. https://doi.org/10.1177/0148607104028004265.
21. Hirsch TI, Wang SZ, Fligor SC, et al. Fat malabsorption in short bowel syndrome: a review of pathophysiology and management. Nutr Clin Pract. 2024;39 Suppl 1(Suppl 1):S17–28. https://doi.org/10.1002/ncp.11119.
22. Ziegler TR, Evans ME, Fernández-Estívariz C, Jones DP. Trophic and cytoprotective nutrition for intestinal adaptation, mucosal repair, and barrier function. Annu Rev Nutr. 2003;23:229–61. https://doi.org/10.1146/annurev.nutr.23.011702.073036.
23. Pape UF, Maasberg S, Pascher A. Pharmacological strategies to enhance adaptation in intestinal failure. Curr Opin Organ Transplant. 2016;21(2):147–52. https://doi.org/10.1097/MOT.0000000000000296.
24. Matarese LE. Nutrition and fluid optimization for patients with short bowel syndrome. JPEN J Parenter Enteral Nutr. 2013;37(2):161–70. https://doi.org/10.1177/0148607112469818.
25. Lin R, Murtazina R, Cha B, et al. D-glucose acts via sodium/glucose cotransporter 1 to increase NHE3 in mouse jejunal brush border by a Na^+/H^+ exchange regulatory factor 2-dependent process. Gastroenterology. 2011;140(2):560–71. https://doi.org/10.1053/j.gastro.2010.10.042.
26. Parrish CR, DiBaise JK. Short bowel syndrome in adults—part 3. Hydrating the adult patient with short bowel syndrome. Pract Gastroenterol. 2015;39(2):10–8.
27. Jeppesen PB, Lund P, Gottschalck IB, et al. Short bowel patients treated for two years with glucagon-like peptide 2 (GLP-2): compliance, safety, and effects on quality of life. Gastroenterol Res Pract. 2009;2009:425759. https://doi.org/10.1155/2009/425759.

19 Growth-Stimulating Effects of Glucagon-Like Peptide-2, Growth Hormone, and Other Agents

Liana Gheorghe, Roxana Saizu, and Daria Ana Arina Gheorghe

19.1 Introduction

Short bowel syndrome (SBS) is a multifaceted malabsorption disorder, ranging from isolated micronutrient deficiencies to complete intestinal failure. The severity of the condition largely depends on the remaining length and anatomical portion of the intestine, as well as the functional capacity of the remnant bowel [1].

19.1.1 Differentiating SBS with Intestinal Insufficiency Vs. SBS with Intestinal Failure

It is essential to distinguish between short bowel syndrome with intestinal insufficiency and SBS with intestinal failure (IF). Intestinal insufficiency is characterized by a reduced absorptive surface, yet the intestine maintains its autonomy, with deficiencies being manageable through dietary adjustments. In contrast, intestinal failure occurs when absorption is insufficient to maintain homeostasis, requiring parenteral supplementation for survival [2, 3].

L. Gheorghe · R. Saizu (✉) · D. A. A. Gheorghe
Carol Davila University of Medicine and Pharmacy, Bucharest, Romania

Center for Digestive Diseases and Liver Transplant, Fundeni Clinical Institute, Bucharest, Romania

A. Trifan et al. (eds.), *Short Bowel Syndrome in Adults*,
https://doi.org/10.1007/978-3-031-95848-9_19

19.2 Intestinal Adaptation

19.2.1 Phases of Adaptation

Managing short bowel syndrome (SBS) requires understanding its clinical stages: acute, adaptation, and maintenance. The acute phase (lasting weeks to months) involves fluid and electrolyte losses, requiring stabilization and reassessment, often with fasting. As stability improves, parenteral nutrition (PN) is introduced. The adaptation phase (lasting up to 2 years) focuses on reducing PN dependence through progressive nutritional support and intestinal adaptation. The maintenance phase marks the end of spontaneous adaptation, with intestinal failure deemed permanent if PN remains necessary. However, aggressive management may still enable PN weaning [4].

19.2.2 Structural and Functional Changes

However, the adaptation process begins as early as 48 h after surgery, during which the intestine undergoes both structural and functional modifications under the influence of internal and external stimuli, including nutrients (fiber, short-chain fatty acids, and glutamine), bile and pancreatic secretions, and hormones. Among these hormones are trophic factors like growth hormone (GH), glucagon-like peptide-2 (GLP-2), epithelial growth factor (EGF), and transforming growth factor-α (TGF-α), alongside those that regulate intestinal motility, such as GLP-1, GLP-2, and peptide YY (PYY) [1, 5].

Structurally, the intestine undergoes dilation and elongation, leading to an increase in its overall mass, crypt hyperplasia with increased crypt cell depth, villus elongation, microvillus expansion, enterocyte proliferation, and angiogenesis. Functionally, intestinal transit slows down, enzymatic activity and brush border membrane activity change, crypt differentiation accelerates, and nutrient transporter levels increase, expanding the absorptive surface [6].

19.2.3 The Role of Anatomical Configuration in Adaptation

Among the anatomical types of anastomoses—Type 1 (end-jejunostomy), Type 2 (jejuno-colonic anastomosis), and Type 3 (jejuno-ileo-colic anastomosis)—Type 3 appears to have the most favorable prognosis due to the preservation of the terminal ileum and the ileocecal valve [7]. The ileocecal valve plays a crucial role in motility, and this region contains the highest concentration of L cells, which are the primary source of natural GLP-1 and GLP-2 hormone secretion [3, 8]. Additionally, the ileum is capable of complex adaptive processes, both structural and functional. In contrast, Type 1 anastomosis is associated with the least favorable prognosis, as the jejunum lacks adaptive capacity. The colon also appears to undergo adaptive processes following major intestinal resections [9].

19.2.4 The Role of Gastrointestinal Hormones in Adaptation

As previously mentioned, the repair of the intestinal mucosa, its functional maintenance, and adaptation in the context of intestinal impairment occur through the influence of both internal and external stimuli, including the action of gastrointestinal peptide hormones.

19.2.4.1 GLP-2 and Growth Factors

Glucagon-like peptide-1 (GLP-1) belongs to the incretin family, alongside secretin, vasoactive intestinal peptide (VIP), pituitary adenylate cyclase-activating peptide (PACAP), gastric inhibitory polypeptide (GIP), glucagon, GLP-2, calcitonin, calcitonin gene-related peptide (CGRP), parathyroid hormone, corticotropin-releasing factor (CRF), and growth hormone-releasing factor (GHRF). Incretins are gastrointestinal peptide hormones secreted by K and L endocrine cells within the intestinal epithelium. These open-type cells have an apical process equipped with microvilli, allowing direct communication with the intestinal lumen [10].

GLP-1, a peptide composed of 30–31 amino acids, is secreted by L enteroendocrine cells in the terminal ileum, alpha cells in the pancreas, and the central nervous system. Its effects include slowing gastric emptying, promoting satiety, and enhancing insulin secretion in response to oral glucose intake [11, 12].

Thus, its influence on adaptation processes in SBS patients translates into slowed gastric emptying, allowing for increased nutrient absorption in the intestine. This process is driven by GLP-1 secretion from the terminal ileum, either through a neurohumoral feedback mechanism or direct stimulation by luminal carbohydrates. Consequently, resection of the terminal ileum leads to accelerated gastrointestinal motility [13].

Glucagon-like peptide-2 (GLP-2) is a 33-amino acid peptide hormone, member of the PACAP (pituitary adenylate cyclase-activating peptide) glucagon superfamily, that has been proven to have a trophic effect on the entire gastrointestinal tract [14]. It is primarily secreted by enteroendocrine L cells in the distal ileum and proximal colon in response to nutrient ingestion [14, 15]. It is produced through the post-translational processing of proglucagon, a process that also releases the related glucagon-like peptide-1 (GLP-1). In addition to its intestinal origin, GLP-2 is also synthesized in the central nervous system, particularly by neurons in the brainstem and hypothalamus, indicating its broader physiological roles beyond the gastrointestinal tract [16, 17].

Within the intestine, this hormone plays a crucial role in maintaining homeostasis by promoting crypt cell proliferation, inhibiting enterocyte apoptosis, suppressing gastric acid secretion, enhancing nutrient absorption, and regulating gastric emptying. Additionally, it increases intestinal blood flow, slows gastric emptying, and reduces intestinal motility. GLP-2 also plays a key role in stimulating crypt cell proliferation, further supporting intestinal adaptation and function [15].

These properties make GLP-2 a significant target for therapeutic strategies addressing conditions such as short bowel syndrome and other gastrointestinal disorders.

In patients with distal intestinal resections, where there is a deficiency of hormones secreted as a pro-adaptive feedback response in the terminal ileum (GLP-1, GLP-2, peptide YY, oxyntomodulin, and fibroblast growth factor (FGF)), the pro-secretory and pro-motility effects of hormones released proximally (gastrin, cholecystokinin, secretin, and motilin) is not counteracted. Consequently, accelerated intestinal transit, hypersecretion, and disturbances in blood and lymphatic flow occur [18].

Growth hormone (GH), composed of 191 amino acids, is secreted by the pituitary gland and plays a well-known role in promoting postnatal growth in mammals. In the intestine, its receptors are widely distributed, from epithelial cells to the deeper layers, including the muscularis propria.

Beyond its direct effect on stimulating the growth of intestinal wall cells, GH also promotes the secretion of other growth-related hormones, such as insulin-like growth factor 1 (IGF-1) [19]. Additionally, previous studies have shown that in animal models, hypophysectomy reduces intestinal adaptation processes [20]. For these reasons, GH analogues have been proposed as a potential treatment option for patients with SBS-IF.

19.3 Aim of Treatment

The goal of treating patients with intestinal failure (IF) due to short bowel syndrome (SBS) is to optimize the function of the remaining intestine while ensuring adequate nutritional and fluid support, thereby maintaining proper nutritional and hydroelectrolytic balance. This approach aims to alleviate gastrointestinal symptoms and reduce the need for supplemental nutrition and hydration [21].

The definitive aim of the adaptation process is to discontinue home parenteral nutrition (HPN), which has long been considered the standard of care in SBS with intestinal failure. However, despite its effectiveness, HPN has a significant impact on quality of life and poses substantial risks, such as steatohepatitis, IF-associated liver disease, and catheter-related complications, such as recurrent sepsis and thrombosis [22, 23].

Therefore, the key objectives in treating SBS include enhancing the absorptive surface, preventing and managing complications related to nutritional deficiencies, easing symptoms, and, most importantly, facilitating the successful cessation of HPN.

19.4 Patient Selection

This treatment is primarily intended for patients who, despite optimized dietary measures and conventional therapy, have not achieved enteral independence during the adaptation period [7].

Although the intestine should normally be given sufficient time for physiological adaptation before treatment is initiated, in cases where rapid adaptation is desired, treatment may begin earlier. In patients with extensive resections and anastomoses and a guarded prognosis, early intervention is indicated. For example, in patients with a group I jejuno- or ileostomy anastomosis—where adaptation and gradual weaning from HPN occur in fewer than 20% of cases 1 year after intervention—treatment with hormonal analogues is justified [24].

It should be borne in mind that, in patients with SBS, complete weaning off HPN is unlikely (<10%) if 2–3 years have elapsed since the most recent intestinal resection [2].

19.4.1 Recommendations for Initiating Treatment with Hormonal Analogues

The initiation of treatment with hormonal analogues should be guided by an assessment of natural intestinal adaptation and the optimal timing of intervention. In most cases, it is advisable to allow sufficient time for physiological adaptation before starting therapy. However, in patients with extensive resections and a guarded prognosis, early initiation of hormonal analogue treatment may be beneficial to promote intestinal adaptation (see Table 19.1).

It is essential that patients receive comprehensive information regarding their pathology, therapeutic options, and the associated risks. Conventional treatment is generally associated with lower costs, and its adverse reactions are better understood. Prior to considering hormonal analogue therapy, it is advisable to stabilize the patient using individualized conventional therapeutic measures. Additionally, patients should be informed about the potential benefits and risks associated with growth factor therapy, including the likelihood of successfully discontinuing HPN, the possibility of improved quality of life, the estimated duration of treatment, potential adverse reactions, and relevant cost considerations [7, 24].

Table 19.1 Adaptation rates and indications for hormonal analogue therapy by anastomosis type

Type	Adaptation rate	Hormonal analogue therapy
Jejuno-ileostomy (group I)	Low adaptation rate (<20% weaned at 1 year)	Recommended to accelerate adaptation
Jejuno-colonic anastomosis (group 2)	Progressive adaptation (~50% weaned by 5 years, minimal progress at 2–3 years)	Considered based on clinical status and need to speed up adaptation
Jejuno-Ileo-colonic anastomosis (group 3)	Majority achieve adaptation (75% weaned by 5 years)	Considered case-by-case if additional support is needed

19.5 Growth Factors Treatment

Currently, only two molecules have been approved for the treatment of SBS: somatotropin (growth hormone), available only in the US, and teduglutide (a glucagon-like peptide-2 analogue), approved in both the US and Europe [25].

19.5.1 GLP-2 Analogues

Teduglutide, a glucagon-like peptide-2 (GLP-2) analog, is the treatment of choice for patients with short bowel syndrome (SBS) who have not attained intestinal autonomy during the adaptation phase and remain dependent on parenteral nutrition despite intensive conventional therapy. This recombinant is a long-acting GLP-2 analog offering the advantage of a longer half-life (2–6 h), enabling convenient, once-daily subcutaneous administration. In contrast, human GLP-2 (h-GLP2) has a significantly shorter half-life of only 7 min [26, 27].

Teduglutide's prolonged duration of action is due to its resistance to degradation by the enzyme dipeptidyl-peptidase IV (DPP-IV) [28].

GLP-2 is released in response to enteral nutrient stimulation, a process regulated by the vagus nerve that, at the cellular level, activates G-protein-coupled receptors. Exogenous administration of GLP-2 to an intact intestine promotes gastrointestinal mucosal hypertrophy, leading to increased villus height, crypt deepening, greater intestinal mass, enhanced blood flow, and improved glucose absorption [29, 30].

After proximal intestinal resection, GLP-2 secretion from the distal ileum rises, facilitating enhanced nutrient absorption. Moreover, research indicates that GLP-2 can stimulate adaptation pathways in the remaining ileum, even in the absence of enteral nutrient stimulation [31].

In adults, exogenous GLP-2 administration promotes adaptation of the remaining jejunum, despite previous studies suggesting its limited capacity to adapt. The induced changes include increased crypt cell proliferation, an improved villus height-to-crypt depth ratio, an expansion of the total mucosal surface area, and enhanced glucose absorption [27].

Following resection, GLP-2 secretion increases significantly, especially when the colon remains intact, with its levels directly linked to the extent of intestinal adaptation. In this setting, phase 3 studies have shown that teduglutide administration effectively reduces the dependency on parenteral nutrition and intravenous fluids [32, 33].

A 2009 prospective longitudinal observational study [34] on 11 patients treated with teduglutide 400 μg TID for 2 years found that fecal wet weight decreased by ~1 L/day, averaging 811 g/day in year 1 and 1081 g/day in year 2, stabilizing after week 13. After treatment cessation, fecal weight returned to baseline but was fully regained within 13 weeks of reinitiation. Oral intake declined gradually, reaching full adaptation by week 52 in year 1 but much faster (by week 13) in year 2.

Intestinal absorption efficiency improved, but total absorption remained unchanged. No significant morphological changes were observed, with villus height

($P = 0.37$) and crypt depth ($P = 0.44$) showing no overall change. Among electrolytes, magnesium absorption increased, while sodium, potassium, and calcium remained unchanged. GLP-2 alone had minimal effects on the energy balance, but when combined with cholylsarcosine, it significantly reduced fecal fat excretion and slightly increased energy absorption, though not significantly. Doubling the GLP-2 dose had no added benefits.

A randomized placebo-controlled study performed on 85 patients over a period of 24 weeks, published in 2011 [35], evaluated teduglutide's impact on parenteral support reduction. When administered at 0.05 mg/kg/day, the treatment was more effective than 0.10 mg/kg/day, significantly reducing parenteral volume, increasing urine output, and enhancing enterocyte mass. While 0.10 mg/kg/day showed no significant difference from placebo ($P = 0.16$), 0.05 mg/kg/day demonstrated a significant improvement ($P = 0.007$).

More patients in the 0.05 mg/kg/day group achieved ≥20% PN reduction (46% vs. 6%, $P = 0.005$), with two fully weaned from PN. Parenteral energy needs dropped the most at 0.05 mg/kg/day (−912 kJ/day, $P = 0.001$), though intergroup differences were not significant.

Both doses increased lean body mass, while bone mineral content improved at 0.10 mg/kg/day ($P = 0.046$). Villus height increased in both groups, but colonic crypt depth increased only at 0.10 mg/kg/day ($P = 0.016$). Plasma citrulline levels improved at both doses, indicating intestinal adaptation. Despite these positive effects, quality of life remained unchanged.

The STEPS-2 placebo-controlled study [36] evaluated the long-term safety and efficacy of teduglutide in 88 patients, with 74% completing the study. Among teduglutide-treated patients, 89% achieved ≥20% reduction in parenteral support (PS) volume, compared to 46% in the placebo group and 50% in the not treated group, with greater reductions in those treated longer. Thirteen patients achieved full enteral autonomy, mostly in the teduglutide-treated group. Plasma citrulline increased by 71% in the teduglutide, indicating enhanced intestinal adaptation.

Teduglutide was well tolerated, with 95% of patients reporting mild-to-moderate adverse events and no significant changes in kidney function, electrolytes, or malignancy risk. Teduglutide-specific antibodies were found in 43% of patients but had no clinical impact. Liver enzymes declined in responders, and "slow responders" showed improvements with continued treatment.

Teduglutide demonstrated sustained benefits in reducing PS volume, with some patients achieving complete independence. It was safe and effective over long-term use, with no major safety concerns.

In the combined phase III studies [37], 16 of 134 patients (12%) treated with teduglutide 0.05 mg/kg/day achieved complete independence from PN after a median of 5 years. Most (75%) had partial colon-in-continuity, though four reached independence without a colon, with no significant difference between the groups.

PN reductions began within days to months, but 75% required at least 1 year for enteral autonomy. By week 24, the teduglutide group reduced PN by 4.4 L, compared to 2.3 L in the placebo group. Fifteen patients (11%) across phase III trials and extensions achieved full independence within 12–130 weeks (median 89 weeks).

Plasma citrulline increased by 28.3%, reflecting intestinal adaptation, while body weight, albumin, and creatinine remained stable. All independent patients had mild-to-moderate adverse events, mainly abdominal pain, nausea, diarrhea, and injection site reactions. Serious AEs occurred in 13 patients, mostly catheter infections, with no neutralizing antibodies detected.

Summarizing the study results, teduglutide effectively *reduces dependence on parenteral support,* with 12% of patients achieving complete independence. While some required over a year of treatment before reaching enteral autonomy, reductions began within days to months, and long-term treatment provided sustained benefits.

Regarding *intestinal absorption and adaptation*, villus height increased in the small intestine, while colonic crypt depth expanded at higher doses. These structural changes enhanced nutrient and fluid absorption, leading to reduced oral fluid intake and increased urine output.

In terms of *body weight and composition*, data indicate that *teduglutide promotes an increase in lean body mass and overall body weight.*

In the pediatric population, a 24-week phase 3 clinical trial conducted on 59 patients [38] evaluated teduglutide's efficacy and safety in reducing PN dependence. Fifty patients received teduglutide (24 at 0.025 mg/kg, 26 at 0.05 mg/kg), and nine received standard care (SOC).

Teduglutide significantly reduced PN volume, with 69% (0.05 mg/kg) and 54% (0.025 mg/kg) achieving ≥20% reduction, compared to 11% in SOC. PN volume decreased by 23.3 mL/kg/day (0.05 mg/kg), 16.2 mL/kg/day (0.025 mg/kg), and 6.0 mL/kg/day (SOC). PN calories, infusion duration, and frequency also declined. By week 24, five teduglutide patients (8–12%) achieved full enteral autonomy, while none in the SOC group did. Enteral nutrition (EN) increased significantly, with EN volume rising by ~77–79% and EN calories by ~83–86%, compared to minimal SOC changes.

Teduglutide was well tolerated, with mostly mild-to-moderate AEs including pyrexia, vomiting, diarrhea, and abdominal pain. Serious AEs (TESAEs) were more common in teduglutide groups but did not lead to treatment discontinuation. Teduglutide-specific antibodies appeared in 13–20% of patients, but neutralizing antibodies were found in only 4%, with no cases of intestinal stenosis, heart failure, or drug absorption issues. No deaths occurred.

Therefore, teduglutide effectively reduced PS needs in pediatric patients, with higher doses achieving greater reductions. Some patients achieved full enteral autonomy, and PS volume, calories, and infusion time decreased significantly. The treatment was well tolerated, with manageable AEs and no major safety concerns.

Teduglutide (Revestive in Europe and Canada; Gattex in the United States of America) was approved in 2012 for the treatment of SBS patients who need parenteral support, in adults and children 1 year of age and older. In adults, the recommended dose is 0.05 mg/kg SubQ once daily. A treatment period of 6 months is recommended, after which the treatment effect should be evaluated. In children below the age of 2 years, treatment should be evaluated after 12 weeks. The dosage for children is calculated on a mg/kg basis (see https://www.ema.europa.eu/documents/product-information/revestive-epar-product-information_en.pdf).

19.5.1.1 Safety

The most commonly reported adverse effects (AEs) in the studies were abdominal pain, nausea, gastrointestinal stoma complication, and abdominal distension. Treatment-emergent serious AEs were acute cholecystitis and small intestinal stenosis. A small percentage of patients developed antibodies, without these being neutralizing or causing systemic hypersensitivity [33]. In the randomized placebo-controlled trial published by B. Jeppesen in 2011 [35], the most frequent AEs were abdominal pain, nausea, vomiting, and nasopharyngitis. There were no deaths reported during the study. In the group studied by Lauren K. Schwartz [36], gastrointestinal AEs and catheter-related complications were the most common (abdominal pain, nausea, constipation, catheter sepsis). In addition, three patients developed neoplasms, all of whom had significant risk factors. Two heavy smokers were diagnosed with lung cancer, while one patient with a history of Hodgkin's lymphoma, previously treated with chemotherapy and radiotherapy, was found to have metastatic adenocarcinoma.

19.5.1.2 Special Considerations

Given that teduglutide is a growth factor capable of stimulating intestinal and colonic mucosal growth and polyp formation, pretreatment upper gastrointestinal endoscopy and colonoscopic screening are recommended, with polyp resection if necessary. In children under 12 years old, a fecal hemoccult test should be performed before starting therapy. Additionally, caution should be exercised in patients at risk of intestinal obstruction, such as those with a narrowed stoma opening.

In adults, a follow-up colonoscopy is advised 2 years after treatment initiation, followed by regular surveillance every 5 years. In pediatric patients, a colonoscopy should be performed 1 year after starting treatment, with continued monitoring every 5 years.

If neoplasms are detected during treatment, therapy must be discontinued.

The only contraindication to teduglutide is active gastrointestinal neoplasia. Therefore, the GLP-2 analogue should not be used in patients suspected or diagnosed with malignancies or those with a history of gastrointestinal diseases within the past 5 years, including hepatic and pancreaticobiliary disorders.

Novel long-acting GLP-2 analogues (glepaglutide and apraglutide), which would allow greater spacing between administrations, were developed, but their efficacy on intestinal adaptation and their safety profile still need more studies [39, 40].

19.5.2 GLP-1 Analogues

Originally developed for diabetes management, GLP-1 analogues show promise in reducing gastrointestinal motility, increasing transit time, and improving fluid balance in SBS patients. While research on their use in SBS is still evolving, early findings suggest that GLP-1 analogues could play a valuable role in enhancing intestinal adaptation and improving quality of life in affected patients.

A study on five SBS patients [13], which included manometric studies, found that exenatide significantly improved bowel function, nutrient absorption, and quality of life. Patients experienced a notable reduction in bowel movements (from up to 12 per day to as few as 3), allowing for better continence, improved sleep, and increased daily activity. Post-meal bowel movements were delayed from 15 min to 2–6 h, suggesting enhanced nutrient absorption. Albumin, total protein, and vitamin levels increased, and two patients successfully discontinued PN while maintaining stable weight and hydration. Manometry findings indicated that exenatide suppressed continuous antral contractions, slowing gastric emptying and motility, which may contribute to improved absorption. The treatment was well tolerated, with minimal side effects, as only one patient reported nausea, which resolved with dose adjustment. These findings suggest that exenatide could be a promising therapy for reducing PN dependence and improving overall SBS management.

A study of eight SBS-IF [41] patients with end-jejunostomy found that liraglutide reduced ostomy wet weight output by 13%, leading to a 50% increase in urine output and improved intestinal fluid absorption. Energy absorption increased by 9%, with higher carbohydrate uptake (53% → 62%), while lipid and protein absorption showed minor improvements.

Liraglutide was well tolerated, causing mild nausea and appetite reduction but no serious side effects. Body weight, composition, bone mineral content, and hormone levels remained unchanged, and quality of life scores showed no significant improvement. Despite no effect on gastric emptying, liraglutide enhanced fluid balance and absorption efficiency, suggesting potential benefits for SBS-IF patients.

A placebo-controlled study on nine SBS patients [42] (seven with end-jejunostomies, two with partial colon continuity) evaluated the effects of GLP-1, GLP-2, and their combination on fluid balance, nutrient absorption, and body composition.

GLP treatments significantly reduced fecal wet weight output compared to placebo (GLP-1: −295 g/day, GLP-2: −387 g/day, GLP-1 + 2: −503 g/day), with GLP-2 and GLP-1 + 2 improving absolute wet weight absorption. Urine volume remained unchanged. Sodium and potassium excretion decreased with all treatments, but only GLP-1 + 2 significantly increased sodium absorption (42.5%). Energy absorption improved, with GLP-1 + 2 leading to the largest relative increase (+7.0%).

GLP-1 + 2 increased total fat mass (1.8 kg) and total body mass (2.2 kg), but no significant changes were observed in lean mass, bone mineral content, or weighed body weight. GLP-1 reduced appetite, while GLP-2 decreased the perception of fecal production. GLP-1 also tended to increase nausea. Altogether, GLP-1, GLP-2, and their combination improved wet weight absorption and reduced fecal losses, with GLP-1 + 2 showing the most benefits in energy absorption and body composition changes.

GLP-1 analogues show promising results in SBS treatment by slowing gastrointestinal motility, improving fluid balance, and enhancing nutrient absorption. The two molecules have an additive effect, amplifying their benefits while potentially mitigating each other's adverse effects.

19.5.3 Growth Hormone Analogues

Growth hormone was initially explored as a supplementary therapy for short bowel syndrome (SBS) due to its potential to enhance intestinal adaptation and reduce dependence on parenteral nutrition. However, inconsistent efficacy and safety concerns prevented its approval for SBS treatment. While GH therapy may provide short-term benefits for some patients, its long-term effectiveness and safety remain uncertain. Further research is needed to clarify GH therapy's role in both adult and pediatric SBS populations and determine its potential as a viable treatment option [7, 20].

In the studies available to date, the observed positive effects of GH include a reduction in PN dependence, which was enhanced by the addition of glutamine, as well as weight gain, though accompanied by increased fluid intake, likely compensating for PN reductions. Reported adverse effects include peripheral edema, musculoskeletal complaints, and gastrointestinal symptoms. GH was temporarily discontinued in four patients due to chest pain (two patients), severe edema, headaches, and vomiting [43].

In children and adolescents, growth hormone (GH) therapy has shown significant benefits in reducing parenteral nutrition (PN) dependence, increasing lean body mass, and promoting weight gain, with effects sustained even after treatment discontinuation. GH therapy maintains stable hematologic and organ function, making it a promising option for managing intestinal adaptation. However, adverse effects such as peripheral edema (94%), musculoskeletal pain (44%), and gastrointestinal symptoms (75%) are common, necessitating careful monitoring and dose adjustments. While chest pain, headaches, and rare cases of intracranial hypertension have been reported, symptoms typically resolve upon temporary discontinuation or dose reduction. Given these findings, GH therapy offers a viable but closely monitored approach to improving outcomes in patients requiring PN support [44].

Nevertheless, the effects of GH on nutrient absorption diminished after discontinuation in other studies, raising concerns about its long-term efficacy [19].

References

1. Massironi S, Cavalcoli F, Rausa E, Invernizzi P, Braga M, Vecchi M. Understanding short bowel syndrome: current status and future perspectives. Dig Liver Dis. 2020;52(3):253–61. https://doi.org/10.1016/j.dld.2019.11.013.
2. Pironi L, et al. ESPEN endorsed recommendations. Definition and classification of intestinal failure in adults. Clin Nutr. 2015;34(2):171–80. https://doi.org/10.1016/j.clnu.2014.08.017.
3. Reiner J, et al. Dapiglutide, a novel dual GLP-1 and GLP-2 receptor agonist, attenuates intestinal insufficiency in a murine model of short bowel. J Parenter Enter Nutr. 2022;46(5):1107–18. https://doi.org/10.1002/jpen.2286.

4. Yamada's textbook of gastroenterology, 6th ed., vol. 1. Wiley; 2016.
5. Thiesen A, et al. Adaptation following intestinal resection: mechanisms and signals. Best Pract Res Clin Gastroenterol. 2003;17(6):981–95. https://doi.org/10.1016/s1521-6918(03)00097-0.
6. Pizzoferrato M, Puca P, Ennas S, Cammarota G, Guidi L. Glucagon-like peptide-2 analogues for Crohn's disease patients with short bowel syndrome and intestinal failure. World J Gastroenterol. 2022;28(44):6258–70. https://doi.org/10.3748/wjg.v28.i44.6258.
7. Iyer K, DiBaise JK, Rubio-Tapia A. AGA clinical practice update on management of short bowel syndrome: expert review. Clin Gastroenterol Hepatol. 2022;20(10):2185–94.e2. https://doi.org/10.1016/j.cgh.2022.05.032.
8. Messing B, Crenn P, Beau P, Boutron-Ruault MC, Rambaud JC, Matuchansky C. Long-term survival and parenteral nutrition dependence in adult patients with the short bowel syndrome. Gastroenterology. 1999;117(5):1043–50. https://doi.org/10.1016/s0016-5085(99)70388-4.
9. Kong W, et al. A potential anatomic subtype of short bowel syndrome: a matched case-control study. BMC Gastroenterol. 2016;16(1):12. https://doi.org/10.1186/s12876-016-0425-4.
10. Holst JJ. The incretin system in healthy humans: the role of GIP and GLP-1. Metabolism. 2019;96:46–55. https://doi.org/10.1016/j.metabol.2019.04.014.
11. Yamada's textbook of gastroenterology. Wiley; 2016.
12. Drucker DJ. The GLP-1 journey: from discovery science to therapeutic impact. J Clin Invest. 2024;134(2) https://doi.org/10.1172/JCI175634.
13. Kunkel D, et al. Efficacy of the glucagon-like peptide-1 agonist exenatide in the treatment of short bowel syndrome. Neurogastroenterol Motil. 2011;23(8):739–e328. https://doi.org/10.1111/j.1365-2982.2011.01723.x.
14. Mayo KE, et al. International Union of Pharmacology. XXXV. The glucagon receptor family. Pharmacol Rev. 2003;55(1):167–94. https://doi.org/10.1124/pr.55.1.6.
15. Zhu C, Li Y. An updated overview of glucagon-like peptide-2 analog trophic therapy for short bowel syndrome in adults. J Int Med Res. 2022;50(3) https://doi.org/10.1177/03000605221086145.
16. Meier JJ, et al. Glucagon-like peptide 2 stimulates glucagon secretion, enhances lipid absorption, and inhibits gastric acid secretion in humans. Gastroenterology. 2006;130(1):44–54. https://doi.org/10.1053/j.gastro.2005.10.004.
17. Guan X. The CNS glucagon-like peptide-2 receptor in the control of energy balance and glucose homeostasis. Am J Physiol Regul Integr Comp Physiol. 2014;307(6):R585–96. https://doi.org/10.1152/ajpregu.00096.2014.
18. Jeppesen PB, Hartmann B, Hansen BS, Thulesen J, Holst JJ, Mortensen PB. Impaired meal stimulated glucagon-like peptide 2 response in ileal resected short bowel patients with intestinal failure. Gut. 1999;45(4):559–63. https://doi.org/10.1136/gut.45.4.559.
19. McMellen ME, Wakeman D, Longshore SW, McDuffie LA, Warner BW. Growth factors: possible roles for clinical management of the short bowel syndrome. Semin Pediatr Surg. 2010;19(1):35–43. https://doi.org/10.1053/j.sempedsurg.2009.11.010.
20. Tappenden KA. Intestinal adaptation following resection. J Parenter Enter Nutr. 2014;38(1S) https://doi.org/10.1177/0148607114525210.
21. Nightingale J. Guidelines for management of patients with a short bowel. Gut. 2006;55(suppl_4):iv1–12. https://doi.org/10.1136/gut.2006.091108.
22. Wallis K, Walters JR, Gabe S. Short bowel syndrome: the role of GLP-2 on improving outcome. Curr Opin Clin Nutr Metab Care. 2009;12(5):526–32. https://doi.org/10.1097/MCO.0b013e32832d23cd.
23. Amiot A, Messing B, Corcos O, Panis Y, Joly F. Determinants of home parenteral nutrition dependence and survival of 268 patients with non-malignant short bowel syndrome. Clin Nutr. 2013;32(3):368–74. https://doi.org/10.1016/j.clnu.2012.08.007.
24. Nightingale JMD, editor. Intestinal failure. Cham: Springer; 2023. https://doi.org/10.1007/978-3-031-22265-8.
25. Cuerda C, et al. ESPEN practical guideline: clinical nutrition in chronic intestinal failure. Clin Nutr. 2021;40(9):5196–220. https://doi.org/10.1016/j.clnu.2021.07.002.

26. Billiauws L, Bataille J, Boehm V, Corcos O, Joly F. Teduglutide for treatment of adult patients with short bowel syndrome. Expert Opin Biol Ther. 2017;17(5):623–32. https://doi.org/10.1080/14712598.2017.1304912.
27. Sigalet DL, et al. Glucagon-like Peptide-2 induces a specific pattern of adaptation in remnant jejunum. Dig Dis Sci. 2006;51(9):1557–66. https://doi.org/10.1007/s10620-006-9077-5.
28. Drucker DJ, Deforest L, Brubaker PL. Intestinal response to growth factors administered alone or in combination with human [Gly^2]glucagon-like peptide 2. Am J Physiol Gastroint Liver Physiol. 1997;273(6):G1252–62. https://doi.org/10.1152/ajpgi.1997.273.6.G1252.
29. Roberge JN, Brubaker PL. Secretion of Proglucagon-derived peptides in response to intestinal luminal nutrients*. Endocrinology. 1991;128(6):3169–74. https://doi.org/10.1210/endo-128-6-3169.
30. Munroe DG, et al. Prototypic G protein-coupled receptor for the intestinotrophic factor glucagon-like peptide 2. Proc Natl Acad Sci U S A. 1999;96(4):1569–73. https://doi.org/10.1073/pnas.96.4.1569.
31. Martin GR, Wallace LE, Sigalet DL. Glucagon-like peptide-2 induces intestinal adaptation in parenterally fed rats with short bowel syndrome. Am J Physiol Gastrointest Liver Physiol. 2004;286(6):G964–72. https://doi.org/10.1152/ajpgi.00509.2003.
32. Tappenden KA, Edelman J, Joelsson B. Teduglutide enhances structural adaptation of the small intestinal mucosa in patients with short bowel syndrome. J Clin Gastroenterol. 2013;47(7):602–7. https://doi.org/10.1097/MCG.0b013e3182828f57.
33. Jeppesen PB, et al. Teduglutide reduces need for parenteral support among patients with short bowel syndrome with intestinal failure. Gastroenterology. 2012;143(6):1473–81.e3. https://doi.org/10.1053/j.gastro.2012.09.007.
34. Jeppesen PB, et al. Short bowel patients treated for two years with glucagon-like peptide 2: effects on intestinal morphology and absorption, renal function, bone and body composition, and muscle function. Gastroenterol Res Pract. 2009;2009:1–12. https://doi.org/10.1155/2009/616054.
35. Jeppesen PB, Gilroy R, Pertkiewicz M, Allard JP, Messing B, O'Keefe SJ. Randomised placebo-controlled trial of teduglutide in reducing parenteral nutrition and/or intravenous fluid requirements in patients with short bowel syndrome. Gut. 2011;60(7):902–14. https://doi.org/10.1136/gut.2010.218271.
36. Schwartz LK, et al. Long-term teduglutide for the treatment of patients with intestinal failure associated with short bowel syndrome. Clin Transl Gastroenterol. 2016;7(2):e142. https://doi.org/10.1038/ctg.2015.69.
37. Iyer KR, et al. Independence from parenteral nutrition and intravenous fluid support during treatment with teduglutide among patients with intestinal failure associated with short bowel syndrome. J Parenter Enter Nutr. 2017;41(6):946–51. https://doi.org/10.1177/0148607116680791.
38. Kocoshis SA, et al. Safety and efficacy of teduglutide in pediatric patients with intestinal failure due to short bowel syndrome: a 24-week, phase III study. J Parenter Enter Nutr. 2020;44(4):621–31. https://doi.org/10.1002/jpen.1690.
39. Naimi RM, et al. Glepaglutide, a novel long-acting glucagon-like peptide-2 analogue, for patients with short bowel syndrome: a randomised phase 2 trial. Lancet Gastroenterol Hepatol. 2019;4(5):354–63. https://doi.org/10.1016/S2468-1253(19)30077-9.
40. Slim GM, et al. Novel long-acting GLP-2 analogue, FE 203799 (Apraglutide), enhances adaptation and linear intestinal growth in a neonatal piglet model of short bowel syndrome with total resection of the ileum. J Parenter Enter Nutr. 2019;43(7):891–8. https://doi.org/10.1002/jpen.1500.
41. Hvistendahl M, et al. Effect of liraglutide treatment on jejunostomy output in patients with short bowel syndrome: an open-label pilot study. J Parenter Enter Nutr. 2018;42(1):112–21. https://doi.org/10.1177/0148607116672265.
42. Madsen KB, et al. Acute effects of continuous infusions of glucagon-like peptide (GLP)-1, GLP-2 and the combination (GLP-1+GLP-2) on intestinal absorption in short bowel syndrome (SBS) patients. A placebo-controlled study. Regul Pept. 2013;184:30–9. https://doi.org/10.1016/j.regpep.2013.03.025.

43. Byrne TA, et al. Growth hormone, glutamine, and an optimal diet reduces parenteral nutrition in patients with short bowel syndrome. Ann Surg. 2005;242(5):655–61. https://doi.org/10.1097/01.sla.0000186479.53295.14.
44. Bamba V, Kanakatti Shankar R. Approach to the patient: safety of growth hormone replacement in children and adolescents. J Clin Endocrinol Metab. 2022;107(3):847–61. https://doi.org/10.1210/clinem/dgab746.

Surgical Management of Short Bowel Syndrome: Ostomy, Fistula, Autologous Gastrointestinal Reconstruction

20

Viorel Scripcariu, Dragos Viorel Scripcariu,
Gheorghe G. Balan, and Catalin Victor Sfarti

20.1 Introduction

Short bowel syndrome (SBS) is a complex condition characterized by a significant loss of functional small intestine, leading to malabsorption, diarrhea, electrolyte imbalances, and nutritional deficiencies [1, 2]. It commonly arises following extensive intestinal resection due to conditions such as mesenteric ischemia, Crohn's disease, volvulus, trauma, or congenital disorders, such as gastroschisis and necrotizing enterocolitis [3]. While medical and nutritional therapies, including total parenteral nutrition (TPN), play a crucial role in managing SBS, surgical interventions are often necessary to optimize bowel function, enhance nutrient absorption, and reduce complications associated with long-term parenteral support [4].

Surgical management of SBS is tailored to the individual patient's intestinal anatomy, functional capacity, and clinical status. The primary objectives include preserving and maximizing existing bowel function, restoring intestinal continuity when possible, and slowing intestinal transit to improve absorption [5]. Various procedures are available, ranging from bowel-lengthening techniques—such as the Bianchi procedure and Serial Transverse Enteroplasty (STEP)—to reconstructive strategies, such as strictureplasty and bowel tapering [1, 3]. In severe cases where intestinal failure is irreversible, intestinal transplantation remains a viable option,

V. Scripcariu · D. V. Scripcariu
Grigore T. Popa University of Medicine and Pharmacy, Iaşi, Romania

Department of Surgery, Regional Oncology Institute, Iaşi, Romania
e-mail: viorel.scripcariu@umfiasi.ro

G. G. Balan (✉) · C. V. Sfarti
Grigore T. Popa University of Medicine and Pharmacy, Iaşi, Romania

St. Spiridon Emergency Hospital, Institute of Gastroenterology and Hepatology, Iaşi, Romania

A. Trifan et al. (eds.), *Short Bowel Syndrome in Adults*,
https://doi.org/10.1007/978-3-031-95848-9_20

particularly in patients with TPN-related complications such as liver dysfunction or recurrent sepsis [2, 4].

A multidisciplinary approach involving surgeons, gastroenterologists, dietitians, and transplant specialists is essential for optimizing outcomes in patients with SBS. The decision to pursue surgical intervention is influenced by factors such as residual bowel length, presence of the ileocecal valve, degree of bowel dilation, and dependence on parenteral nutrition (PN) [3]. With advances in surgical techniques and perioperative care, many patients can achieve significant improvements in nutrient absorption and quality of life, with some even attaining enteral autonomy [5].

In nearly every intestinal failure (IF) team, a gastroenterologist takes on a pivotal role, complemented by nursing assistance and, often, contributions from a dietitian. In many of the more advanced programs, there is typically a specialized surgeon who dedicates a significant portion of their practice to IF and associated issues. The surgeon's responsibility involves collaborating closely with the entire interdisciplinary team, participating actively in clinic sessions, and addressing all surgical concerns that emerge within the SBS patient group [6, 7].

In many patients, SBS typically emerges in emergency conditions, due to incidents like midgut volvulus, trauma, or mesenteric ischemia. Alternatively, it can develop gradually following multiple surgical resections, often related to inflammatory bowel disease or intricate adhesions. In acute scenarios, such as the former, a general on-call surgeon usually addresses the issue, while chronic, latter cases may require the expertise of a colorectal specialist [8].

Surgical treatment of SBS addresses issues such as intraoperative management of conditions predisposing to SBS in the instances stated above, ostomy management (local treatment of a dysfunctional ostomy, closure of ostomy), management of fistular complications, autologous gastrointestinal (GI) reconstruction, and intestinal transplantation [9, 10]. While minimally invasive methods may be applicable in certain instances, the intricate nature of surgery and the common history of multiple abdominal procedures often necessitate the use of traditional open techniques.

20.2 Patient Selection for Surgical Management of SBS

Surgical intervention in SBS is not universally indicated for all patients and must be carefully tailored based on clinical presentation, residual bowel anatomy, and dependence on PN. The ideal candidates for surgical management include patients with significant bowel dilation, those with potential for bowel rehabilitation, and those experiencing complications related to their anatomy or dependence on PN [3].

Patients who may benefit from bowel lengthening procedures—such as the STEP procedure or the Bianchi procedure—are typically those with severe bowel dilation and poor motility, as these procedures can increase surface area and improve transit time, thereby enhancing nutrient absorption [11]. Additionally, individuals with segmental strictures due to conditions such as Crohn's disease may require strictureplasty or resection to restore bowel continuity while preserving as much functional intestine as possible [2].

Another category of patients requiring surgical intervention includes those with persistent high-output enterostomies or malabsorptive diarrhea that cannot be adequately controlled with medical therapy. These patients may benefit from intestinal continuity restoration surgeries that reconnect remaining bowel segments to improve fluid and electrolyte balance [1]. In contrast, patients with chronic complications of PN, such as parenteral nutrition–associated liver disease (PNALD) or recurrent catheter-related bloodstream infections, may require intestinal transplantation, particularly if they have irreversible intestinal failure and cannot transition to enteral feeding [4].

Ultimately, the decision to pursue surgery is highly individualized and should involve a multidisciplinary team, including surgeons, gastroenterologists, and nutritionists, to assess the risks and benefits of the procedure and determine the likelihood of achieving enteral autonomy [5]. Surgical strategies are most effective when combined with nutritional rehabilitation and pharmacologic interventions aimed at optimizing bowel adaptation and function.

20.3 Surgical Management of SBS

Table 20.1 summarizes the main surgical options currently available for the management of SBS. Daily practice also faces the need for hybrid procedures depending on patient characteristics that stress the need for tailored therapy. Throughout the current section, we approach the main SBS management strategies currently backed by evidence.

20.3.1 Intraoperative Management of Conditions Predisposing to SBS

A crucial intraoperative approach is to refrain from extensive resection unless it is unequivocally warranted. Decisions regarding resection margins and the management of intestinal lesions should be made only after a comprehensive evaluation of the entire situation. Approaches such as stricturoplasty, intestinal tapering, and

Table 20.1 Surgical options in SBS

Correction of slow transit	• Diagnosis and surgical treatment of strictures, partial obstructions, blind loops, or enteroenteric fistulas
Improvement of intestinal motility in dilated bowel	• Tapering enteroplasty • Longitudinal intestinal lengthening and tailoring (Bianchi LILT procedure) • Serial transverse enteroplasty (STEP)
Decrease in intestinal transit in non-dilated bowel	• Segmental reversal of the small bowel (SRSB) • Isoperistaltic colonic interposition
Increase of mucosal surface	• Sequential intestinal lengthening • Controlled tissue expansion

serosal patching can be advantageous in addressing particular lesions that would typically necessitate resection. Most strictures can be effectively managed using a stricturoplasty technique in a Heineke–Mikulicz pyloroplasty fashion. This involves a longitudinal incision directly over the narrowed segment, followed by a transverse closure to widen the lumen. To ensure adequate patency, the incision should extend approximately 1 cm beyond both the proximal and distal ends of the stricture. Closure of the enterotomy may be performed using either a single-layer or two-layer suture technique, depending on the surgeon's preference and the condition of the bowel. Additionally, care should be taken to avoid the creation of blind loops, which can contribute to stasis and complications such as bacterial overgrowth [12].

Serosal patching offers a valuable surgical option for addressing localized intestinal problems such as persistent fistulas, strictures, or small defects, especially when the affected bowel segment is difficult to mobilize. The technique involves suturing a healthy segment of adjacent bowel—typically another loop of small intestine or colon—so that its serosal surface lies flush against the damaged area. A seromuscular-to-seromuscular anastomosis is fashioned using either interrupted or continuous sutures, creating a stable patch over the lesion. Over time, mucosal regeneration occurs, as epithelial cells from the surrounding intestine migrate laterally to cover the serosal graft, effectively integrating it into the native mucosa [13].

Intestinal ischemia presents a significant intraoperative challenge that necessitates immediate evaluation and intervention. The alleviation of mesenteric obstruction or constriction should be the primary focus, and the affected bowel should be enveloped in warm, moist packs to facilitate reperfusion. Signs of intestinal viability include enhanced coloration, observable peristalsis, and the reestablishment of mesenteric pulsations. Direct palpation of mesenteric vessels can aid in identifying the root cause of the ischemia. Doppler ultrasonography and indocyanine green (ICG) fluorescence angiography can aid the surgeon in assessing perfusion. If possible, efforts should be made to undertake revascularization to preserve potentially viable bowel segments. Clearly necrotic areas must be excised, while segments of uncertain viability should be scheduled for a second-look laparotomy after stabilization.

The creation of an ostomy should be evaluated in patients who are unstable, in situations where bowel viability is in doubt, or when the remaining length of the small intestine is less than 60 cm. In cases where a second-look surgery is expected, temporary discontinuity via stapled bowel ends may be suitable. Whenever a viable distal segment exists, efforts should be made to restore intestinal continuity [9, 10].

20.3.2 Ostomy Management

20.3.2.1 Preoperative Planning of the Stoma Site

Preoperative stoma site marking is a critical step in surgical planning for patients undergoing bowel diversion. A joint position statement by the American Society of Colon and Rectal Surgeons and the Wound, Ostomy, and Continence Nurses Society (WOCN) emphasizes its importance in reducing postoperative complications.

Although the guidelines primarily focus on patients without prior ostomies or enterocutaneous fistulas, the same principles can be adapted to cases with existing stomas or fistulas. Studies consistently show that patients who are marked preoperatively by a trained ostomy specialist experience fewer stoma-related complications and improved functional outcomes [9, 10].

Key elements of effective stoma site selection include placing the stoma within the rectus abdominis muscle, evaluating the site in multiple patient positions (sitting, standing, supine), and avoiding areas of scarring, skin folds, or interference with clothing and belts. While access to certified ostomy nurses may not always be available, it is essential that surgeons are familiar with these core principles. Ultimately, intraoperative judgment determines final stoma placement, but incorporating proper preoperative marking techniques—especially in complex cases—can significantly improve long-term management and quality of life for patients [9, 10].

20.3.2.2 Ostomy Care Principles

Basic ostomy care begins with maintaining healthy peristomal skin. The area should be gently cleaned using plain water or a pH-balanced soap, rinsed with tap water, and dried by patting—never scrubbing. Harsh substances such as alcohol, betadine, or hydrogen peroxide should be avoided. Adhesive residue can be removed with specialized adhesive remover wipes or sprays; if oil-based, these products should be washed off thoroughly to ensure adequate adhesion. Patients should be cautioned against picking or aggressively removing barrier material from the skin, as this can lead to damage. During pouch changes on an active stoma, a bedside suction device with a Yankauer tip can help manage effluent stool, but care must be taken to avoid direct contact with the bowel [1, 9, 10].

Supply management is an important aspect of long-term ostomy care. Ostomy products are generally covered by medical insurance, but specific coverage varies, and copays may apply. When a home health agency is involved, they typically provide supplies during the active care period. Patients with SBS or complex ostomies often benefit from working with agencies experienced in such conditions. Supply costs can escalate quickly when there are persistent issues such as leakage or skin breakdown [6, 7].

Complex ostomy cases demand a methodical, individualized approach to finding the most effective pouching system. Delayed intervention in the face of peristomal complications can lead to skin deterioration, infection, or hospitalization. Early involvement of ostomy care specialists is recommended in difficult cases to optimize management before conditions worsen. In scenarios where pouching remains problematic despite best efforts, referral to a surgeon for evaluation of potential surgical revision or intervention should be considered to restore function and improve quality of life [9, 10, 14].

20.3.2.3 Ostomy Care for High-Output Stomas

High-output stomas are a common challenge in patients with short bowel syndrome (SBS), particularly in the early postoperative period. Output is typically liquid and high in both digestive enzymes and alkaline, making it caustic to the skin. The amount and consistency of effluent are influenced by the type and length of remaining bowel, patient adherence to the treatment plan, and the phase of intestinal adaptation. High output is generally defined as exceeding 2 L/day and is often associated with symptoms such as dehydration, electrolyte imbalances, and early weight loss, with malnutrition becoming a concern in the longer term [6, 7].

While the core principles of ostomy care remain the same, patients with ABS require more intensive management due to the high volume and irritant nature of the effluent. A key goal is to identify a pouching system that provides consistent wear time and maintains skin integrity. Average wear times for standard colostomies and ileostomies range from 3 to 4 days, but no standard exists for high-output stomas due to variability in effluent volume and stoma anatomy. Regular assessment of barrier seal performance is essential. During pouch changes, the wafer should be examined for signs of erosion, moisture absorption, or leakage to guide reinforcement with barrier rings or caulking agents [9, 10, 15].

The physical characteristics of the stoma—such as height, location, and lumen orientation—play a major role in appliance effectiveness. Ideally, the stoma should protrude approximately 2 cm above the skin surface, with the lumen at the apex to allow efficient flow into the pouch. Stomas positioned within skin folds, near scars, or with low profiles increase the risk of leakage and skin breakdown. Although these anatomical features cannot easily be altered postoperatively, recognizing their impact can guide pouching strategies and the need for additional supportive materials [16].

Patients with SBS often present with challenging abdominal contours due to prior surgeries and weight loss, resulting in soft, doughy, or fibrotic skin. To properly assess pouching system fit, it is important to evaluate the peristomal area in multiple patient positions—lying, sitting, standing, and bending—to identify potential stress points on the barrier. These dynamic assessments allow for more personalized and effective management plans, minimizing the risk of barrier failure and improving patient outcomes [17].

20.3.2.4 Barrier Products and Wafers

Barrier products play a critical role in protecting the peristomal skin, especially in patients with SBS, where stoma effluent is typically high in volume and enzymatically active. Moisture-associated skin damage, rashes, and erosions are not expected outcomes of an ostomy and often indicate a compromised pouch seal. Barrier products are designed to maintain the integrity of the skin, smooth uneven peristomal surfaces, and support a secure wafer attachment. These include liquid skin barriers, powders for denuded or weeping skin, and caulking agents, such as pastes, strips, or rings that help create an even, sealed surface around the stoma. When treating irritated skin, alcohol-free products should be used to minimize pain and further trauma [9, 10].

Wafers, which serve as the adhesive base for the ostomy pouch, come in flat or convex forms and in standard or extended-wear options. Convex wafers are useful when the peristomal skin is uneven, scarred, or pliable, as they help improve stoma protrusion and seal integrity. Convexity can range from soft and flexible to rigid, with selection based on the firmness and contour of the abdominal wall. Extended-wear wafers are typically recommended for high-output ostomies, as they contain additional substances to resist breakdown from frequent or liquid effluent. Wafers should be cut to fit within 3 mm of the stoma margin and resized periodically, especially if the stoma changes due to weight fluctuation or surgical recovery [9, 10].

Proper fit and barrier performance should be evaluated with every pouch change. The back of the wafer should be inspected for signs of leakage, erosion, or excessive moisture absorption, which may suggest a need for additional reinforcement or a different barrier configuration. An ostomy belt may enhance convex wafer performance if the stoma lies at the natural waistline. For stomas above or below this level, belts may shift with movement and cause leaks, requiring alternative support solutions [9, 10, 18].

20.3.2.5 Ostomy Pouches and High-Output Considerations

Ostomy pouches are designed to be odor-proof and water-resistant and are available in one-piece or two-piece systems. One-piece pouches have the wafer and pouch fused together, while two-piece systems allow the pouch to detach from the wafer using mechanical or adhesive couplings. Features such as built-in filters, tail closures, and varying pouch sizes are generally selected based on patient preference and output type. Pouches are usually changed every 2–3 days, in coordination with wafer changes [9, 10, 19].

In patients with high-output ostomies, larger-capacity pouches with drainage spouts are recommended to handle the volume and weight of liquid effluent. Allowing the pouch to overfill can stress the wafer seal and contribute to peristomal breakdown. Patients should be educated to empty their pouch when it reaches one-third to one-half capacity. For extremely high volumes, connecting the pouch to a dependent drainage system—such as a bedside collection bag—can reduce strain on the seal and improve comfort. These systems are typically changed monthly and should be disinfected regularly with a diluted bleach solution [20].

20.3.2.6 Restoring Intestinal Continuity

Determining the appropriate timing and necessity of restoring intestinal continuity in patients with a distal small bowel or colonic remnant is a critical component in the management of SBS. More than 50% of patients initially receive an ostomy during their primary resection, frequently due to the urgent nature of the surgical procedure, doubts regarding the perfusion of the remaining bowel, preexisting colonic conditions, or concerns about immediate postoperative functionality [9, 10, 21].

From a functional standpoint, restoring continuity offers several potential benefits. Reintegrating segments of residual small bowel or colon can enhance nutrient absorption and overall intestinal function. In appropriate cases, this can help reduce or eliminate the need for long-term parenteral nutrition (PN). Additional advantages include elimination of the stoma, increasing the patient's quality of life.

However, this decision must be carefully individualized, considering several key factors: (i) length of the remaining small intestine (generally, ≥60–90 cm is favorable); (ii) presence and function of the ileocecal valve; (iii) condition and functional capacity of the colon; and (iv) patient's overall health and surgical risk profile. Although functional improvements may be achievable, it is important to acknowledge the possible disadvantages. Restoring continuity might result in complications, including diarrhea induced by bile acids, breakdown of the perianal skin, and an elevated risk of kidney stones, particularly when there is an increase in oxalate absorption within the colon. In certain situations, these negative outcomes could overshadow the advantages, especially in patients with limited bowel length or notable comorbidities [22].

In practice, only a limited percentage (approximately 25%) of patients with SBS who initially receive a stoma ultimately achieve a successful reversal. For certain individuals, the stoma is retained permanently due to elevated surgical risks or anticipated suboptimal postoperative function. In specific instances, transitioning a high-output proximal stoma to a more distal location may serve as a viable compromise, enhancing nutritional absorption while minimizing the risk of severe diarrhea [23].

While the traditional approach has been to delay reentry into the abdomen for 6 months or more, following complex surgery, clinical experience now suggests that repeat operations are often safely feasible after approximately 3 months, and in some cases, even earlier. The timing of reoperation, however, requires careful surgical judgment, considering the specific circumstances and complications of previous procedures. If a surgeon determines that a longer delay is necessary, the patient should be considered for referral to a specialized center with expertise in complex intestinal reconstruction [24].

20.3.3 Surgical Management of Enterocutaneous Fistulas

Enterocutaneous fistulas (EFs) most commonly occur as a postoperative complication, with up to 90% arising after abdominal surgery. Unlike surgically planned stomas, EFs develop unpredictably, often emerging in anatomically challenging locations, such as skin folds, wound edges, or over scar tissue—areas that complicate appliance adherence and effluent control. EFs are classified based on their output volume, anatomical origin, underlying cause, and number of fistula tracts, all of which influence management strategy. Successful care requires coordination between the surgical team, WOC nurses, nutritionists, and bedside clinicians, particularly in patients with high-output fistulas and short bowel syndrome [6, 7, 25].

The primary surgical management goals mirror those of ostomy care: protect the perifistular skin, contain effluent, manage odor, and establish a secure pouching system when needed. Low-output fistulas (<100 mL/day) may be managed conservatively using absorptive dressings like gauze, foam, or hydrofiber, with careful skin protection using ointments or zinc-based pastes. Fistulas with higher output generally require a pouching system, tailored to the location, number, and configuration of the fistula(s). Evaluating the patient in multiple positions helps anticipate how skin creases and body contours may affect seal integrity and wear time [9, 10, 26].

For high-output or complex EFs, pouching begins with leveling the skin around the fistula. This may involve the use of caulking materials or custom fillers, such as a paste-and-powder mixture, to fill in surface irregularities and accommodate movement. Standard ostomy appliances, commercial fistula management systems, or custom-cut barriers can be used, depending on the availability of intact skin around the fistula (typically requiring at least 2–3 in. for adequate adhesion). Templates are created to guide cutting of the appliance, ensuring a margin of intact skin is preserved. Internal dressings can be maintained within wound managers using systems that feature access windows, extending the functional life of the pouch and minimizing the frequency of full appliance changes [9, 27, 28].

Advanced drainage options may be necessary for patients with high-volume or continuous fistula output. Many pouch systems include a drainable spout or port that can be connected to dependent drainage (e.g., Foley bag) or suction systems. For suction, a drain (e.g., red rubber catheter, JP tube) may be inserted into the pouch port and secured with a stabilizer, allowing continuous evacuation of liquid effluent. Solid food intake may need to be limited, as particulate matter can clog tubing. When not on drainage, the pouch should be emptied when one-third to one-half full in order to avoid excessive weight on the wafer, which could compromise seal integrity and increase the risk of skin breakdown or leakage [29].

Negative pressure wound therapy (NPWT) can be used in conjunction with an ostomy pouch to manage open abdominal wounds complicated by enterocutaneous fistulas (EFs). The key principle is the isolation of the fistula from the surrounding wound bed to allow simultaneous control of fistula output and promotion of granulation and healing. This is achieved by first applying barrier products around the fistula to protect the skin and create separation. The open wound is then dressed with NPWT foam or gauze, typically layered over a protective nonadherent mesh to prevent direct contact with exposed bowel or viscera. A transparent occlusive drape is applied to create an airtight seal, and negative pressure is initiated [9, 10, 30].

Once suction is established, a small opening is cut in the drape directly over the isolated fistula, and an ostomy pouch is applied to collect effluent. This technique is most effective when the fistula is stomatized, well defined, and positioned in a way that allows for clear separation from the wound. It is crucial to understand that NPWT is not suitable for directly managing fistula effluent, as thick drainage can clog the suction system and compromise function. Instead, NPWT should focus on wound healing while effluent is diverted through a separate, appropriately fitted pouching system. Proper implementation of this combined approach can reduce complications, improve skin integrity, and enhance healing in complex abdominal wounds involving EFs [9, 10, 29, 30].

20.3.4 Surgical Management of Percutaneous Enteral Tube Sites

Percutaneous enteral tubes, such as gastrostomy or jejunostomy tubes, are frequently associated with minor complications including skin irritation, leakage, bleeding, infection, and hypergranulation tissue formation. These issues are often exacerbated by poor tube positioning, excess movement, or incorrect dressing practices. From a surgical standpoint, proper tube placement and secure anchoring are critical in preventing stoma site enlargement and subsequent leakage. The external retention bumper should sit lightly on the skin—typically 0.5–1 cm above the surface—to prevent pressure injuries while minimizing mobility. Excessive tightening or looseness can result in pressure ulcers or leaks, both of which compromise skin integrity and can increase the risk of infection or need for tube revision [31].

Routine site care and inspection are essential to identify early signs of breakdown, such as moisture-associated dermatitis, denudation, or infection. Daily gentle cleaning with mild soap and water under the retention bumper, without shifting or sliding the bumper, helps prevent damage over time. Use of harsh chemicals or routine topical antibiotics should be avoided, as they may worsen skin conditions. For minor irritation, alcohol-free barrier wipes and oil-based ointments may provide adequate protection. Leakage should be managed promptly, as gastric or enteric effluent is caustic and can rapidly break down the surrounding skin. Frequent dressing changes and minimizing moisture retention are key to preventing further complications.

Pressure injuries and hypergranulation tissue are common with improperly secured tubes or when retention bumpers apply constant pressure. Thin foam or alginate dressings may help relieve localized pressure, but the underlying cause—such as a tight bumper or short tube length—must be corrected. Hypergranulation can lead to persistent drainage, pain, and bleeding, and may require treatment with silver nitrate, topical steroids, moisture-managing dressings, or surgical excision under local anesthesia. Surgical teams should monitor tube site healing closely, particularly in high-risk patients (e.g., obese, immunocompromised, diabetic), and intervene early to prevent chronic wound complications [32].

Correct tube anchoring is one of the most effective strategies to reduce stoma complications. Tubes lacking built-in retention devices should be immobilized using adhesive patches, commercial tube holders, or custom solutions, such as anchoring with a modified ostomy wafer and baby bottle nipple setup. These methods provide cost-effective, patient-specific stabilization to prevent in/out motion of the tube, which can enlarge the stoma tract and perpetuate leakage. Simply upsizing the tube to manage leakage is not a definitive solution and may worsen the problem if mobility persists.

From a surgical management perspective, minimizing complications begins with proper placement technique, appropriate site selection, and careful attention to abdominal wall anatomy. Follow-up should include patient and caregiver education on daily care, recognition of early signs of skin compromise, and maintenance of tube positioning. When persistent site issues occur despite optimal care, referral to a wound care specialist or surgical re-evaluation may be necessary to prevent escalation to more serious wound or infectious complications.

20.3.5 Autologous Gastrointestinal Reconstruction

Autologous gastrointestinal reconstruction pertains to the surgical alteration of the existing small or large intestine in patients with short bowel syndrome. This process typically employs surgical methods designed to address intestinal dilation, thereby enhancing the exposure of the mucosal absorptive surface to the enteric flow. Candidates for autologous reconstruction must not have responded to standard medical treatment and present with small intestine dilation exceeding 3.5 cm. A range of surgical techniques is available for modifying the dilated intestine, aiming to enhance overall functionality. The outcomes associated with these techniques, both in the short and long term, are generally comparable [6, 7].

One of the consequences of SBS is the progressive dilation of the residual small intestine, often occurring without a clear mechanical obstruction. While the exact mechanism remains uncertain, this dilation may be part of the natural intestinal adaptation process. In some cases, however, it results from partial obstructions, which can be surgically relieved to allow the bowel to return to a more normal caliber. In certain instances, some surgical approaches have been proposed to intentionally induce near-complete obstruction to promote dilation, serving as a preparatory step for autologous bowel reconstruction procedures [33].

These autologous reconstruction techniques, often referred to as "lengthening procedures," are aimed not only at increasing intestinal length but more importantly at normalizing luminal diameter. Dilated bowel segments often exhibit poor motility and are prone to bacterial overgrowth due to stasis and remixing of intestinal contents, which impairs tolerance of enteral feeding. Surgical tapering or enteroplasty addresses these issues by reducing the diameter of the bowel, improving motility, enhancing nutrient absorption, and potentially enabling weaning from parenteral nutrition. The perceived lengthening effect is thus secondary to the functional benefits achieved through reshaping the bowel [34].

There remains some debate in the surgical community regarding the role of dilation as a potentially beneficial adaptation. Some advocate for promoting or preserving dilation to maximize mucosal surface area, followed by planned enteroplasty. This approach suggests that dilation can be harnessed rather than reversed to improve long-term outcomes. Others argue for early intervention to restore normal diameter and function. At present, the optimal strategy remains uncertain, and surgical decisions must be individualized based on patient anatomy, symptoms, and nutritional goals.

20.3.6 The Longitudinal Intestinal Lengthening and Tapering Procedure

The Longitudinal Intestinal Lengthening and Tapering (LILT) procedure, also known as the Bianchi procedure, is a surgical technique developed in the 1980s to address bowel dilation and insufficient intestinal length in patients with short bowel syndrome. The procedure takes advantage of the mesenteric blood supply, which fans out to each side of the intestine, allowing for safe longitudinal division of the bowel into two parallel, well-vascularized segments. LILT is typically applied to moderately or severely dilated segments of small intestine, excluding short segments (<10 cm), the duodenum, and areas that have previously undergone enteroplasty (with some exceptions) [6, 7, 35].

The surgery begins by opening the dilated segment longitudinally along its antimesenteric border. The surgeon then develops the plane between the two mesenteric vascular pedicles. With careful dissection and traction, the bowel is divided into two equal halves, each supported by its own mesenteric blood supply. These segments are then tubularized and reconnected in a looped "lazy S" configuration, which maintains isoperistalsis. This reconstruction aims not only to lengthen the intestine but also to normalize luminal diameter and improve motility, reducing complications like bacterial overgrowth and poor nutrient absorption.

There are variations in surgical technique. In the original description, the bowel was divided manually using electrocautery and sutured by hand. A modified approach uses a longitudinal stapler to divide the bowel more rapidly, but this method has been associated with a higher rate of certain complications, such as staple-line breakdown or intraloop fistula formation, especially if not executed with meticulous technique.

Surgical risks include the standard complications of major gastrointestinal surgery—such as anastomotic leak, bleeding, and infection—as well as unique risks like segmental ischemia or necrosis due to compromised blood supply. Long-term issues may include stricture formation and fistulas between adjacent loops, particularly when stapling is used instead of hand sewing. These risks emphasize the need for careful patient selection, surgical expertise, and close postoperative monitoring. Long-term outcomes following LILT are highly variable, largely influenced by patient anatomy, and the expertise of the surgical center. Reported success rates for complete weaning from parenteral nutrition range widely—from as low as 4% to as high as 100%—with an average of around 70%. Most patients who achieve enteral autonomy do so within 1–2 years postoperatively. Ultimately, LILT remains a valuable option for select patients with SBS and dilated small bowel, particularly when performed in experienced centers with a multidisciplinary approach to postoperative care [36, 37].

20.3.7 The Serial Transverse Enteroplasty Procedure

The STEP procedure, introduced in 2003 by Kim et al., has become the most commonly performed bowel-lengthening surgery worldwide for the treatment of short bowel syndrome. STEP involves applying a series of alternating transverse staple lines along a dilated segment of bowel using a gastrointestinal anastomosis stapler. This zigzag pattern effectively reduces the luminal diameter to approximately 2 cm while simultaneously increasing the overall length of the intestine—sometimes by more than 100%, depending on the segment's initial diameter. This is a key advantage over the LILT (Longitudinal Intestinal Lengthening and Tapering) procedure, which typically cannot achieve more than a 100% length gain [5, 6, 36].

Surgical precision is critical during the STEP procedure. Staple lines must cross the longitudinal midline of the bowel in an alternating pattern to form an effective and uniform zigzag. The orientation of the bowel must be carefully maintained throughout the operation to ensure symmetrical tapering and avoid twisting or misalignment. While staple firings can be performed either transversely or in a mesenteric-to-antimesenteric fashion, the latter may offer better control of alignment. A small incision in the mesentery is often required to facilitate proper stapler placement while avoiding vascular injury. Once complete, all staple lines should be inspected and reinforced as needed [37].

One of STEP's advantages is its versatility and adaptability. The procedure can be repeated in segments that have previously undergone STEP or even a LILT procedure, and it can be applied to short dilated segments or, with caution, portions of the duodenum. However, repeat operations can be challenging if the initial staple lines were poorly aligned or placed off-axis. In such cases, restoring uniform luminal diameter may require a combination of extending staple lines, adding new ones, or performing excisional tapering. Nevertheless, repeat STEP procedures have shown outcomes comparable to primary surgeries when performed by experienced hands.

A more recent extension of the STEP technique involves its use in infants during their initial surgery, such as in cases of intestinal atresia. This is intended to address discrepancies in diameter between a dilated proximal bowel and a narrower distal segment, which can impair anastomotic function. Historically, proximal tapering enteroplasty was used in such cases, but surgeons now sometimes opt for STEP. However, the short staple lines typical of these neonatal procedures often fail to maintain a reduced diameter long term. When reoperation is needed, these previously stapled segments can complicate subsequent attempts at effective tapering, and long-term outcomes for this indication remain unclear. This application should therefore be reserved for centers with expertise in complex intestinal reconstruction [38].

In terms of operative safety, STEP can generally be performed with low morbidity when done by skilled surgeons. Complication rates are similar to those observed with LILT, though STEP appears to have a lower risk of intraloop fistulization, possibly due to the standardized stapling technique. Following a successful STEP, patients often show gradual reduction in dependence on parenteral nutrition over 6–12 months, with a corresponding increase in enteral intake. Reported rates of parenteral nutrition weaning vary widely, from 20% to 100%, with an average of 60–70%, which is similar to outcomes seen with LILT [38, 39].

Long-term complications of STEP include recurrent bowel dilation, stricture formation, and delayed gastrointestinal bleeding. Recurrent dilation may result from technical inadequacies during the initial procedure or from progressive underlying bowel pathology. Strictures are typically the result of overcorrection—narrowing the lumen too aggressively in an effort to lengthen the bowel—leading to impaired flow and feeding intolerance. These often require surgical revision, such as stricturoplasty or segmental resection. Delayed GI bleeding is less common but may also necessitate intervention.

An additional concern observed in some cases is the development of an unexplained inflammatory response in distal segments of the small intestine, often near the colon. These segments do not show ischemia and are not associated with similar changes elsewhere in the bowel. The etiology is unclear but may involve altered microbial populations following bowel reconstruction. In select cases, this inflammatory response has recurred even after resection and may respond to immunomodulatory therapy. This highlights the need for long-term follow-up and individualized management in patients undergoing STEP.

20.3.8 The Spiral Intestinal Lengthening and Tapering Procedure

The Spiral Intestinal Lengthening and Tapering (SILT) procedure is a recently developed enteroplasty technique designed for use in dilated bowel segments, particularly those that are appropriate for LILT but may be too short to allow traditional longitudinal division. It is not typically suited for reoperations following prior enteroplasty. The surgical technique involves marking the bowel orientation and creating a series of alternating 60° spiral incisions along the length of the dilated segment. This configuration enables the surgeon to apply longitudinal traction, effectively lengthening the bowel and tapering its diameter. The cut edges are then reanastomosed to form a narrowed, isoperistaltic segment, preserving the natural direction of peristalsis [40].

Unlike the STEP procedure, which creates a zigzag configuration and may alter peristaltic flow, SILT aims to maintain the bowel's native longitudinal alignment, potentially offering better physiological motility. While early technical results are promising, and perioperative morbidity appears comparable to that of other enteroplasty procedures, published outcome data remain limited due to the novelty of the technique. Further studies are needed to evaluate its long-term impact on enteral tolerance and nutritional autonomy in patients with short bowel syndrome [41].

20.3.9 The Excisional Tapering Enteroplasty

The tapering enteroplasty is a valuable surgical option for managing bowel dilation, particularly when the goal is to reduce luminal diameter without altering the native orientation of smooth muscle fibers or the myenteric plexus. The most widely used method is the longitudinal excisional tapering enteroplasty, which involves resecting a strip of the antimesenteric bowel wall along the dilated segment, typically using a stapler [42]. This reduces the diameter of the bowel to a more physiologic size, thereby improving the volume-to-surface area ratio, which enhances motility and nutrient transit. The procedure preserves the bowel's longitudinal structure, allowing for the later application of other enteroplasty techniques (e.g., STEP, SILT, or LILT) if needed.

This technique is most appropriate when bowel length is sufficient and further lengthening would not significantly improve function. It is especially effective in the duodenum, where dilation can hinder gastric emptying, and in short, dilated segments, particularly in areas previously modified by STEP where additional transverse staple lines cannot be placed. Although tapering results in a modest loss of absorptive surface, this trade-off is usually acceptable when it leads to improved luminal uniformity and function. In certain rare disorders like intestinal myopathies or idiopathic dilation, tapering can be performed over long segments—sometimes up to 200 cm—requiring careful attention to avoid over-narrowing and to maintain bowel orientation.

A nonexcisional variation of the tapering enteroplasty exists, where the antimesenteric surface is imbricated rather than resected. This technique reduces the diameter by folding excess tissue inward, minimizing the risk of leaks. However, it is less effective in bulky bowel segments and has a tendency to re-dilate over time, potentially compromising long-term outcomes. While it may have selected use—such as in high-risk duodenal segments where leak avoidance is critical—excisional tapering remains the preferred and more reliable technique in most cases due to its durable and functional results [43].

20.3.10 Operations to Slow Intestinal Transit in the Absence of Bowel Dilatation

In patients with SBS but without significant bowel dilation, certain surgical procedures aim to slow intestinal transit to enhance nutrient absorption. One of the most promising techniques is segmental reversal of the small bowel (SRSB), which involves reversing a 10–12 cm segment of small intestine to create an antiperistaltic segment, typically placed just upstream of a stoma or small bowel-colon anastomosis. Factors associated with better outcomes include earlier timing after enterectomy, longer reversed segments, and extended care within a nutrition-focused program [44, 45].

Another less commonly performed option is isoperistaltic colonic interposition, in which a segment of colon is inserted into the small bowel while maintaining the direction of peristalsis. Although initially described in animal models, limited human data exist. The largest series followed six infants, three of whom achieved enteral autonomy within 4 months. However, the remaining three failed to wean from PN and died within 2 years. Given the mixed outcomes and the advancement of intestinal transplantation, this approach is considered experimental and should be approached cautiously, especially in infants with severe SBS [46, 47].

20.4 The Future of Surgical Management of SBS

The future of surgical management of SBS is evolving with advancements in regenerative medicine, bioengineering, and innovative surgical techniques, aiming to improve long-term outcomes and reduce dependence on PN. One of the most promising developments is tissue engineering and bioartificial intestine fabrication, where researchers are exploring the use of stem cells, scaffold-based tissue regeneration, and intestinal organoids to grow functional intestinal tissue for transplantation [48]. This approach has the potential to restore absorptive function without the need for traditional transplantation and immunosuppression.

Additionally, refinements in intestinal lengthening procedures, such as robot-assisted and minimally invasive techniques may allow for more precise anastomotic reconstruction, reducing postsurgical complications such as strictures, dysmotility, and bacterial overgrowth [49]. Advances in intestinal transplantation are also making significant strides, with improvements in immunosuppressive protocols, tolerance induction strategies, and gene editing, potentially reducing the risk of graft rejection and long-term complications [50].

Furthermore, the integration of AI and precision medicine into surgical planning and postoperative monitoring is expected to enhance decision-making and predict individualized patient outcomes, leading to more personalized and effective interventions [51]. As these technologies continue to develop, the future of SBS surgery is moving toward less invasive, more regenerative, and highly personalized treatment approaches, ultimately improving quality of life and enteral autonomy for patients.

20.5 Conclusions

The surgical management of short bowel syndrome (SBS) presents a complex and evolving challenge, requiring a highly individualized, multidisciplinary approach. Surgeons play a critical role, from initial emergency interventions to intricate bowel reconstruction and continuity restoration. Despite significant advances in techniques such as longitudinal and transverse enteroplasty, autologous gastrointestinal reconstruction, and improved ostomy and fistula care, many patients continue to face substantial hurdles in achieving long-term intestinal autonomy.

Key challenges remain in determining the optimal timing and selection of reconstructive procedures, particularly in the setting of severe bowel dilation or high-output stomas. While methods like STEP and LILT have improved outcomes, the risk of complications, such as strictures, fistulization, and recurrent dilation, persists. Furthermore, managing high-output stomas and enterocutaneous fistulas still relies heavily on specialized wound and ostomy care, which may not be universally accessible.

Another unresolved issue lies in predicting which patients will benefit from restorative procedures and which may ultimately require intestinal transplantation. Functional outcomes vary widely, and there is currently no standardized algorithm to guide surgical decision-making across diverse patient presentations. The role of novel techniques, such as SILT, and the long-term implications of reversing intestinal segments or utilizing colonic interpositions also require further validation through clinical trials and long-term studies.

Ultimately, the goal of surgical care in SBS is not only to restore anatomy but also to optimize function, preserve quality of life, and reduce dependence on parenteral nutrition. Continued innovation, improved access to multidisciplinary teams, and more robust outcome data are essential for addressing the persistent gaps in care and improving prognosis for this complex patient population.

References

1. Iyer KR. Surgical management of short bowel syndrome. JPEN J Parenter Enteral Nutr. 2014;38(1 Suppl):53S–9S.
2. Bering J, DiBaise JK. Short bowel syndrome in adults. Am J Gastroenterol. 2022;117(6):876–83.
3. Billiauws L, Maggiori L, Joly F, Panis Y. Medical and surgical management of short bowel syndrome. J Visc Surg. 2018;155(4):283–91.
4. Muff JL, Sokolovski F, Walsh-Korb Z, Choudhury RA, Dunn JC, Holland-Cunz SG, Vuille-dit-Bille RN. Surgical treatment of short bowel syndrome—the past, the present and the future: a descriptive review of the literature. Children (Basel). 2022;9(7):1024.
5. Caporilli C, Giannì G, Grassi F, Esposito S. An overview of short-bowel syndrome in pediatric patients: focus on clinical management and prevention of complications. Nutrients. 2023;15(10):2341.
6. Thompson JS, Rochling FA, Mercer DF, Weseman R. Postoperative short bowel syndrome. J Am Coll Surg. 2005;201:85–9.
7. Berke CT, Brown C. Surgical considerations in the short bowel syndrome. In: DiBaise JK, Parrish CR, Thompson JS, editors. Short bowel syndrome: practical approach to management. Boca Raton (FL): CRC Press; 2016. p. 277–92.
8. Thompson JS, Mercer DF, Mangus RS. Mesenteric ischemia: acute mesenteric arterial ischemia. In: Schein M, Wise L, editors. Critical controversies in surgery. New York: Springer; 2001. p. 167–74.
9. Wound Ostomy and Continence Nurse Society. Management of the patient with a fecal ostomy: best practice guideline for clinicians. Mount Laurel (NJ): Author; 2010. p. i–44.
10. Gray M, Colwell JC, Doughty D, Black P. Peristomal moisture-associated skin damage in adults with fecal ostomies. J Wound Ostomy Continence Nurs. 2013;40(4):389–99.
11. Kim HB, Fauza D, Garza J, Oh JT, Nurko S, Jaksic T. Serial transverse enteroplasty (STEP): a novel bowel lengthening procedure. J Pediatr Surg. 2003;38(3):425–9.
12. Thompson JS. Strategies for preserving intestinal length in the short-bowel syndrome. Dis Colon Rectum. 1987;30:208–13.
13. Thompson JS, Mercer DF, Haase GM, et al. Morphologic and nutritional responses to intestinal patching following intestinal resection. Surgery. 1988;103:79–86.
14. Carlsson E, Persson E, Eeg-Olofsson K, Hallén A-M. Living with an ostomy and short bowel syndrome: practical aspects and impact on daily life. J Wound Ostomy Continence Nurs. 2001;28(2):96–105.
15. McDonald A. Orchestrating the management of patients with high-output stomas. Br J Nurs. 2014;23(12):645–9.
16. Diamond IR, de Silva N, Pencharz PB, Kim JH, Wales PW. Advantages of the distal sigmoid colostomy in the management of infants with short bowel syndrome. J Pediatr Surg. 2008;43:1464–7.

17. Thompson JS, Mercer DF, Sudan D. Predicting outcome of procedures to slow intestinal transit. Transplant Proc. 2006;38:1838–9.
18. Colwell JC. Principles of stoma management. In: Colwell JC, Goldberg MT, Carmel JE, editors. Fecal & urinary diversions: management principles. St. Louis: Mosby; 2004. p. 240–62.
19. Sica J, Callan E, Hegarty J. Management of intestinal failure and high-output stomas. Br J Nurs. 2007;16(13):772–7.
20. Baker ML, Williams RN, Nightingale JM. Causes and management of a high-output stoma. Color Dis. 2010;13:191–7.
21. Mercer DF. Surgical considerations in the management of short bowel syndrome. Nutr Clin Pract. 2023;38:S88–97.
22. Guillen B, Atherton NS. Short bowel syndrome. In: StatPearls. Treasure Island (FL): StatPearls Publishing; 2023.
23. Vantini I, Zancan L, Rosti L, et al. Survival rate and prognostic factors in patients with intestinal failure. Dig Liver Dis. 2004;36:46–55.
24. Ball CG, Feliciano DV. The art and craft of reoperative abdominal surgery after prior trauma or acute care surgery operation. J Am Coll Surg. 2020;231(5):e1–6.
25. Hoedema RE, Andrews JS. Enterostomal therapy and wound care of the enterocutaneous fistula patient. Clin Colon Rectal Surg. 2010;23(3):161–8.
26. Gribovskaja-Rupp I, Melton GB. Enterocutaneous fistula: proven strategies and updates. Clin Colon Rectal Surg. 2016;29(2):130–7.
27. Evenson AR, Fischer JE. Current management of enterocutaneous fistula. J Gastrointest Surg. 2006;10(3):455–64.
28. Wound Ostomy and Continence Nurses Society. WOCN Society and ASCRS position statement on preoperative stoma site marking for patients undergoing colostomy or ileostomy surgery. Mount Laurel (NJ): Author; 2014.
29. Haffejee AA. Surgical management of high-output enterocutaneous fistulae: a 24-year experience. Curr Opin Clin Nutr Metab Care. 2004;7(3):309–16.
30. Llanos S, Danilla S, Barraza C, et al. Effectiveness of negative pressure closure in the integration of exposed enteric fistula in the open abdomen. Wound Repair Regen. 2006;14(3):320–5.
31. Blumenstein I, Shastri YM, Stein J. Gastroenteric tube feeding: techniques, problems and solutions. World J Gastroenterol. 2014;20(26):8505–24.
32. Wound Ostomy and Continence Nurse Society. Management of gastrostomy tube complications for the pediatric and adult patient. Mount Laurel (NJ): Author; 2008.
33. Mercer DF. Autologous gastrointestinal reconstruction. In: DiBaise JK, Parrish CR, Thompson JS, editors. Short bowel syndrome: practical approach to management. Boca Raton (FL): CRC Press; 2016. p. 293–300.
34. Panis Y, Le Gall C, Meurette G, et al. Segmental reversal of the small bowel as an alternative to intestinal transplantation in patients with short bowel syndrome. Ann Surg. 1997;225:401–7.
35. Frongia G, Kessler M, Weih S, et al. Comparison of LILT and STEP procedures in children with short bowel syndrome: a systematic review of the literature. J Pediatr Surg. 2013;48(8):1794–805.
36. van Praagh JB, Hofker HS, Haveman JW. Comparing bowel lengthening procedures: which, when, and why? Curr Opin Organ Transplant. 2022;27(2):112–8.
37. Jones BA, Hull MA, Potanos K, et al. Report of 111 consecutive patients enrolled in the International Serial Transverse Enteroplasty (STEP) Data Registry: a retrospective observational study. J Am Coll Surg. 2013;216(3):438–46.
38. Khalil AI, Abbass AA, El Monaem AHEDA, Yousef Salem AAA. Serial transverse enteroplasty (STEP) versus longitudinal intestinal lengthening and tailoring (LILT): systematic review and meta-analysis of outcomes and complications. QJM. 2024;117(Suppl 1):hcae070-228.
39. Shah AA, Petrosyan M, Franklin AL, et al. Autologous intestinal reconstruction: a single institution study of the serial transverse enteroplasty (STEP) and the longitudinal intestinal lengthening and tailoring (LILT). Pediatr Surg Int. 2019;35:649–55.

40. Cserni T, Nagy E, Kalmár-Nagy K, et al. The first clinical application of the spiral intestinal lengthening and tailoring (SILT) in extreme short bowel syndrome. J Gastrointest Surg. 2014;18(10):1852–7.
41. Fujiki M, Armanyous SR, ElSherif A, et al. Serial transverse enteroplasty and the re-establishment of enteral autonomy among the adult population: new insights with advanced clinical practice and novel outcome predictive model. Ann Surg. 2025; https://doi.org/10.1097/SLA.0000000000006072.
42. Wales PW, de Silva N, Kim J, Lecce L, To T, Moore A. Delayed primary serial transverse enteroplasty as a novel management strategy for infants with congenital ultra-short bowel syndrome. J Pediatr Surg. 2013;48(5):993–9.
43. Vaghiri S, Alipouriani A, Knoefel WT, et al. Extended mesenteric resection reduces the rate of surgical recurrence in Crohn's disease: a systematic review and meta-analysis. Int J Color Dis. 2025;40(1):51.
44. Beyer-Berjot L, Dabadie A, Cosse C, et al. Segmental reversal of the small bowel can end permanent parenteral nutrition dependency: an experience of 38 adults with short bowel syndrome. Ann Surg. 2012;256:739–44.
45. Thompson JS, Rochling FA, Weseman R, Mercer DF. Effect of reversed intestinal segments on intestinal structure and function. J Surg Res. 1995;58:19–27.
46. Diamond IR, de Silva N, Pencharz PB, Kim JH, Wales PW. Does the colon play a role in intestinal adaptation in infants with short bowel syndrome? A multiple variable analysis. J Pediatr Surg. 2010;45(5):975–9.
47. Boroni G, Parolini F, Stern MV, Moglia C, Alberti D. Autologous intestinal reconstruction surgery in short bowel syndrome: which, when, and why. Front Nutr. 2022;9:861093.
48. Deutsch L, Cloutier A, Lal S. Advances in chronic intestinal failure management and therapies. Curr Opin Gastroenterol. 2020;36(3):223–9.
49. Frau T, El Khatib M, De Dreuille B, et al. Emerging drugs for the treatment of short bowel syndrome. Expert Opin Emerg Drugs. 2024;29(3):277–88.
50. Di Cocco P, Martinino A, Pinto F, et al. Living donor intestinal transplantation. Gastroenterol Clin N Am. 2024;53(3):441–52.
51. Kenig N, Monton Echeverria J, Muntaner Vives A. Artificial intelligence in surgery: a systematic review of use and validation. J Clin Med. 2024;13(23):7108.

Intestinal Transplantation in Short Bowel Syndrome

21

Daniel Timofte, Sebastian Zenovia, and Cristina Muzica

21.1 Introduction

Short bowel syndrome (SBS) occurs when the small intestine reaches less than 180–200 cm, following intestinal resection, when the typical length ranges from 275 to 850 cm. It is the most common cause of intestinal failure (IF), which the European Society for Clinical Nutrition and Metabolism defines as a condition where the gut's functionality is insufficient to absorb essential macronutrients, water, or electrolytes, making intravenous supplementation necessary to sustain health or support growth [1].

The number of hospitalizations for patients with chronic intestinal failure (CIF) caused by SBS increased in one decade by 55%, from 4037 in 2005 to 6265 in 2014. This increase was primarily due to complications such as fluid and electrolyte imbalances (52.5%), catheter-related bloodstream infections leading to sepsis (41.4%), and malnutrition (40.1%) [2]. CIF is a severe condition in which the body is unable to absorb the necessary nutrients and fluids to sustain vital functions and patients with CIF rely on parenteral nutrition (PN), administered intravenously, to receive carbohydrates, proteins, fats, water, electrolytes, trace elements, and essential vitamins needed for maintaining health. PN is delivered daily over several hours and requires a long-term central venous catheter (CVC) [3].

D. Timofte
Surgery Department, Grigore T. Popa University of Medicine and Pharmacy, Iaşi, Romania

St. Spiridon Emergency Hospital, General Surgery Clinic, Iaşi, Romania
e-mail: daniel.timofte@umfiasi.ro

S. Zenovia (✉) · C. Muzica
Gastroenterology Department, Grigore T. Popa University of Medicine and Pharmacy, Iaşi, Romania

Institute of Gastroenterology and Hepatology, St. Spiridon Emergency Hospital, Iaşi, Romania

A. Trifan et al. (eds.), *Short Bowel Syndrome in Adults*,
https://doi.org/10.1007/978-3-031-95848-9_21

A recently approved drug, teduglutide (a glucagon-like peptide-2 (GLP-2) analog), offers some patients with SBS-related intestinal failure the possibility of reducing or discontinuing PN. However, this treatment comes at a high cost, estimated at $300,000/year, and carries significant risks, including the potential development of colonic polyps and cancers [4, 5]. The only definitive cure for CIF is intestinal transplantation (ITx), which enables patients who can no longer tolerate PN due to complications to regain the ability to eat and drink normally. ITx has been a recognized treatment for over three decades and was initially offered to patients with IF who could no longer receive intravenous nutrition due to end-stage venous access loss or advanced liver disease. However, with costs exceeding $1 million per transplant and the risks associated with lifelong immunosuppression—including severe complications and even mortality—ITx is reserved for patients facing life-threatening PN-related complications [6].

According to the Intestinal Transplant Registry, a total of 4103 intestinal transplant procedures, with or without a liver graft, have been performed worldwide up to 2019 since the registry was established in 1985 [7]. Recent advancements in surgical techniques and immunosuppressive therapies have led to better short-term outcomes for ITx patients, including improved survival rates and digestive independence. However, this procedure should be reserved for a highly specific group of SBS patients who experience severe, irreversible complications from PN and have no prospects for intestinal recovery [6]. ITx can be categorized into several types: isolated small bowel, combined liver-intestine, multivisceral transplantation (MVT), and modified MVT, having, over the years, transitioned from being an experimental procedure to a vital, life-saving treatment for patients with intestinal failure. Although it is often performed as a standalone procedure, ITx can also be combined with a liver transplant (orthotopic liver transplantation [OLT] + ITx); or with the liver, stomach, and pancreas MVT; or with just the stomach and pancreas (modified MVT) [8]. The causes of intestinal failure, the choice of graft type, surgical approaches, outcomes, and the achievement of nutritional independence vary between adults and children. Children generally respond well to long-term parenteral nutrition; both parents and physicians aim to support children's growth into adulthood before considering a transplant, and only if complications make it absolutely necessary, the procedure can be performed, though with high risk. It is advisable to refer patients for an early evaluation for intestinal transplantation in order to address those with a high risk of mortality, enhance the chances of discontinuing parenteral nutrition, and avoid complications associated with its failure.

21.2 Indications for Intestinal Transplantation

The degree of nutrient absorption directly correlates with the length of the remaining bowel.

Patients at the highest risk of malnutrition—and thus candidates for ITx—typically include those with a duodenostomy or jejunoileal anastomosis and ≤35 cm of residual small intestine, those with a jejunocolic or ileocolic anastomosis and

≤60 cm of residual small intestine, and those with an end jejunostomy and ≤115 cm of residual small intestine. In 2002, the Centers for Medicare and Medicaid Services officially recognized ITx for adult patients as a standard treatment rather than an experimental procedure, later extending approval to pediatric patients. When establishing eligibility criteria for ITx, Medicare acknowledged the high survival rates of patients with CIF receiving PN, with 1-year survival exceeding 90% and 4-year survival ranging from 80% to 85% [9, 10]. Medicare criteria for ITx can be summarized as the presence of irreversible CIF, effectively defined as permanent dependence on PN along with the development of PN-related complications (Table 21.1). The most common complications include intestinal failure–associated liver disease, catheter-related issues such as recurrent life-threatening sepsis, a single episode of fungal sepsis, or metastatic infections like endocarditis or osteomyelitis. Additionally, ITx may be indicated when central venous access is lost due to central venous stenosis or thrombosis. The time from the decision to refer a patient for ITx evaluation to the actual transplant date varies and is often prolonged (Table 21.2). Several factors contribute to these delays, including the patient's medical complexity, the need to travel long distances to a specialized referral center, and extended wait times after being placed on the transplant list due to the availability of a suitable donor [11].

As a result, delays in referral for ITx evaluation can lead to many patients with CIF requiring simultaneous liver transplantation at the time of ITx, which is associated with significantly higher mortality while on the waiting list [12].

The American Society for Transplantation established guidelines for appropriate indications for ITx in both adults and pediatric patients. They identified three categories of patients who should be considered for ITx: those with complications of intestinal failure, those with a low likelihood of survival, and those with significantly reduced quality of life [13]. Complications of intestinal failure include severe liver disease, recurring sepsis, and impending loss of vascular access. Patients with a low likelihood of survival include those with extremely short bowel syndrome (defined as less than 10 cm of small bowel distal to the ligament of Treitz without an ileocecal valve), as well as enterocyte defects like microvillus inclusion disease and tufting enteropathy. The final category, reduced quality of life, includes patients with high output requiring challenging fluid management and those with

Table 21.1 Criteria for intestinal transplantation based on international consensus

Severe and irreversible intestinal failure accompanied by significant complications: • Frequent or life-threatening septic episodes • Loss of at least 50% of central venous access sites • Persistent and uncontrollable fluid balance disturbances • Liver disease accompanied by portal hypertension
The consensus criteria of the working group for consultation or referral (in addition to the above): • Children who have undergone extensive small bowel resection • Children with severely damaged intestines and significant morbidity • Ongoing uncertainty in prognosis or diagnosis • Microvillus inclusion disease or intestinal epithelial dysplasia

Table 21.2 Criteria for waiting list inclusion of patients for intestinal transplantation[a]

Signs of advanced or worsening liver disease related to intestinal failure: • Bilirubin >75 μmol/L (4.5 mg/dL), despite intravenous lipid modification methods, lasting for more than 2 months[b] • Any combination of raised bilirubin, altered synthesis function (evidenced by low albumin or an increased international normalized ratio), and indications of portal hypertension and hypersplenism, especially a low platelet count, persisting for over 1 month in the absence of any complicating infectious events
Thrombosis in three out of four distinct upper body central veins (left subclavian and internal jugular, right subclavian and internal jugular) or blockage of a brachiocephalic vein in children. In adults, this criterion should be assessed on a case-by-case basis
Patients who are indefinitely dependent on parenteral nutrition face life-threatening morbidity, whether stemming from anatomical or functional causes, as indicated by the following: • In pediatric patients, two admissions to an intensive care unit after initial recovery from the event leading to IF occur due to cardiorespiratory failure, necessitating mechanical ventilation or inotrope infusion, resulting from sepsis or other complications associated with IF • In adults, this should be evaluated on a case-by-case basis
Invasive intra-abdominal desmoid tumors in adolescents and adults
Acute diffuse intestinal infarction accompanied by hepatic failure
Failure of the first intestinal transplant

[a]Patients are presumed to have undergone evaluation by a multidisciplinary team, rehabilitation options have been considered, and they are in a condition of permanent or life-limiting intestinal failure

[b]A total serum bilirubin level of 62 or 70 μmol/L is associated with increased mortality rates. A bilirubin level of 75 μmol/L serves as a useful consensus marker for progressive liver disease; however, it must be evaluated alongside other clinical parameters

pseudo-obstruction who experience recurrent bowel dilation and pain [13, 14]. Advancements in parenteral nutrition management and the reduction of complications have significantly changed the field of intestine transplantation. As a result, in 2019, a new consensus panel re-evaluated the existing criteria for intestine transplant indications. The working group of transplant experts critically examined the original indications to assess whether updates were necessary. Specifically, the group questioned whether the loss of two access sites and recurrent sepsis, in the absence of life-threatening episodes, should be sufficient to justify an intestine transplant [14] (Table 21.2).

Demographic factors and the underlying disease may influence decisions related to placement on the transplant waiting list. In contrast to the variable clinical progression typically observed in short bowel syndrome, certain conditions warrant early listing for transplantation due to their consistently unfavorable prognosis. IF resulting from SBS in infants and children is now linked to prolonged survival on PN for varying lengths of time in approximately 85–100% of patients, while in adults, the 5-year survival rate on PN ranges from 58% to 83%, with an increased risk of death associated with the patient's age and the specific underlying condition causing the IF [15]. Historically, patients with ultrashort bowel—defined as less than 10 cm in children and less than 20 cm in adults—have been considered appropriate candidates for immediate listing. This is due to the low probability of discontinuing parenteral nutrition (PN) and the elevated risk of severe infections and chronic liver failure, either individually or collectively. However, in modern practice, patients with ultrashort bowel can remain on PN for extended periods, which raises questions about the continued appropriateness of this traditional approach [6, 15, 16]. Although conclusions are limited due to the small number of cases reported, it appears that those who cannot have enterocolonic continuity restored have a worse prognosis than those who can, and in the absence of more definitive evidence, they may still be considered on a case-by-case basis for early placement on the transplant waiting list.

21.2.1 Indications for Intestinal Retransplantation

ITx is a high-risk procedure with a small, yet real, possibility of graft loss, and a high mortality rate.

Early graft loss can occur due to technical issues like graft ischemia or severe, irreversible acute rejection [17]. However, as with all organ transplants, as long-term survival rates improve for ITx recipients, it has become evident that late-stage graft loss, caused by chronic allograft enteropathy or chronic rejection, happens in 7–10% of cases [18]. In these cases, meticulous immunosuppressive management and retransplantation in appropriately selected patients can result in successful long-term survival with a functioning second graft. Additionally, in well-selected patients, strategically planned retransplantation can achieve outcomes similar to those of first-time ITx. Managing immunosuppression during the transition and induction of the second graft, addressing risks of sepsis and allosensitization (with the development of preformed antibodies), and technical factors such as planning the vascular reconstruction for the second graft are key aspects that influence patient survival [19].

21.3 Preemptive Intestinal Transplantation

As the outcomes of intestinal rehabilitation improve, particularly with the addition of teduglutide to the range of available multimodal treatments, the justification for "preemptive" intestinal transplant may become more difficult to justify. However, in this context, "preemptive" should be understood as "prior to the development of significant complications" related to PN or chronic IF [20]. A reasonable approach might suggest that different thresholds for considering intestinal transplant should be established, based on the underlying cause of CIF and the potential for intestinal rehabilitation, which can depend on the diagnosis and, in the case of SBS, the remaining gastrointestinal anatomy. For example, a patient with global gastrointestinal dysmotility caused by pseudo-obstruction, who has a poor quality of life on PN, cannot eat or drink, and needs ongoing gastrointestinal decompression through ostomies or enteric tubes, could be considered for early intestinal transplant even before significant complications arise. Similarly, a patient with extreme SBS who has a stapled-off foregut and requires foregut decompression through a gastrostomy tube while on PN, with no potential for PN weaning, should be considered for early transplant as well, potentially even preemptively. A proposed approach could offer a rational, multimodal care plan for CIF, with timely consideration of intestinal transplantation. Ultimately, a more enlightened perspective might regard ITx as a critical tool in the growing field of intestinal rehabilitation, one that should be used at the right time for patients who still have the potential for good long-term survival and quality of life [21].

21.4 Surgical Approach

The definition of SBS relies on an accurate measurement and reporting of the remaining bowel length. Surgeons performing extensive bowel resections should report the length of the residual bowel, not just the length of bowel that was removed. The outcome of the condition is determined by the remaining bowel length, which cannot be accurately predicted if only the resected bowel length is known. Typically, the residual bowel length is measured during surgery along the antimesenteric border of the unstretched bowel, from the duodenojejunal flexure to the ileocecal junction, or to the site of any small bowel–colon anastomosis or end-ostomy. Patients with short SBS can be categorized into three types based on the presence of residual colon: Type 1 includes patients with an end-jejunostomy; Type 2 consists of patients with a jejunum anastomosed to a partial colon (jejunocolonic anastomosis); and Type 3 encompasses patients with a jejuno-ileocolic anastomosis, retaining the entire colon and ileocecal valve. The relationship between residual bowel anatomy and prognosis has been thoroughly outlined. Type 3 represents the most favorable anatomical outcome for SBS, while Type 1 represents the most severe form, with patients having high-output end-jejunostomies being the most difficult to manage. The degree of nutrient absorption directly correlates with the length of the remaining bowel. Patients at the highest risk of malnutrition typically include those with a duodenostomy or jejunoileal anastomosis and ≤35 cm of residual small intestine, those with a jejunocolic or ileocolic anastomosis and ≤60 cm of residual small intestine, and those with an end jejunostomy and ≤115 cm of residual small intestine. Historically, SBS patients were categorized into two distinct subgroups: those with the colon in continuity and those without. In individuals with SBS, the colon assumes a crucial compensatory role in digestion and fluid absorption, helping to mitigate nutrient and electrolyte losses [22].

21.4.1 Intestinal Transplantation Techniques

The terminology used to describe the technical aspects of intestinal transplantation has been inconsistent in medical literature, especially when additional organs are transplanted alongside the intestinal graft [8]. There are three primary types of intestinal transplants: (I) isolated intestinal transplant, (II) combined liver-intestine transplant, and (III) MVT [23]. The most frequently performed procedure is the isolated intestinal transplant, which involves transplanting the entire jejunum and ileum from a deceased donor. This procedure is typically indicated for patients with intestinal failure confined to the small intestine. The arterial connection is established using the recipient's superior mesenteric artery or a jump graft from the infrarenal aorta. Venous drainage is usually achieved by connecting the superior mesenteric vein of the graft to the recipient's native superior mesenteric vein or splenic vein; in some cases, systemic venous drainage to the inferior vena cava is necessary. Gastrointestinal continuity is restored through an anastomosis between the recipient's and donor's proximal jejunum, along with the creation of a distal Bishop-Koop or loop ileostomy, with or without anastomosis to the recipient's colon. In living donor transplants or cases where there is a significant size discrepancy between the donor and recipient (such as an adult deceased donor to a pediatric recipient), a 200-cm segment of the distal small intestine is used, with blood supply provided by the ileocolic artery and drainage through the ileocolic vein. For patients with concurrent pancreatic dysfunction, such as those with cystic fibrosis, type 1 diabetes, or chronic pancreatitis, the pancreas may also be included in the intestinal transplant [23].

The second most commonly performed technique involves transplanting the liver and pancreas along with the intestine [8]. In this procedure, the liver, pancreas, and intestine (including the duodenum) are retrieved as a single unit from the donor and transplanted en bloc into the recipient. The arterial supply for this combined graft is derived from an aortic conduit that includes both the celiac trunk and the superior mesenteric artery, while venous drainage is managed through the hepatic veins or the inferior vena cava. During the recipient's surgery, the arterial connection is established between the donor's aortic conduit and the recipient's suprarenal or infrarenal aorta.

Venous drainage is facilitated either through a standard caval replacement or via the piggyback technique. Gastrointestinal continuity is restored by creating a direct anastomosis between the proximal donor and recipient jejunum or duodenum, while a distal Bishop-Koop or loop ileostomy is created, with or without a connection to the recipient's colon. Additionally, in this type of transplant, a portocaval shunt is necessary to manage venous outflow from the remaining native organs, including the stomach, pancreas, duodenum, and spleen. The third type of intestinal transplant is the MVT, which involves transplanting additional gastrointestinal organs along with the intestine. These may include the donor's stomach, duodenum, pancreas, and colon, with or without the liver. MVT is commonly indicated for conditions such as hollow visceral myopathy or neuropathy, pseudo-obstruction syndrome, extensive gastrointestinal polyposis, neuroendocrine tumors, and symptomatic total splanchnic vascular thrombosis. The procedure requires complete removal of the recipient's splanchnic organs, followed by the en bloc transplantation of the stomach, duodenum, pancreas, liver, and small intestine, sometimes including the right and transverse colon (full MVT) [23]. If the stomach is removed during upper abdominal organ removal, gastrointestinal continuity is restored by connecting the donor's stomach to the recipient's distal esophagus or remaining gastric tissue. For patients with preserved liver function, a modified MVT may be performed, where the native liver is left intact. In cases where the patient has chronic or impending renal failure, a kidney transplant (typically the right kidney) can also be incorporated into the procedure [24]. While earlier studies suggested that including the colon increased the risk of infections, more recent findings indicate that colon inclusion is not only safe but may also enhance water absorption, reducing dehydration episodes and hospital readmissions. The inclusion of the stomach remains a debated topic, with some transplant centers routinely incorporating it while others rarely or never do. Currently, there is limited evidence to definitively determine the risks or benefits of including the stomach in an MVT [8].

The recipient's surgery can be particularly complex due to factors such as abdominal adhesions from previous surgeries, existing stomas, gastrojejunostomies, limited intra-abdominal space, and, in cases requiring a liver transplant, significant portal hypertension. One unique challenge in intestinal transplantation is the loss of abdominal domain, which is generally not an issue unless the patient has substantial ascites due to liver failure or conditions like hollow visceral myopathy or neuropathy (e.g., pseudo-obstruction syndrome) [8]. Several innovative approaches have been developed to address this issue, including abdominal wall transplantation, the use of tissue expanders, staged closure techniques, and musculocutaneous free flaps. Gastrojejunostomy tubes are almost always inserted during surgery to allow for gastric decompression and early enteral nutrition [25]. A Bishop-Koop or loop ileostomy is also created to decompress the terminal ileum and enable endoscopic access for biopsies, which are crucial for monitoring the graft and detecting acute rejection. These ileostomies are typically reversed within a year posttransplant if ongoing monitoring is no longer necessary. Additionally, prophylactic appendectomy and cholecystectomy—whether of the donor or recipient—are routinely performed to minimize the risk of postoperative infections. In MVT, a donor pyloroplasty is recommended to promote proper gastric emptying [8].

21.5 Post-surgical Immunosuppressive Management

Immunosuppressive therapy should commence immediately after surgery. Various protocols have been established for this purpose. According to the OPTN/SRTR 2013 Annual Data Report, T-cell depleting agents were used in 54% of intestinal transplant recipients, while 11% received interleukin-2 receptor antagonists as induction therapy. Notably, 38% of recipients did not receive any induction therapy. The most commonly prescribed maintenance immunosuppressants included tacrolimus (95%), corticosteroids (73%), mycophenolate (35%), and mTOR inhibitors (15%). One year after transplantation, 70% of recipients were still on oral steroid therapy. Tacrolimus blood concentration targets are typically 12–15 ng/mL during the first postoperative month, then adjusted to 8–12 ng/mL over the following 3 months. Despite immunosuppressive regimens, intestinal transplants remain highly susceptible to rejection. The OPTN/SRTR 2013 report indicated that among adults undergoing isolated intestinal transplants, 45% experienced acute rejection within the first year, increasing to 53% by the second year. While induction therapy and tacrolimus-based maintenance regimens have reduced rejection episodes, steroid-resistant rejection continues to pose a significant risk, carrying a 50% mortality rate in adult recipients, primarily due to sepsis [26]. Traditionally, acute rejection has been managed by suppressing T-cell activity with corticosteroid pulses or anti-lymphocyte therapy. However, growing attention is being directed toward antibody-mediated rejection (AMR) in intestinal transplantation. AMR remains challenging to treat, as it does not respond well to steroids. The detection of donor-specific antibodies (DSA) has gained importance with the implementation of advanced immunological techniques, such as single-antigen fluorescent bead assays. The presence of preformed or newly developed DSAs correlates with rejection episodes and graft failure. Patients with DSAs before and after transplantation tend to have the lowest long-term graft survival, primarily due to both acute rejection episodes and chronic allograft enteropathy [27]. Chronic allograft enteropathy is characterized by mucosal atrophy, ulceration, mesenteric lymphoid depletion, fibrosis, and sclerosis, often linked to mesenteric vasculopathy influenced by DSAs. While CD4 activity and antibody-mediated complement activation in mesenteric vasculopathy are not well documented—largely due to reliance on mucosal rather than full-thickness intestinal biopsies—complement activation plays a crucial role in late graft dysfunction. DSAs can bind to the C1q component of complement, triggering the complement cascade and contributing to chronic graft deterioration. Interestingly, the inclusion of a liver graft alongside the intestinal transplant appears to offer protective benefits, potentially promoting immune tolerance through antigen-presenting cells in the liver or by sequestering sensitized T-cells and antibodies targeting the intestine. Further large-scale studies are needed to refine immunosuppressive strategies targeting different mediators of rejection, including plasmapheresis and immunoglobulin for preformed DSAs, infliximab for cytokine inhibition, rituximab for B-cell suppression, bortezomib for plasma cell depletion, and eculizumab for early complement cascade inhibition [27].

21.6 Outcomes

Studies have shown that transplants containing the liver offer the highest survival rates [6].

Additionally, the small intestine presents unique challenges as a transplant organ due to its strong immunogenicity, the high concentration of donor immune cells within the graft, and its non-sterile environment, all of which contribute to an increased risk of rejection and infection [28].

Advancements in immunosuppressive therapy have significantly improved short-term outcomes, leading to better survival rates and digestive autonomy. However, long-term success remains hindered by chronic rejection and complications related to immunosuppressive treatment.

At present, the 1-year survival rate for intestinal transplantation is approximately 80%, while the 5-year survival rate stands at around 50% [28]. Most long-term survivors achieve independence from PN. A recent study conducted by Ceulemans et al., based on The Intestinal Transplant Registry, reported that there are no significant differences in rejection or survival between living donor ITx and deceased donor ITx, highlighting that living donor ITx has been rarely performed worldwide [29]. However, ITx should be reserved for a highly specific group of SBS patients who suffer from severe, irreversible PN-related complications and have no potential for intestinal rehabilitation.

21.7 Conclusions

Traditionally, ITx has been reserved for patients with irreversible intestinal failure who develop complications from PN. In most cases, the necessity for an MVT indicates a delayed referral for transplantation. Patients awaiting a combined liver-intestinal transplant face higher mortality rates on the waiting list compared to those awaiting an isolated intestinal transplant. However, referring patients with intestinal failure at an earlier stage—particularly those at high risk for complications related to PN or experiencing a significantly reduced quality of life—may lead to better transplant outcomes. Despite its benefits, ITx remains limited to a specific SBS group of patients with total and irreversible intestinal failure accompanied by complications from PN.

References

1. Pironi L. Definitions of intestinal failure and the short bowel syndrome. Best Pract Res Clin Gastroenterol. 2016;30:173–85.
2. Siddiqui MT, Al-Yaman W, Singh A, et al. Short-bowel syndrome: epidemiology, hospitalization trends, in-hospital mortality, and healthcare utilization. JPEN J Parenter Enteral Nutr. 2021;45(7):1441–55.
3. Pironi L, Arends J, Baxter J, et al. Home Artificial Nutrition & Chronic Intestinal Failure; Acute Intestinal Failure Special Interest Groups of ESPEN. ESPEN endorsed recommendations. Definition and classification of intestinal failure in adults. Clin Nutr. 2015;34(2):171–80.
4. Pape UF, Iyer KR, Jeppesen PB, et al. Teduglutide for the treatment of adults with intestinal failure associated with short bowel syndrome: pooled safety data from four clinical trials. Ther Adv Gastroenterol. 2020;13:1756284820905766.
5. Jeppesen PB, Pertkiewicz M, Messing B, et al. Teduglutide reduces need for parenteral support among patients with short bowel syndrome with intestinal failure. Gastroenterology. 2012;143(6):1473–81, e3.
6. Grant D, Abu-Elmagd K, Mazariegos G, et al. Intestinal Transplant Association. Intestinal transplant registry report: global activity and trends. Am J Transplant. 2015;15(1):210–9.
7. International Intestinal Transplant Registry. IRTA international intestinal transplant report: general characteristics. Available at Terasaki.org/itr. Accessed 5 Jan 2025.
8. Sudan D. The current state of intestinal transplantation: indications, techniques, outcomes and challenges. Am J Transplant. 2014;14:1976–84.
9. https://www.cms.gov/medicare-coverage-database/view/ncd.aspx?ncdid5280. Accessed 15 Jan 2025.

10. Howard L, Heaphey L, Fleming CR, et al. Four years of North American registry home parenteral nutrition outcome data and their implications for patient management. JPEN J Parenter Enteral Nutr. 1991;15(4):384–93.
11. Ivanics T, Vianna R, Kubal CA, et al. Impact of the acuity circle model for liver allocation on multivisceral transplant candidates. Am J Transplant. 2022;22(2):464–73.
12. Horslen SP, Smith JM, Weaver T, et al. OPTN/SRTR 2020 annual data report: intestine. Am J Transplant. 2022;22(Suppl 2):310–49.
13. Kaufman SS, Atkinson JB, Bianchi A, et al. Indications for pediatric intestinal transplantation: a position paper of the American Society of Transplantation. Pediatr Transplant. 2001;5(2):80–7.
14. Kaufman SS, Avitzur Y, Beath SV, et al. New insights into the indications for intestinal transplantation: consensus in the year 2019. Transplantation. 2020;104(5):937–46.
15. Pironi L, Goulet O, Buchman A, et al. Home Artificial Nutrition and Chronic Intestinal Failure Working Group of ESPEN. Outcome on home parenteral nutrition for benign intestinal failure: a review of the literature and benchmarking with the European prospective survey of ESPEN. Clin Nutr. 2012;31:831–45.
16. Pither C, Duncan S, Gao R, et al. Quality of life and performance status before and after small intestinal transplantation. Transplant Proc. 2014;46:2109–13.
17. Huard G, Schiano TD, Moon J, et al. Severe acute cellular rejection after intestinal transplantation is associated with poor patient and graft survival. Clin Transpl. 2017;31(5)
18. Iyer K, Moon J. Adult intestinal transplantation in the United States. Curr Opin Organ Transplant. 2020;25(2):196–200.
19. Ekser B, Kubal CA, Fridell JA, et al. Comparable outcomes in intestinal retransplantation: single-center cohort study. Clin Transpl. 2018;32(7):e13290.
20. Lauro A, Marino IR, Iyer KR. Pre-emptive intestinal transplant: the surgeon's point of view. Dig Dis Sci. 2017;62(11):2966–76.
21. Iyer KR. Indications for intestinal transplantation. Gastroenterol Clin N Am. 2024;53(2):233–44. https://doi.org/10.1016/j.gtc.2024.02.001. Epub 2024 Apr 3. PMID: 38719375.
22. American Gastroenterological Association. American Gastroenterological Association medical position statement: short bowel syndrome and intestinal transplantation. Gastroenterology. 2003;124(4):1105–10. https://doi.org/10.1053/gast.2003.50139. PMID: 12671903.
23. Abu-Elmagd KM, Costa G, Bond GJ, et al. Five hundred intestinal and multivisceral transplantations at a single center. Ann Surg. 2009;250(4):567–81.
24. Bremner AR, Gupte G. Management of short bowel syndrome. Paediatr Child Health. 2011;(21) 9:411–7.
25. Moon J, Iyer K. Intestinal rehabilitation and transplantation for intestinal failure. Mt Sinai J Med. 2012;79:256–66.
26. Smith JM, Skeans MA, Horslen SP, et al. OPTN/ SRTR 2013 annual data report: intestine. Am J Transplant. 2015;15(Suppl 2):1–16.
27. Berger M, Zeevi A, Farmer DG, et al. Immunologic challenges in small bowel transplantation. Am J Transplant. 2012;12:S2–8.
28. Nightingale J, Woodward JM, Gastroenterology Small Bowel and Nutrition Committee of the British Society of Gastroenterology. Guidelines for management of patients with a short bowel. Gut. 2006;55:1–12.
29. Ceulemans LJ, Dubois A, Clarysse M, Canovai E, Venick R, Mazariegos G, Vanuytsel T, Hibi T, Avitzur Y, Hind J, Horslen S, Gondolesi G, Benedetti E, Gruessner R, Pirenne J. Outcome after intestinal transplantation from living versus deceased donors: a propensity-matched cohort analysis of the international intestinal transplant registry. Ann Surg. 2023;278(5):807–14.

Multidisciplinary Approach in Short Bowel Syndrome

22

Anca Trifan, Cristian Lupascu, Ramona Cadar, Ana-Maria Trofin, Mihaela Blaj, Cristina Muzica, Irina Girleanu, and Tudor Cuciureanu

22.1 The Role of Gastroenterologists

The gastroenterologist plays a central and continuous role in the multidisciplinary management of short bowel syndrome (SBS), from initial diagnosis through long-term follow-up. Their involvement begins with a comprehensive evaluation of the patient's condition, including identification of the underlying cause of SBS, such as Crohn's disease, mesenteric ischemia, surgical resection, or congenital anomalies [1, 2]. Through clinical assessment, imaging studies, endoscopic evaluations, and laboratory investigations, the gastroenterologist determines the length and functional capacity of the remaining bowel, assesses the degree of malabsorption, and establishes a baseline for nutritional and metabolic status [2].

Following initial stabilization, the gastroenterologist oversees the monitoring and promotion of intestinal adaptation, a key physiological process by which the remnant bowel attempts to increase its absorptive efficiency [3]. This is supported by targeted medical therapies, such as proton pump inhibitors or H2 blockers to

A. Trifan · C. Muzica · I. Girleanu (✉) · T. Cuciureanu
Gastroenterology Department, Grigore T. Popa University of Medicine and Pharmacy, Iaşi, Romania

Institute of Gastroenterology and Hepatology, St. Spiridon Emergency Hospital, Iaşi, Romania

C. Lupascu · R. Cadar · A.-M. Trofin
Surgery Department, Grigore T. Popa University of Medicine and Pharmacy, Iaşi, Romania

General Surgery and Liver Tranplantation, St. Spiridon Emergency Hospital, Iaşi, Romania

M. Blaj
Intensive Care Department, Grigore T. Popa University of Medicine and Pharmacy, Iaşi, Romania

Intensive Care Unit, St. Spiridon Emergency Hospital, Iaşi, Romania

A. Trifan et al. (eds.), *Short Bowel Syndrome in Adults*,
https://doi.org/10.1007/978-3-031-95848-9_22

reduce gastric acid secretion, antimotility agents to slow intestinal transit and enhance absorption, and bile acid binders when appropriate [4, 5]. In selected cases, newer therapies like glucagon-like peptide-2 (GLP-2) analogues are used to stimulate mucosal growth and reduce reliance on parenteral nutrition [6]. The gastroenterologist must closely monitor clinical parameters, including fluid and electrolyte balance, nutritional markers, and bowel function, to tailor interventions effectively.

In addition to supporting adaptation, the gastroenterologist is responsible for identifying and managing complications commonly associated with SBS. These include small intestinal bacterial overgrowth (SIBO), which often presents with bloating, diarrhea, and malnutrition and requires clinical vigilance and appropriate antibiotic therapy [7]. Hepatic complications related to long-term parenteral nutrition—collectively referred to as intestinal failure–associated liver disease (IFALD)—necessitate regular liver function monitoring and adjustments in nutrition and lipid intake [8]. Other complications, such as metabolic bone disease and nephrolithiasis, arise from chronic deficiencies in calcium, vitamin D, magnesium, and fluid imbalances, requiring routine surveillance and supplementation guided by the gastroenterologist.

Nutritional management is another critical area of oversight. While clinical dietitians calculate daily caloric and micronutrient needs and plan enteral or parenteral nutrition regimens, the gastroenterologist determines the appropriate route of nutrition and ensures that the patient's hydration, electrolyte, and vitamin needs are being met [9]. They oversee the transition from parenteral to enteral nutrition when feasible and monitor for complications such as refeeding syndrome during this process. The gastroenterologist ensures that patients receive adequate supplementation of fat-soluble vitamins, vitamin B12, trace elements, and essential minerals, adjusting regimens based on clinical progress [9].

In cases where intestinal rehabilitation is no longer sufficient and complications from parenteral nutrition become life-threatening, the gastroenterologist initiates referral for intestinal transplantation [10]. They are responsible for identifying suitable candidates—typically those with progressive liver disease, loss of central venous access, recurrent catheter-related sepsis, or severely impaired quality of life—and for coordinating the necessary pretransplant evaluations. Close communication with transplant centers is vital to optimize timing, manage expectations, and provide ongoing support during the pre- and posttransplant periods.

A key component of the gastroenterologist's role is long-term patient education and follow-up [11, 12]. They educate patients and caregivers on dietary modifications, symptom recognition, medication adherence, and signs of dehydration or infection. Regular outpatient monitoring, including laboratory tests and clinical assessments, ensures that emerging issues are addressed promptly and that therapy remains individualized and responsive to the patient's evolving needs.

In summary, the gastroenterologist serves as both a clinician and coordinator in the care of patients with SBS, navigating the complex interplay between medical therapy, nutrition, and surgical considerations. Their active involvement across all stages of disease management is essential to improving outcomes and ensuring comprehensive, patient-centered care.

22.2 The Role of the Anesthesiologist and Perioperative Team

In the multidisciplinary management of SBS, the anesthesiologist plays a critical role during surgical interventions, including primary enterectomy, surgical procedures to restore intestinal continuity, or intestinal transplantation. These operations are often complex due to the patient's compromised physiological state, chronic malnutrition, and systemic effects of long-term inflammation. Perioperative morbidity and mortality are significantly increased in this population and are influenced by the severity of the underlying pathology, comorbidities, and the urgency and extent of the surgical procedure. Effective perioperative planning and optimization are essential to improving outcomes.

Surgical intervention for patients with inflammatory bowel disease (IBD), one of the leading causes of SBS, remains common despite advancements in biological therapy [13]. Approximately 70–80% of patients with Crohn's disease will require bowel surgery within 20 years of diagnosis, and up to 30% of them may require a second operation [14]. In ulcerative colitis, colectomy is needed in around 20–30% of patients after 25 years, although this percentage has declined due to more effective therapies [15]. However, surgical emergencies still occur due to complications such as bowel perforation, severe hemorrhage, or toxic megacolon. These emergencies often involve septic shock, severe hypovolemia, and multi-organ dysfunction, significantly raising perioperative risk.

A recent Danish study involving 394 patients with IBD reported that 31.2% of surgical interventions were performed emergently, with the remainder being elective [15]. Despite improvements in perioperative management, these patients remain at risk for prolonged hospital stays, complications, and intensive care requirements.

Patients with IBD often present with a range of systemic complications. These include malnutrition, sarcopenia, anemia (due to iron deficiency or chronic inflammation), fluid and electrolyte imbalances, and a dysregulated immune system. Many are colonized by multidrug-resistant organisms due to repeated hospital exposure. Additionally, IBD is associated with an increased risk of thromboembolic events, cardiovascular disease, and major adverse cardiac events (MACE), including myocardial injury after noncardiac surgery (MINS), particularly in younger patients under 50 years old [16].

In elective surgeries, the anesthesiologist plays a key role in preoperative assessment and optimization. This includes evaluation of functional status, cardiovascular risk, fluid and electrolyte balance, and anemia. Iron supplementation is recommended in cases of iron deficiency anemia. Nutritional rehabilitation and muscular conditioning should be coordinated with dietitians and physiotherapists. Corticosteroid and biologic therapy must be reviewed in collaboration with the gastroenterologist to reduce the risk of postoperative infections and impaired wound healing. Early counseling by colorectal surgeons and stoma nurses improves patient readiness and postoperative recovery.

Preoperative preparation follows Enhanced Recovery After Surgery (ERAS) protocols, which have shown promise in promoting early mobilization, reducing complications, and shortening hospital stays. ERAS includes preoperative carbohydrate loading, maintaining oral intake up to 2 h before surgery, and clear, consistent patient education [17].

Intraoperatively, general anesthesia using short-acting agents is standard. Multimodal analgesia—particularly the use of epidural anesthesia—is encouraged, barring contraindications, to reduce opioid consumption and enhance postoperative recovery. Intraoperative fluid therapy should be guided by invasive monitoring and echocardiographic assessment when available, maintaining mean arterial pressure above 65 mmHg. Central venous access and large-bore intravenous lines may be necessary for fluid and blood product administration. Preventing hypothermia through core temperature monitoring and active warming is a key component of ERAS.

Minimally invasive surgical techniques and the avoidance of unnecessary abdominal drains are preferred to limit surgical trauma and promote faster recovery. Prophylactic antibiotics should be administered according to protocol.

Postoperatively, ERAS continues with early removal of nasogastric tubes and urinary catheters, rapid reintroduction of oral intake (as early as the evening of the day of surgery), and mobilization within the first 24 h. If oral intake is inadequate by postoperative day 3, nutritional screening should guide the initiation of parenteral nutrition. Patients are encouraged to chew gum to reduce postoperative ileus, and daily monitoring of stoma output is crucial to detect high-output states.

Pain control is maintained through multimodal strategies, and respiratory therapy is initiated with positive expiratory pressure devices to prevent pulmonary complications. Thromboprophylaxis with low molecular weight heparin and compression stockings is standard.

A comparison of ERAS to traditional perioperative care in IBD surgery found a reduced median ICU stay (from 6 to 4 days) and faster recovery, although it did not significantly impact serious postoperative complications or readmission rates. The rate of complications was slightly lower in the ERAS group (15.0% vs. 20.8%), though this did not reach statistical significance [15].

In emergency surgeries for causes such as intestinal ischemia, perforation, strangulated hernia, or obstructing malignancy, patients often arrive hemodynamically unstable with acute electrolyte disturbances, metabolic acidosis, and renal dysfunction. These situations require aggressive resuscitation, close intraoperative monitoring, and multidisciplinary collaboration to stabilize the patient and reduce the risk of perioperative death.

In summary, anesthesiologists are integral to the multidisciplinary management of patients with SBS requiring surgery. Their involvement in preoperative optimization, intraoperative management, and postoperative recovery—guided by ERAS principles—contributes substantially to improving outcomes in this vulnerable population.

22.3 Surgical Management in Short Bowel Syndrome

Surgical therapy for patients with short bowel syndrome (SBS) typically begins prior to or during the initial operation, with the objective of employing all feasible strategies to prevent extensive intestinal resection and the subsequent development of SBS. This approach involves adopting a conservative strategy in cases of uncertain intestinal ischemia, planning second-look surgeries when necessary, and minimizing the risk of abdominal compartment syndrome and further bowel ischemia by avoiding premature or inappropriate abdominal closure [18].

In contrast to intestinal transplantation, definitive guidelines for non-transplant surgical procedures in SBS patients have not been fully established. The timing and role of bowel-lengthening procedures remain topics of ongoing debate. Current expert opinion suggests that surgery should be reserved for patients who are unable to discontinue parenteral nutrition after all conservative measures have been exhausted. Surgical intervention is generally recommended for those who fail to achieve at least 50% of their daily caloric needs enterally after 6 months of optimized treatment [19].

Some specialists recommend that bowel-lengthening surgery be considered only for long-term parenteral nutrition (PN)-dependent patients who exhibit significant bowel dilation. The primary indication for such surgery includes patients who have reached a stable phase of intestinal adaptation or those experiencing persistent complications, such as small intestinal bacterial overgrowth (SIBO) [20].

End-stage liver disease is a well-known contraindication to bowel-lengthening procedures, as patients in this condition typically benefit more from intestinal transplantation [20, 21].

Although uncommon, some patients with SBS may exhibit delayed intestinal transit. In such cases, it is essential to thoroughly investigate underlying causes, including partial obstructions, blind loops, or intestinal fistulas [22].

Patients who do not respond to medical therapy may be candidates for surgical procedures known as "narrowing enteroplasty" or "bottleneck enteroplasty." This technique involves resecting the dilated portion of the bowel along its antimesenteric border, with the goal of restoring peristaltic efficiency while preserving overall intestinal length. Such surgery is appropriate when the residual bowel length is sufficient to ensure adequate nutrient absorption despite the reduced surface area [23, 24].

Surgical interventions can be categorized into three main approaches [25, 26]:

1. **Restoration of intestinal transit**
2. **Enhancement of intestinal motility by addressing bowel dilation**

3. **Slowing intestinal transit without inducing bowel dilation**

22.3.1 Surgeries to Correct Intestinal Transit

This surgical approach must adhere to anatomical principles, promoting the transition from jejunostomy or ileostomy to colon-in-continuity procedures, with the goal of improving long-term prognosis [27]. In cases where intestinal length is not a limiting factor, segmental intestinal dilatation can be effectively addressed by a straightforward tapering enteroplasty. This involves resecting a portion of the bowel along the antimesenteric border to restore normal luminal diameter [28].

In patients with short bowel syndrome (SBS) and marked bowel dilatation, the primary objective is to taper the intestine without compromising the mucosal surface area available for absorption. Two major surgical techniques are used in this context: the Longitudinal Intestinal Lengthening and Tailoring (LILT) procedure, originally described by Bianchi, and the Serial Transverse Enteroplasty (STEP) procedure, introduced by Kim [28, 29].

The LILT technique is especially useful when intestinal length is critically short. It creates a narrower intestinal configuration while preserving the absorptive surface area. The procedure begins by identifying a longitudinal, avascular segment approximately 5 cm along the mesenteric border of the dilated bowel [30, 31]. The intestine is then divided longitudinally into two separate channels, which are reconstructed to form a single, narrower, iso-peristaltic segment—effectively doubling the length of the absorptive surface.

Alternatively, this procedure can be performed using a gastrointestinal anastomosis stapler to divide the bowel into two narrower tubes, which are then reconnected in an end-to-end, iso-peristaltic fashion [32]. LILT should be performed cautiously, particularly in patients with severely reduced bowel length or those with end-stage liver disease.

The success of the LILT technique depends on careful anatomical identification of the mesenteric vasculature, specifically the bifurcation of the mesenteric arteries into anterior and posterior branches before entering the intestinal wall. This step ensures adequate blood flow to both segments during the longitudinal division [33].

Potential complications associated with LILT include anastomotic fistula, sepsis, redilatation, strictures, adhesions, and perforation [34, 35]. Among these, intestinal necrosis remains the most feared and severe complication [36].

The Serial Transverse Enteroplasty (STEP) procedure is another surgical technique used in the management of short bowel syndrome. It was first described by Kim et al. in 2003 [37]. The method involves applying surgical staplers in a zigzag pattern perpendicular to the longitudinal axis of the intestine [38]. These transverse staple lines alternate from either side of the bowel, effectively reducing the diameter of dilated segments while simultaneously increasing overall bowel length [39].

The STEP procedure can be repeated multiple times if necessary, a strategy known as re-STEP, to further reduce intestinal diameter and improve functional outcomes [40, 41]. It is particularly suited for cases where the bowel is significantly dilated but sufficiently long. By contrast, the Longitudinal Intestinal Lengthening and Tailoring (LILT) procedure may be more appropriate for anatomically complex segments, such as the duodenum, or when bowel length is critically short.

Although the STEP technique is associated with lower mortality and is generally less technically demanding than LILT, patients undergoing STEP are more likely to eventually require intestinal transplantation [42]. Complications associated with STEP include staple-line leaks, intra-abdominal abscesses, sepsis, bowel obstructions, bleeding, and recurrent intestinal dilatation [43, 44].

On average, the STEP procedure achieves a bowel lengthening of approximately 49%, and about 45% of patients successfully wean off parenteral nutrition. The overall mortality rate associated with STEP is around 7%, which contributes to its reputation as a safer and more accessible alternative to LILT in appropriately selected patients [45].

While STEP offers advantages in simplicity and lower operative risk, the decision between LILT and STEP should be based on individual patient characteristics, bowel anatomy, and the experience of the surgical team [46]. LILT has been associated with improved long-term outcomes, including higher survival rates, increased independence from PN, and a lower likelihood of requiring intestinal transplantation. However, it also carries a higher risk of postoperative complications compared to STEP, which has led to wider adoption of the STEP procedure in many centers [47].

A more recent surgical innovation, Spiral Intestinal Lengthening and Tailoring (SILT), was developed specifically for patients with severely dilated bowel. In this technique, a spiral-shaped incision is made at a 45°–60° angle relative to the longitudinal axis of the bowel, followed by re-tubularization into a longer, narrower segment [48]. Unlike STEP, SILT preserves the natural orientation of the intestinal muscle fibers and requires less manipulation of the mesentery compared to the Bianchi (LILT) procedure [49, 50].

22.3.2 Surgeries to Extend Intestinal Transit

22.3.2.1 Reversed Segmental Small Intestine (RSSI)

This surgery involves the creation of an antiperistaltic segment of small intestine as distally as possible—ideally near the terminal stoma or the small intestine–colon junction. This reversed segment promotes retrograde peristalsis distally while simultaneously inhibiting motility in the proximal intestine. The result is a suppression of intrinsic nerve plexus activity, which in turn delays the propagation of myoelectric activity in the distal segment [30, 31]. By slowing intestinal transit and enhancing nutrient absorption, this technique can significantly reduce or even eliminate the need for parenteral nutrition in selected patients. To optimize enteral autonomy, it is critical to minimize the time between the initial enterectomy and RSSI surgery. Furthermore, the reversed segment should be at least 10 cm in length to achieve meaningful physiological benefit [51].

22.3.2.2 Colon Interposition

This technique involves interposing a colonic segment within the residual small intestine, in either an iso- or antiperistaltic orientation, to slow intestinal transit while preserving peristaltic coordination. Some patients undergoing this procedure have achieved enteral autonomy from PN within 4 months [52, 53].

22.3.2.3 Valves and Sphincters

This can be surgically constructed using several techniques, including external intestinal constriction, segmental denervation, or, most commonly, intussusception of an intestinal segment. These methods aim to create a partial obstruction that disrupts normal intestinal motility patterns and prevents retrograde reflux [47].

22.3.3 Transplantation of the Intestinal Organs

A combined liver–intestine transplant can be performed simultaneously and is generally reserved for patients in whom autologous gastrointestinal reconstruction has failed or who remain fully dependent on parenteral nutrition [54]. Intestinal transplantation, however, is not suitable for every patient, as several contraindications exist. A combined liver–intestinal transplant is typically required when short bowel syndrome is accompanied by advanced liver disease [55, 56], particularly in cases of severe portal hypertension or irreversible hepatic dysfunction. In some patients with complex multiorgan involvement or total splenic vein thrombosis, multivisceral transplantation—sometimes including the pancreas—may be indicated [57]. While most organ donations are from deceased donors, living-related intestinal transplantation has been explored, especially in pediatric populations. In these cases, the terminal ileum is often favored over the jejunum due to its technical accessibility and superior adaptive capacity. Recent advances in surgical techniques and immunosuppressive therapy have led to improved short-term outcomes, including increased survival rates and better digestive autonomy [58].

Over the past two decades, immunosuppression protocols have significantly evolved. Tacrolimus-based maintenance therapy remains the global standard, though adjunctive immunosuppressants such as corticosteroids, azathioprine, mycophenolate mofetil, sirolimus, or everolimus may be employed during rejection episodes [26, 31].

A highly selective subgroup of SBS patients may be candidates for intestinal transplantation—those with irreversible complications from long-term PN and no potential for intestinal rehabilitation. It is crucial to refer these patients for transplant evaluation early, before liver dysfunction progresses to the point of necessitating a liver transplant. Due to stringent eligibility criteria for liver transplantation, patients requiring combined transplants often face worse outcomes compared to those needing isolated intestinal grafts [31].

Reported 1-year survival rates after intestinal transplantation are approximately 89%, with a graft survival rate of 79%. These numbers decline to 72% and 69%, respectively, in patients undergoing combined liver–intestinal transplantation.

Interestingly, long-term survival following isolated small bowel transplantation is slightly lower than with combined procedures, largely due to a higher incidence of chronic rejection. This disparity is attributed to the greater immunological tolerance conferred by hepatic lymphocytes compared to intestinal lymphocytes [26, 59].

Despite current challenges, outcomes following intestinal transplantation have improved considerably and are now approaching those seen with long-term PN dependence. It is important to recognize that for many candidates, lifelong PN is associated with near-universal mortality in the midterm [60].

It is estimated that 50–60% of patients undergoing autologous gastrointestinal reconstruction may eventually achieve independence from PN. However, no single surgical procedure can offer a definitive cure for SBS. All surgical strategies must be considered within the framework of comprehensive, multidisciplinary care [31, 59].

22.3.4 Other Methods of Surgical Procedures

A modified technique known as duodenal lengthening has recently been introduced for patients diagnosed with "no gut" syndrome and duodenal dilation [61]. This method applies a variation of the STEP procedure, involving sequential transverse applications of an endoscopic stapler to the anterior and posterior walls of the duodenum. The procedure must be performed with great caution to avoid injury to the biliopancreatic structures. This approach has been used successfully in patients with a mega-duodenal stump, re-establishing digestive continuity through an end-to-side anastomosis between the duodenum and colon [62].

An alternative strategy for prolonging intestinal transit time involves the use of a reversed antiperistaltic segmental bowel loop, which functions by delaying content progression through the intestine. While bowel-lengthening operations inherently slow transit, this technique can further enhance absorption, particularly in patients with sufficient residual bowel length. Clinical studies have reported that, following this procedure, the median rate of oral autonomy can reach approximately 100% ± 38%, significantly reducing or eliminating the need for parenteral nutrition [63, 64].

The combination of successive bowel-lengthening procedures with controlled tissue expansion (CTE) has shown promising yet limited improvements in clinical outcomes [64]. Despite these gains, stimulating neo-mucosal growth remains a major challenge. Recent preclinical experiments in pigs have reinforced the theoretical basis of CTE in non-dilated bowel segments, designed to prepare the intestine for later lengthening procedures. These studies demonstrated mucosal hypertrophy and measurable increases in both bowel length and diameter following partial obstruction [65].

A novel direction in SBS surgery involves the use of intestinal organoids, in which epithelial tissue derived from stem cells is implanted into larger segments of intestine to restore function. This technique aims to improve mucosal absorptive capacity and long-term prognosis. Although it represents a highly innovative approach, several hurdles remain—particularly in generating functional organoids that possess vascular networks and coordinated peristaltic activity [66].

Additionally, biomimetic approaches inspired by shark intestines have been explored in experimental models. These involve the creation of spiral valves within the gut using external sutures and STEP techniques to mimic the natural resistance and absorption enhancement observed in certain aquatic species [67].

References

1. Jeppesen PB, Gabe SM, Seidner DL, et al. Short bowel syndrome and intestinal failure: consensus definitions and overview. Clin Gastroenterol Hepatol. 2022;20(4):498–511.e1.
2. Aksan A, Farrag K, Blumenstein I, Schröder O, Dignass AU, Stein J. Chronic intestinal failure and short bowel syndrome in Crohn's disease. World J Gastroenterol. 2021;27(24):3440–65. https://doi.org/10.3748/wjg.v27.i24.3440. PMID: 34239262; PMCID: PMC8240052.
3. Pironi L, Arends J, Baxter J, Bozzetti F, Peláez RB, Cuerda C, Forbes A, Gabe S, Gillanders L, Holst M, Jeppesen PB, Joly F, Kelly D, Klek S, Irtun Ø, Olde Damink SW, Panisic M, Rasmussen HH, Staun M, Szczepanek K, Van Gossum A, Wanten G, Schneider SM, Shaffer J, Home Artificial Nutrition & Chronic Intestinal Failure. Acute Intestinal Failure Special Interest Groups of ESPEN. ESPEN endorsed recommendations. Definition and classification of intestinal failure in adults. Clin Nutr. 2015;34(2):171–80.
4. Wall EA. An overview of short bowel syndrome management: adherence, adaptation, and practical recommendations. J Acad Nutr Diet. 2013;113(9):1200–8. https://doi.org/10.1016/j.jand.2013.05.001. Epub 2013 Jul 3. PMID: 23830324.
5. Ubesie AC, Kocoshis SA, Mezoff AG, Henderson CJ, Helmrath MA, Cole CR. Multiple micronutrient deficiencies among patients with intestinal failure during and after transition to enteral nutrition. J Pediatr. 2013;163(6):1692e6.
6. Pizzoferrato M, Puca P, Ennas S, Cammarota G, Guidi L. Glucagon-like peptide-2 analogues for Crohn's disease patients with short bowel syndrome and intestinal failure. World J Gastroenterol. 2022;28(44):6258–70. https://doi.org/10.3748/wjg.v28.i44.6258.
7. Dibaise JK, Young RJ, Vanderhoof JA. Enteric microbial flora, bacterial overgrowth, and short-bowel syndrome. Clin Gastroenterol Hepatol. 2006;4(1):11–20. https://doi.org/10.1016/j.cgh.2005.10.020. PMID: 16431299.
8. Żalikowska-Gardocka M, Przybyłkowski A. Review of parenteral nutrition-associated liver disease. Clin Exp Hepatol. 2020;6(2):65–73. https://doi.org/10.5114/ceh.2019.95528. Epub 2020 May 21. PMID: 32728621; PMCID: PMC7380469.
9. Iyer K, DiBaise JK, Rubio-Tapia A. AGA clinical practice update on management of short bowel syndrome: expert review. Clin Gastroenterol Hepatol. 2022;20(10):2185–94.e2. https://doi.org/10.1016/j.cgh.2022.05.032. Epub 2022 Jun 11. PMID: 35700884.
10. Kahn AB, Tulla KA, Tzvetanov IG. Indications of intestinal transplantation. Gastroenterol Clin N Am. 2019;48(4):575–83. https://doi.org/10.1016/j.gtc.2019.08.010. Epub 2019 Oct 4. PMID: 31668184.
11. Friedman AJ, Cosby R, Boyko S, Hatton-Bauer J, Turnbull G. Effective teaching strategies and methods of delivery for patient education: a systematic review and practice guideline recommendations. J Cancer Educ. 2010;26(1):12–21.
12. Paterick TE, Patel N, Tajik AJ, Chandrasekaran K. Improving health outcomes through patient education and partnerships with patients. Proc (Bayl Univ Med Cent). 2017;30(1):112–3.
13. Cosnes J, Gower-Rousseau C, Seksik P, Cortot A. Epidemiology and natural history of inflammatory bowel diseases. Gastroenterology. 2011;140:1785–94.
14. John TK. Surgical treatment of inflammatory bowel disease: from the gastroenterologist's stand-point. World J Gastrointest Surg. 2024;16(5):1235–54.

15. Lin V, Poulsen JK, Juvik AF. The implementation of an inflammatory bowel disease-specific enhanced recovery after surgery protocol: an observational cohort study. Tech Coloproctol. 2024;28:58. https://doi.org/10.1007/s10151-024-02933-3.
16. Hao Wu , Tingzi Hu, Hong Hao, Inflammatory bowel disease and cardiovascular diseases: a concise review, Eur Heart J Open (2021) 2, 1–9, https://doi.org/10.1093/ehjopen/oeab029.
17. Melnyk M, Casey RG, Black P, Koupparis AJ. Enhanced recovery after surgery (ERAS) protocols: time to change practice? Can Urol Assoc J. 2011;5(5):342–8. https://doi.org/10.5489/cuaj.11002. PMID: 22031616; PMCID: PMC3202008.
18. Amiot A, Messing B, Corcos O, et al. Determinants of home parenteral nutrition dependence and survival of 268 patients with non-malignant short bowel syndrome. Clin Nutr. 2013;32:368–74.
19. Cuerda C, Pironi L, Arends J, et al. ESPEN practical guideline: clinical nutrition in chronic intestinal failure. Clin Nutr. 2021;40:5196–220.
20. Shah AA, Petrosyan M, Franklin AL, et al. Autologous intestinal reconstruction: a single institution study of the serial transverse enteroplasty (STEP) and the longitudinal intestinal lengthening and tailoring (LILT). Pediatr Surg Int. 2019;35:649–55.
21. Hommel MJ, Van Baren R, Haveman JW. Surgical management and autologous intestinal reconstruction in short bowel syndrome. Best Pract Res Clin Gastroenterol. 2016;30:263–80.
22. Hernandez F, Andres AM, Lopez-Santamaria M. Long term results of surgery for bowel lengthening: how many transplants are avoided, for which patients? Curr Opin Organ Transplant. 2018;23:207–11.
23. Van Praagh JB, Sijbrand Hofker H, Haveman JW. Comparing bowel lengthening procedures: which, when, and why? Curr Opin Organ Transplant. 2022;27(2):112–8.
24. Kishore RI. Surgical management of short bowel syndrome. J Parenter Enter Nutr. 2014;20:1–7.
25. Malcolm KR, Wilmore DW. Short bowel syndrome. JPEN J Parenter Enteral Nutr. 2014;38:427–37.
26. Furtado AJL. Transplantacão de órgão abdominais em Coimbra; 2010. 272 j coloproctol (rio j). 2016;36(4):262–72.
27. Iyer KR. Surgical management of short bowel syndrome. JPEN J Parenter Enteral Nutr. 2014;38:53S–9S.
28. Bianchi A. From the cradle to enteral autonomy: the role of autologous gastrointestinal reconstruction. Gastroenterology. 2006;130:S138–46.
29. Lauro A, Santoro A, Cirocchi R, et al. Serial transverse enteroplasty (STEP) in case of short bowel syndrome: did we achieve our goal? A systematic review. Updates Surg. 2022;74(4):1209–23.
30. Baxter JP, Fayers PM, Mckinlay AW. A review of the quality of adult patients treated with long-term parenteral nutrition. Clin Nutr. 2006;25:543–53.
31. Fishbein TM. Intestinal transplantation. N Engl J Med. 2009;361:998–1008.
32. Bianchi A. Longitudinal intestinal lengthening and tailoring: results in 20 children. J R Soc Med. 1997;90:429–32.
33. Coletta R, Morabito A. Non-transplant surgical management of short bowel syndrome in children: an overview. Curr Pediatr Rev. 2019;15:106–10.
34. Frongia G, Kessler M, Weih S, et al. Comparison of LILT and STEP procedures in children with short bowel syndrome—a systematic review of the literature. J Pediatr Surg. 2013;48:1794–805.
35. Ramos-Gonzalez G, Kim HB. Autologous intestinal reconstruction surgery. Semin Pediatr Surg. 2018;27:261–6.
36. Coletta R, Mussi E, Uccheddu F, et al. Preoperative planning of spiral intestinal lengthening and tailoring: a geometrical approach. Bioengineering. 2021;8:20.
37. Kim HB, Fauza D, Garza J, Oh JT, Nurko S, Jaksic T. Serial transverse enteroplasty (STEP): a novel bowel lengthening procedure. J Pediatr Surg. 2003;38:425–9.
38. Pakarinen MP, Kurvinen A, Koivusalo AI, et al. Long-term controlled outcomes after autologous intestinal reconstruction surgery in treatment of severe short bowel syndrome. J Pediatr Surg. 2013;48:339–44.

39. Abu-Elmagd KM, Armanyous SR, Fujiki M, et al. Management of five hundred patients with gut failure at a single center: surgical innovation versus transplantation with a novel predictive model. Ann Surg. 2019;270:656–74.
40. Lemoine C, Larkin K, Brennan K, et al. Repeat serial transverse enteroplasty procedure (reSTEP): is it worth it? J Pediatr Surg. 2021;56:951–60.
41. Jones BA, Hull MA, Potanos KM, et al. International STEP Data Registry. Report of 111 consecutive patients enrolled in the International Serial Transverse Enteroplasty (STEP) Data Registry: a retrospective observational study. J Am Coll Surg. 2013;216:438–46.
42. Cserni T, Biszku B, Guthy I, et al. The first clinical application of the spiral intestinal lengthening and tailoring (silt) in extreme short bowel syndrome. J Gastrointest Surg. 2014;18:1852–7.
43. Mehrabi V, Mehrabi A, Jamshidi SH, et al. Modified spiral intestinal lengthening and tailoring for short bowel syndrome. Surg Innov. 2016;23:30–5.
44. Fitzgeral K, Muto M, Belza C, et al. The evolution of the serial transverse enteroplasty for pediatric short bowel syndrome at a single institution. J Pediatr Surg. 2019;54:993–8.
45. Nagelkerke SCJ, Poelgeest MYV, Wessel LM, et al. Bowel lengthening procedures in children with short bowel syndrome: a systematic review. Eur J Pediatr Surg. 2021;9:301.
46. Umar S. Intestinal stem cells. Curr Gastroenterol Rep. 2010;12:340–8.
47. Ec R, Barbosaa E. Short bowel syndrome: treatment options, j coloproctol (rio j). 2016;36(4):262–72.
48. Alberti D, Boroni G, Giannotti G, et al. "Spiral intestinal lengthening and tailoring (SILT)" for a child with severely short bowel. Pediatr Surg Int. 2014;30:1169–72.
49. Layec S, Beyer L, Corcos O, et al. Increased intestinal absorption by segmental reversal of the small bowel in adult patients with short-bowel syndrome: a case control study. Am J Clin Nutr. 2013;97:100–8.
50. Thompson JS. Reversed intestinal segment revisited. Transplant Proc. 2016;48:453–6.
51. Seetharam P, Rodrigues G. Short bowel syndrome: a review of management options. Saudi J Gastroenterol. 2011;17:229–35.
52. Murphy F, Khalil BA, Gozzini S, et al. Controlled tissue expansion in the initial management of the short bowel state. World J Surg. 2011;35:1142–5.
53. Gondolesi GE, Ortega M, Martinez MI, et al. Autologous gastrointestinal reconstruction surgery for short bowel syndrome: the cornerstone for intestinal rehabilitation. Curr Opin Organ Transplant. 2022;27(2):148–53.
54. Sudan D. Long-term outcomes and quality of life after intestine transplantation. Curr Opin Organ Transplant. 2010;15(3):357–60.
55. Kong W, Wang J, Ying R, et al. A potential anatomic subtype of short bowel syndrome: a matched case-control study. BMC Gastroenterol. 2016;16:12.
56. Matsumoto CS, Subramanian S, Fishbein TM. Adult intestinal transplantation. Gastroenterol Clin N Am. 2018;47:341–54.
57. Ueno T, Wada M, Ogawa E, et al. Present state of intestinal transplantation in Japan. Pediatr Surg Int. 2023;39(1):276.
58. Kobayashi E. A new stage of experimental surgery for organoid based intestinal regeneration—a review of organoid research and recent advance. Magy Seb. 2022;75(4):261–4.
59. Pascher A. Indikation und Ergebnisse der Darmtransplantation bei Kurzdarmsyndrom nach mesenterialer Ischämie [Indications and results of intestinal transplantation for short bowel syndrome after mesenteric ischemia]. Chirurgie (Heidelb). 2024;95(5):375–81.
60. Bueno J, Redecillas S, GarcÍa L, et al. Duodenal lengthening in short bowel with dilated duodenum. J Pediatr Surg. 2015;50:493–6.
61. Bueno J, Burgos R, Redecillas S, et al. Duodenal lengthening in an adult with ultra-short bowel syndrome. A case report. Rev Esp Enferm Dig. 2018;110:59–62.
62. Muff JL, Sokolovski F, Walsh-Korb Z, et al. Surgical treatment of short bowel syndrome—the past, the present and the future, a descriptive review of the literature. Children (Basel). 2022;9(7):1024.

63. Yaprak M, Volkan D, Erdoğan O. Role of serial enteroplasty in the management of adult-type short bowel syndrome: experience from a single tertiary referral hospital in Turkey. Turk J Gastroenterol. 2021;32:11–21.
64. Lauro A, Coletta R, Morabito A. Restoring gut physiology in short bowel patients: from bench to clinical application of autologous intestinal reconstructive procedures. Expert Rev Gastroenterol Hepatol. 2019;13(8):785–96.
65. Urbán D, Kőnig R, Cserni T. A rövidbél-szindróma korszerű sebészi kezelése: autológ rekonstrukció és intestinalis rehabilitáció [Autologous reconstructive surgery and intestinal rehabilitation in the management of short bowel syndrome]. Orv Hetil. 2020;161(7):243–51.
66. Wada M, Watanabe K, Sugimoto S, et al. A novel organoid-based strategy using hybrid colon interposition for short bowel syndrome: a mini review of in vivo models and possible human candidates. Gastroenterol Clin N Am. 2024;53(3):481–91.
67. Saeki I, Kurihara S, Kojima M, et al. A new surgical technique for short bowel syndrome. BMC Surg. 2022;22:375.

Education of Patients with Short Bowel Syndrome

23

Camelia Cojocariu, Cristina Muzica, Oana Petrea, and Laura Huiban

23.1 Introduction

Short bowel syndrome (SBS) is a severe malabsorptive disorder associated with considerable morbidity and mortality, a reduced quality of life, and substantial healthcare costs. Short bowel syndrome is defined as a severe clinicopathological entity resulting from the loss of intestinal length due to underlying disease or surgical resection. Functionally, it is characterized by the inability to maintain nutritional, fluid, and electrolyte homeostasis on a standard diet following bowel resection [1].

The most common causes of SBS in adults are mesenteric ischemia, Crohn's disease, complications of abdominal surgery, including bariatric procedures, and various malignancies. Other causes include severe abdominal trauma, volvulus and other types of strangulation of the bowel, radiation enteritis, and multiple bowel fistulas [2].

The severity of SBS depends on the extent and location of intestinal loss, with proximal resections leading to deficiencies in iron, calcium, and fat-soluble vitamins, while distal resections impact vitamin B12 absorption and bile salt reabsorption. Understanding the etiology of SBS is essential for tailoring appropriate medical, nutritional, and surgical interventions to optimize patient outcomes. Moreover, it is crucial to bear in mind that the multidisciplinary treatment of patients diagnosed with SBS also considers the type of SBS. Therefore, based on the presence or absence of the residual colon, patients with SBS can be categorized into three groups: *group 1*—end-jejunostomy; *group 2*—jejunum anastomosed to a

C. Cojocariu · C. Muzica · O. Petrea · L. Huiban (✉)
Gastroenterology Department, Grigore T. Popa University of Medicine and Pharmacy, Iaşi, Romania

Institute of Gastroenterology and Hepatology, St. Spiridon Emergency Hospital, Iaşi, Romania

A. Trifan et al. (eds.), *Short Bowel Syndrome in Adults*,
https://doi.org/10.1007/978-3-031-95848-9_23

partial colon (jejuno-colonic anastomosis); and *group 3*—jejuno-ileo-colic anastomosis, where the entire colon and ileocecal valve are preserved. Patients with jejuno-ileo-colic anastomosis represent the most favorable anatomical phenotype of SBS, whereas those with end-jejunostomy are the most severe. Patients with high-output end-jejunostomies pose the greatest management challenges due to significant fluid and nutrient losses [3].

Recent guidelines emphasize a multidisciplinary approach involving gastroenterologists, dietitians, surgeons, and specialized healthcare providers. The clinical presentation, prognosis, and management of SBS are influenced by the anatomical configuration of the remaining bowel and its functional capacity. The primary management goals are to minimize reliance on parenteral nutrition (PN), alleviate SBS-related symptoms, prevent complications associated with this condition, and achieve a good quality of life [1].

Survival in patients with SBS is influenced by multiple factors, including the anatomical and functional integrity of the remaining bowel, patient age, underlying disease etiology, coexisting medical conditions, presence of chronic intestinal obstruction, and the expertise of the healthcare management team [2].

The management of patients with SBS differs nationwide. Many individuals, including those with diagnosed or undiagnosed SBS, continue to seek medical care with minimal or no prior education about their condition. That is why these patients need special care and education, and engaging with peers and organizations that have firsthand experience with SBS can significantly enhance patients' understanding of the condition and improve their overall well-being [4]. There are many organizations offering support and education for SBS patients, such as the Oley Foundation and the Short Bowel Syndrome Foundation [2]. Furthermore, actively involving patients with SBS in treatment decisions can enhance their adherence to therapy and contribute to an improved quality of life.

Patients with SBS and their caregivers should receive comprehensive education on essential aspects of the condition. While long-term parenteral nutrition (PN) can impose limitations on daily activities and affect quality of life, it remains a vital, life-sustaining therapy. Over time, with proper guidance and adaptation, individuals receiving PN can adjust their lifestyles to reduce its impact and maintain a greater degree of routine and stability [1].

Effective management of patients with SBS demands diligence, perseverance, and meticulous attention to detail. These patients are fragile and face substantial risks, often leading to a significant decline in quality of life and increased healthcare costs. A thorough understanding of gastrointestinal anatomy and physiology is crucial for identifying these risks and optimizing patient care. A comprehensive, multidisciplinary approach is essential, incorporating dietary and fluid adjustments, symptom-targeted pharmacologic therapy, judicious use of intestinotrophic agents and surgical interventions, and the management of comorbid conditions to enhance outcomes and improve long-term prognosis [1, 2].

The management of SBS patients requires individualized interventions in each particular case and multidisciplinary coordination of dietary, fluid, pharmacologic, and comorbid disease management [5]. The management interventions are vital in both phases of SBS. While the acute phase generally lasts for a few weeks past the intestinal resection and is characterized by increased intestinal fluid losses and metabolic impairment, the adaptation phase could last up to 2 years post-resection. During the adaptation phase, the remaining portions of the intestines and the digestive system undergo structural and functional changes to compensate for the loss by adjusting nutrient absorption and orocecal transit time [6].

As up to 60% of adults and 25% of pediatric patients are lost within 5 years of diagnosis [7, 8], and in most cases, the patients remain on home parenteral nutrition, patient education could be an important component of healthcare, complementary to management interventions.

23.2 The Role of Patient Education in SBS

Recent clinical practice guidelines for SBS patient management recommend that patients and their caregivers should be educated on the most important aspects of SBS. Previous experience showed that patient education successfully improves outcomes, medication adherence, and survival in different chronic and malignant diseases [9–12]. As a result of the important contribution of patient education in disease management, several strategies are also recommended for educating SBS patients. The complexity of this pathological condition and the extensive self and assisted care that includes adherence to medication and dietary adjustments necessitate comprehensive training of the multidisciplinary team, patient, and caregiver (specialized personnel or family members) (Table 23.1).

Current expert opinions suggest that permanent communication between specialists and SBS patients is vital [13]. Additionally, experts highlighted the need for education and specialization for healthcare providers. Both SBS and experts in SBS are relatively rare, thus patients should be advised by the general practitioner to find SBS experts. Iyer et al. [13] cited the example of a New Mexico–based multidisciplinary team that provides educational support for nonspecialist clinicians.

Table 23.1 The targets of SBS patient education

Understanding the anatomy and physiology of SBS
Performing efficient self-monitoring of symptoms and general health status
Understanding the lifestyle changes
Understanding the urge for requesting medical and psychological support, when appropriate
Understanding the importance of clinical monitoring and follow-up
Constantly updating the knowledge on the pathology, management options, and resources
Understanding their participation as active contributors to disease management

Clinical outcomes improvement could be the most important impact of patient education in SBS. Recent studies show that educational interventions directed to SBS patients with intestinal failure could improve awareness and understanding of the disease, facilitate timely diagnosis, and standardize management practices as well as reduce the occurrence of complications requiring hospital admissions, thus reducing the costs of patient management [14, 15].

Since SBS patients are often dependent on partial or total parenteral nutrition, their quality of life could be severely affected. By contrast, being partially or totally disabled could be prevented by patient education in self-management. A systematic review of European and Canadian studies regarding the SBS patients' and caregivers' quality of life concluded that the type of treatment significantly affects the patients' lives [16]. No treatment and dependency on parenteral nutrition were reported as a significant negative influence on quality of life. Iyer et al. [13] established that patients with parenteral nutrition could be educated on how to automate and mobilize logistical support to reduce disability. A recent study shows that self-management techniques could contribute to enhanced coping mechanisms and emotional support [17].

Another important role of SBS patient education is adherence to prescribed treatment. According to the guidelines suggested by Kumpf and Parrish [18], different types of treatments significantly improve patient outcomes. Yet a vital component of treatment approaches that ensures efficiency is patient adherence [19].

23.3 Common Practices in SBS Patient Education

In SBS, patient education should be focused on self-monitoring, self-care, and psychological support. Specifically, several key components include the patient's understanding of the pathology and the particular management interventions recommended for their case. The attending physician should clearly explain the causes, symptoms, and changes in their lives when being diagnosed with SBS. The use of simple terms and visual aids, such as charts, videos, or any digital resource could help patients better understand the condition they are diagnosed with. Clinical practice experience has shown that patients who understand the meaning of their symptoms have increased positive outcomes. These could result from reporting the symptoms to a healthcare provider and dealing with them through interventions previously designed by their medical caregivers [16]. In SBS, patients should be educated to recognize the clinical signs of the most frequent symptoms and complications, such as diarrhea, weight loss, dehydration, anemia, and nutrient deficiencies.

Also, SBS patients could benefit from a good understanding of the medication used for their condition. Besides the long-term treatments, SBS patients should know when to self-administer therapies, such as over-the-counter antidiarrheals, prebiotics, probiotics, vitamins, minerals, electrolytes, and digestion supplements [5].

While SBS patients are dependent on partial or total parenteral nutrition, in many cases, they should be instructed to communicate with their attending physician when changes in overall health status occur. Recently, the dependency on partial or total parenteral nutrition could be corrected by innovative interventions (e.g. intestinal transplantation). Catron et al. [20] reported parenteral nutrition elimination in five young SBS patients following intestinal transplantation, but concluded that the success of the procedure is primarily due to individualized care and frequent patient communication.

Since previous studies have reported that the incidence of nutritional deficits is high when partial or total parenteral nutrition is administered, SBS patients should be instructed to recognize the most common symptoms of various hypovitaminosis and mineral deficits and to search for immediate medical care [19, 21–23]. Similarly, SBS patients should be educated to recognize the symptoms of known complications and early signs of occurrence of comorbidities, such as small intestine bacterial overgrowth, severe dehydration, kidney failure, and liver failure [19, 21, 24]. However, since some of the symptoms may not be recognized by the patient or their caregiver, SBS patient education should focus on the importance of monitoring and follow-up provided by the attending physician. They should understand the particular needs of their condition for regular medical monitoring and self-monitoring of health status. Benefits may arise from using written logs or smart applications.

SBS patients who are not dependent on PN should be instructed on the particular requirements of their diet as well as the benefits that these changes provide. Various studies and resources teach SBS patients that nutrient absorption is more efficient if smaller and repeated meals are administered, while abundant meals and several aliments predispose them to complications, such as intestinal obstruction [5, 25–27]. Similarly, SBS patients should be instructed on how to prevent diarrhea and intestinal bacterial overgrowth by limiting simple carbohydrates and adding foods that are rich in protein content [28, 29].

Consequent to the progress of science and technology, new resources are emerging. As psychological and emotional support was previously provided through support groups and specialized therapy, online resources and widespread multilingual access now enable SBS patients to connect globally [5, 30]. However, caution should be advised when using these resources, as many differences were noted between the populations in several physiological aspects, such as diet particularities [1, 31–34]. An educational paper written by a Polish group of SBS experts [35] comprehensively presented detailed information about the particularities of the digestive system and nutrition in SBS.

Due to the increased psychological burden and decreased quality of life among SBS patients, patient education and management should include efforts to prevent the occurrence of comorbid mental health disorders, such as stress, anxiety, and depression [36, 37]. Consequently, SBS patients should be educated on symptom management options to live a close-to-normal life rather than limiting their activities (travel, work, daily chores, and social interactions) [13, 38].

As described above, almost any resource at the disposal of the gastroenterology expert could be used to educate SBS patients as a part of the more complex process

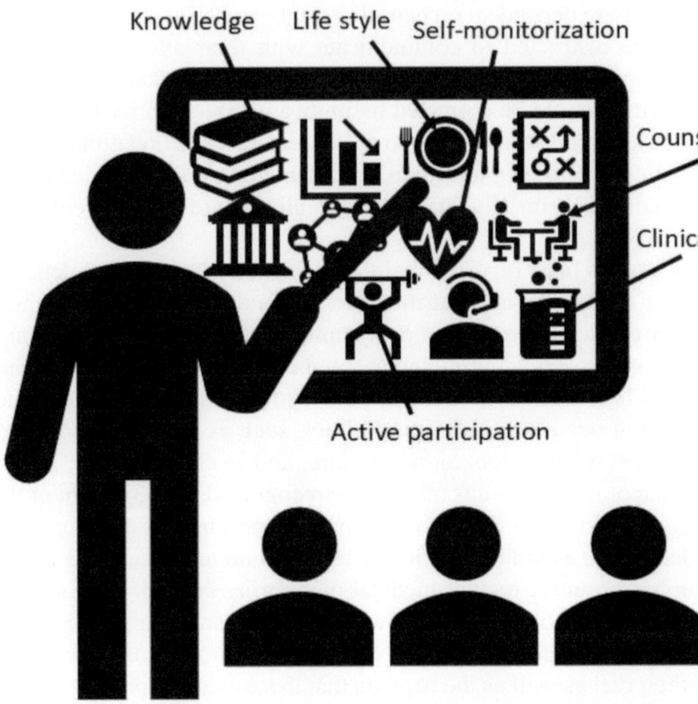

Fig. 23.1 Items of SBS patient education. (Created with BioRender.com)

of disease management (Fig. 23.1). The objective assessment of the patient's clinical spectrum, needs, preferences, limitations, and goals could significantly improve the formulation of individualized management programs. The thorough training of the experts should be accompanied by the willingness to develop trusting relationships with the patients. Modern technological resources (smartphone applications, telehealth, online resources) could also be useful in SBS patient education.

23.4 Limitations and Future Perspectives

Sometimes, SBS patient education could be limited by certain issues, such as limited availability of specialists or time, limited access to educational means, or limited understanding (Table 23.2).

The patient education process often resides in the education of the clinical practitioner who provides healthcare services [39, 40]. Real-world observations based on clinical cases suggested that efficient guidelines for managing the most prevalent symptoms that lead to complications (chronic diarrhea and nutrient loss) could significantly improve the development of best practices for individualized medical care [41]. Furthermore, the reduced number of gastroenterology specialists and the increasing number of patients could prevent extended management processes for

Table 23.2 Limitations of SBS patient education

Limited resources and guidelines for healthcare providers
Limited number of specialists to perform patient education programs
Limited time for counseling and education
Limited access to educational means
Cultural, educational, or cognitive limitations

SBS patients. Since patient education is mainly performed by the clinical practitioner during monitoring visits and follow-ups, counseling and education could take time.

In SBS patients experiencing severe complications, the associated comorbid cognitive disorders, such as depression, anxiety, or decreased performance in content retention, could prevent understanding and participation in educational processes [5]. Also, belonging to vulnerable populations or having limited medical knowledge could decrease the efficiency of patient education programs [42, 43]. Socioeconomic and cultural barriers were also reported as potential limitations of the efficiency of education programs.

The future perspectives of SBS patient education could be correlated with addressing the limitations with continuous research on SBS pathology and management options. The development of novel educational means could also improve the patient education process by adapting innovative resources to the needs of both educators and patients (e.g., artificial intelligence). The increasing number of reports of the significant improvements brought by artificial intelligence use in patient education suggests the encouraging future perspective of artificial intelligence-based resources [44–48]. A prestigious medical school in England is currently offering online programs to train healthcare providers on artificial intelligence as an efficient tool in clinical practice.

Furthermore, long-term educational interventions are less studied for SBS but reported as efficient in the management of other gastrointestinal diseases, with special regard to improving the patient's quality of life [49], improving ergonomics in gastrointestinal endoscopy [50, 51] or preventing the misuse of over-the-counter medication, such as broad-spectrum antibiotics or proton pump inhibitors [52, 53].

23.5 Conclusions

In conclusion, healthcare providers should consider that individualized approaches are often needed in SBS patients based on the particularities of their pathological profiles. In this context, SBS management could imply periodic follow-ups and specialized medical counseling as newer resources are constantly emerging and modern-era pathologies are complexly evolving. Thus, the final role of patient education is to provide comprehensive support and empowerment for SBS patients to maximize outcomes and improve their quality of life. Many resources could be used to educate SBS patients as a part of the more complex disease management. The objective assessment of the patient's clinical tableau, needs, preferences, limitations, and goals could significantly improve the formulation of individualized management programs. The thorough training of the experts should be accompanied by the willingness to develop trusting relationships with the patients. Modern technological resources (smartphone applications, telehealth, online resources) could also be vital in SBS patient education.

References

1. Tappenden KA. Anatomical and physiological considerations in short bowel syndrome: emphasis on intestinal adaptation and the role of enterohormones. Nutr Clin Pract. 2023;38:S27–34.
2. Parrish CR, DiBaise JK. Managing the adult patient with short bowel syndrome. Gastroenterol Hepatol (N Y). 2017;13(10):600–8. PMID: 29230136; PMCID: PMC5718176.
3. Tappenden KA. Pathophysiology of short bowel syndrome: considerations of resected and residual anatomy. JPEN J Parenter Enteral Nutr. 2014;38:14S–22S.
4. Parrish CR, Wall E. The Clinician's Toolkit for the adult short bowel patient part I: nutrition and hydration therapy. Pract Gastroenterol. 2022;46(6):32–8 and 40–41 and 49–53.
5. Ahmed M, Ahmed S. Functional, Diagnostic and Therapeutic Aspects of Gastrointestinal Hormones. Gastroenterol Res. 2019;12(5):233–44.
6. DiBaise JK. Management of short bowel syndrome in adults. In: Connor RF, editor. UpToDate. Wolters Kluwer. Last updated: 6 Feb 2023. Accessed 20 Feb 2025.
7. Schalamon J, Mayr JM, Höllwarth ME. Mortality and economics in short bowel syndrome. Best Pract Res Clin Gastroenterol. 2003;17(6):931–42.
8. Ukkola-Vuoti L, Tuominen S, Pohju A, Kovac B, Lassenius MI, Merras-Salmio L, et al. Expenditure and survival of adult patients with intestinal failure due to short bowel syndrome: real-world evidence from Southern Finland. Scand J Gastroenterol. 2024;59(4):401–10.
9. Underwood PW, Herremans KM, Neal D, Riner AN, Nassour I, Hughes SJ, Trevino JG. Changing practice patterns and improving survival for patients with pancreatic ductal adenocarcinoma. Cancer. 2023;15(18):4464.
10. Friedman AJ, Cosby R, Boyko S, Hatton-Bauer J, Turnbull G. Effective teaching strategies and methods of delivery for patient education: a systematic review and practice guideline recommendations. J Cancer Educ. 2010;26(1):12–21.
11. Paterick TE, Patel N, Tajik AJ, Chandrasekaran K. Improving health outcomes through patient education and partnerships with patients. Proc (Bayl Univ Med Cent). 2017;30(1):112–3.
12. Magee MF, Khan NH, Desale S, Nassar CM. Diabetes to go: knowledge- and competency-based hospital survival skills diabetes education program improves postdischarge medication adherence. Diabetes Educ. 2014;40(3):344–50.
13. Iyer K, DiBaise JK, Rubio-Tapia A. AGA clinical practice update on management of short bowel syndrome: expert review. Clin Gastroenterol Hepatol. 2022;20(10):2185–94.e2.
14. Belcher E, Mercer D, Raphael BP, Salinas GD, Stacy S, Tappenden KA. Management of short-bowel syndrome: a survey of unmet educational needs among healthcare providers. JPEN J Parenter Enteral Nutr. 2022;46(8):1839–46.
15. Adu-Gyamfi KO, Pant C, Deshpande A, Olyaee M. Readmissions related to short bowel syndrome: a study from a national database. J Investig Med. 2019;67(7):1092–4.
16. Chen Y, Yan M, Chen H, Sheng Y, Wang Z, Wu B. A systematic review of quality of life in patients with short bowel syndrome and their caregivers. Patient Prefer Adherence. 2024;18:1217–30.
17. Kumpf VJ, Neumann ML, Kakani SR. Advocating for a patient- and family centered care approach to management of short bowel syndrome. Nutr Clin Pract. 2023;38(Suppl 1):S35–45.
18. Kumpf VJ, Parish CR. The Clinician's Toolkit for the adult short bowel patient part II: pharmacologic interventions. Pract Gastroenterol Nutr Issues Gastroenterol. 2022;222:12–31.

19. Wall EA. An overview of short bowel syndrome management: adherence, adaptation, and practical recommendations. J Acad Nutr Diet. 2013;113(9):1200–8.
20. Catron H, Hanson C, Beerman L, Carney J, Janiak K, Gerhardt B, Rochling F, Mercer D. Sustained elimination of parenteral support in adult patients with under 60 cm of small intestine: a case series. Nutr Clin Pract. 2024;39(1):227–34.
21. Utrilla Fornals A, Costas-Batlle C, Medlin S, Menjón-Lajusticia E, Cisneros-González J, Saura-Carmona P, Montoro-Huguet MA. Metabolic and nutritional issues after lower digestive tract surgery: the important role of the dietitian in a multidisciplinary setting. Nutrients. 2024;16(2):246.
22. Chatzidaki V, Wood R, Alegakis A, Lawson M, Fagbemi A. Parenteral support and micronutrient deficiencies in children with short bowel syndrome: a comprehensive retrospective study. Clin Nutr ESPEN. 2023;58:270–6.
23. Vara-Luiz F, Glória L, Mendes I, Carlos S, Guerra P, Nunes G, Oliveira CS, Ferreira A, Santos AP, Fonseca J. Chronic intestinal failure and short bowel syndrome in adults: the state of the art. GE Port J Gastroenterol. 2024;31(6):388–400.
24. Bering J, DiBaise JK. Short bowel syndrome: complications and management. Nutr Clin Pract. 2023;38(Suppl 1):S46–58.
25. Estívariz CF, Luo M, Umeakunne K, Bazargan N, Galloway JR, Leader LM, Ziegler TR. Nutrient intake from habitual oral diet in patients with severe short bowel syndrome living in the southeastern United States. Nutrition. 2008;24(4):330–9.
26. Akrami M, Sasani MR. Dietary habits affect quality of life: bowel obstruction caused by phytobezoar. Iran J Public Health. 2016;45(8):1080–2.
27. Shah ND, Cornell L, DIGID Short Bowel Syndrome Workgroup. Short bowel syndrome (SBS): Nutrition 101 AGA GI Patient Center Website. https://patient.gastro.org/short-bowel-syndrome-sbs-nutrition-101/. Accessed 19 Feb 2025.
28. Dukowicz AC, Lacy BE, Levine GM. Small intestinal bacterial overgrowth: a comprehensive review. Gastroenterol Hepatol (N Y). 2007;3(2):112–22.
29. Zubair M. Small Intestinal Bacterial Overgrowth (SIBO) MSD manual. Professional version. Patient education page. https://www.msdmanuals.com/professional/gastrointestinal-disorders/malabsorption-syndromes/small-intestinal-bacterial-overgrowth-sibo. Accessed 18 Feb 2025.
30. Short Bowel Syndrome Foundation. Online support groups resources. https://shortbowelfoundation.org/short-bowel-syndrome-support-groups/. Accessed 20 Feb 2025.
31. Bolo A, Verger E, Fouillet H, Mariotti F. Exploring multidimensional and within-food group diversity for diet quality and long-term health in high-income countries. Adv Nutr. 2024;15(9):100278.
32. Bennett G, Bardon LA, Gibney ER. A comparison of dietary patterns and factors influencing food choice among ethnic groups living in one locality: a systematic review. Nutrients. 2022;14(5):941.
33. Singh RB, Fedacko J, Fatima G, Magomedova A, Watanabe S, Elkilany G. Why and how the indo-Mediterranean diet may be superior to other diets: the role of antioxidants in the diet. Nutrients. 2022;14(4):898.
34. Iacovou M, Tan V, Muir JG, Gibson PR. The low FODMAP diet and its application in East and Southeast Asia. J Neurogastroenterol Motil. 2015;21(4):459–70.
35. Szczygiel B, Jonkers-Schuitema CF, Naber T. Basics in clinical nutrition: nutritional support in extensive gut resections (short bowel). e-SPEN. 2010;5:e63–8.
36. Kalaitzakis E, Carlsson E, Josefsson A, Bosaeus I. Quality of life in short-bowel syndrome: impact of fatigue and gastrointestinal symptoms. Scand J Gastroenterol. 2008;43(9):1057–65.
37. Kossewska J, Bierlit K, Trajkovski V. Personality, anxiety, and stress in patients with small intestine bacterial overgrowth syndrome. The Polish Preliminary Study. Int J Environ Res Public Health. 2022;20(1):93.
38. Guillen B, Atherton NS. Short bowel syndrome. [Updated 2023 Jul 17]. In: StatPearls. Treasure Island (FL): StatPearls Publishing; 2025. https://www.ncbi.nlm.nih.gov/books/NBK536935

39. Fradkov E, Goldowsky A, Quiles K, Williams R. A quality improvement educational intervention to increase knowledge of cardiogastroenterology amongst medical trainees and nursing staff. MedEdPORTAL. 2017;13:10642.
40. Sewell JL. A practical approach to disseminating gastroenterology education scholarship. Clin Gastroenterol Hepatol. 2023;21(12):2999–3004.
41. Wall E, Catron H, Delgado A, Greif S, Herlitz J, Moccia L, Lozano E, Mercer D, Vanuytsel T, Berner-Hansen M, Lakananurak N, Gramlich L. A multidisciplinary team evaluation of management guidelines for adult short bowel syndrome. Clin Nutr ESPEN. 2023;54:41–4.
42. Man A, van Ballegooie C. Assessment of the readability of web-based patient education material from major Canadian pediatric associations: cross-sectional study. JMIR Pediatr Parent. 2022;5(1):e31820.
43. Safeer RS, Keenan J. Health literacy: the gap between physicians and patients. Am Fam Physician. 2005;72(3):463–8.
44. Moons P, Van Bulck L. Using ChatGPT and Google Bard to improve the readability of written patient information: a proof-of-concept. Eur J Cardiovasc Nurs. 2024;23(2):122–6.
45. Tariq R, Sahil K. Artificial intelligence–powered patient education for comprehensive and individualized understanding for patients. Clin Gastroenterol Hepatol. 2022;22(7):1550–1.
46. Thorat V, Rao P, Joshi N, Talreja P, Shetty AR. Role of artificial intelligence (AI) in patient education and communication in dentistry. Cureus. 2024;16(5):e59799.
47. Mucci A, Green WM, Hill LH. Incorporation of artificial intelligence in healthcare professions and patient education for fostering effective patient care. In: New directions for adult and continuing education; 2024. p. 51–62.
48. Robinson CL, D'Souza RS, Yazdi C, Diejomaoh EM, Schatman ME, Emerick T, Orhurhu V. Reviewing the potential role of artificial intelligence in delivering personalized and interactive pain medicine education for chronic pain patients. J Pain Res. 2024;17:923–9.
49. Akbari Namvar Z, Mahdavi R, Shirmohammadi M, et al. The effect of group-based education on gastrointestinal symptoms and quality of life in patients with celiac disease: randomized controlled clinical trial. BMC Gastroenterol. 2022;22(18)
50. de Jong JJ, Lantinga MA, Tan ACITL, et al. Web-based educational intervention for patients with uninvestigated dyspepsia referred for upper gastrointestinal tract endoscopy: a randomized clinical trial. JAMA Intern Med. 2021;181(6):825–33.
51. Scaffidi MA, Gimpaya N, Fecso AB, Khan R, Li J, Bansal R, Torabi N, Shergill AK, Grover SC. Educational interventions to improve ergonomics in gastrointestinal endoscopy: a systematic review. Endosc Int Open. 2022;10(9):E1322–7.
52. Lazaridis LD, Rizos E, Bounou L, Theodorou-Kanakari A, Kalousios S, Mavroeidi EA, Roma M, Chatzidakis A, Vlachonicolou G, Miltiadou K, Gkolfakis P, Tziatzios G, Triantafyllou K. An educational intervention to optimize use of proton pump inhibitors in a Greek University Hospital. Ann Gastroenterol. 2021;34(6):781–7.
53. Langdridge D, Virhia J, McMullan R, Banks D, Biard O, Charitonos K, Alunyo JP, Kagoya EK, Olupot-Olupot P. Effectiveness of work-based educational interventions for antimicrobial stewardship: a systematic review. JAC Antimicrob Resist. 2024;6(6):dlae192.

Future Perspectives in Short Bowel Syndrome: Organoid-Based Tissue-Engineered Small Intestine, SIC, and Xenotransplantation

24

Ioana Manea and Liana Gheorghe

24.1 Introduction

The human intestine is a complex structure with multiple functions. In addition to its cardinal role in the final steps of digestion and the absorption of nutrients, it is also pivotal in maintaining a barrier against the contents of the lumen. Harboring the human gut microbiota, immunomodulatory and neurohormonal roles also make the human intestine a key structure in maintaining homeostasis.

Extensive loss of the small intestine, either anatomical (such as short bowel syndrome) or functional (congenital conditions, dysmotility, etc.), leads invariably to intestinal failure (IF). Short bowel syndrome (SBS) is the most severe form of IF, and it is also irreversible. Patients with SBS are dependent on parenteral nutrition and hydration. Intestinal adaptation as a compensatory mechanism can be further stimulated with parenteral nutrition and enhanced with the aid of medication: growth factors (growth hormone, glutamine, glucagon-like peptide 2), antisecretory drugs (H2 receptor antagonists, proton pump inhibitors), antimotility medication (loperamide, cholestyramine), antibiotics, and probiotics to control small intestine bacterial overgrowth (SIBO) [1]. However, current treatment options, including intestine transplantation, seem to be insufficient.

The necessity to overcome the consequences of intestinal failure (digestive incapacity and absorptive dysfunction leading to malnutrition) has brought to attention organoid development and xenografting technologies.

I. Manea (✉)
Carol Davila University of Medicine and Pharmacy, Bucharest, Romania

L. Gheorghe
Carol Davila University of Medicine and Pharmacy, Bucharest, Romania

Center for Digestive Diseases and Liver Transplant, Fundeni Clinical Institute, Bucharest, Romania

A. Trifan et al. (eds.), *Short Bowel Syndrome in Adults*,
https://doi.org/10.1007/978-3-031-95848-9_24

Patient-derived organoids (PDOs) are three-dimensional structures derived from the patient's own cells. The principle behind all organoid generation is that when primary cells isolated from patients are embedded in the proper extracellular matrix-like structure, they have the ability to self-organize into three-dimensional structures that become autonomous and also have the ability, at least in part, to recapitulate the morphology and physiology of the tissue of origin [2]. An essential part of the process is the use of growth media containing, aside from nutrients, the growth factors specific to the tissue of origin.

Thus far, PDOs have been widely used in studies on various types of tissues, both wild-type and tumoral, in order to advance functional studies, disease modeling, pharmacotyping studies [3, 4], etc. When addressing the specific matter of small intestine organoid clinical use, there are several key aspects to be taken into account:

- The type of extracellular matrix extract and growth medium used must be appropriate for organoid grafting/transplantation.
- The amount of organoids generated must be large enough to suffice the grafting/transplantation procedure.
- Organoid models used in basic science studies are usually obtained from intestinal stem cells (ISCs) from the base of the intestinal crypts. Thus, the organoids will not contain the non-epithelial structures present in the original tissue (mesenchymal cells, endothelial cells, immune cells).

Therefore, it is essential to adapt the organoid generation technology to the type of downstream application that follows: basic science studies or clinical studies involving grafting/transplantation.

24.2 Laboratory Requirements for Organoid Culturing

The equipment and general consumables required for organoid generation and biobanking are similar to those used in monolayer cell cultures. The minimal equipment requirements are as follows:

- Safety cabinet—class II
- Centrifuge with temperature control (refrigerated centrifuge)—with rotors suitable for 50 and 15 mL conical tubes (ideally, with swing-out rotors)
- Microcentrifuge
- Incubator with carbon dioxide source (that can be set for 37 °C and 5% carbon dioxide atmosphere)
- Inverted light microscope
- 2–8 °C fridge; −20 °C fridge; −80 °C fridge; liquid nitrogen storing unit
- Freezing containers with a controlled rate of cooling
- Weighing scales (for micrograms, milligrams, and grams)
- Pipettes and micropipettes ranging from 25 mL to 0.1 μL

General consumables are similar for all types of organoids, irrespective of the tissue of origin and are extensively presented in the organoid protocol by Driehuis et al. [5].

24.3 Specimen Collection and Transportation

Organoids can be developed from all kinds of tissues obtained via biopsy or surgical resection. For intestinal organoids, most commonly, the patient undergoes endoscopy and one or several biopsies are taken from the healthy areas of the intestine. The bioptic tissue is then transported to the laboratory (in dedicated transport media) where it is enzymatically digested (using enzymes such as collagenase, Accutase, or various trypsin/trypsin-like enzyme combinations) into small clusters of cells.

A general laboratory good practice rule for any type of cell culture derived from primary cells (patient-derived cell cultures) is that transportation of the biological material to the research laboratory, irrespective of its provenance, should be performed as soon as possible—cell viability decreases over time.

Tissue samples are collected directly in transport medium containing Advanced DMEM/F12, fetal calf serum or fetal bovine serum (FCS or FBS), and several antimicrobial agents [6]. The addition of Rho-kinase inhibitor Y-27632 to the collection and transport medium will decrease anoikis, and thus increase the organoid yield per sample [6].

The sample should be processed immediately upon arrival. However, should extemporaneous processing not be possible, the tissue may be preserved in dedicated cell culture freezing medium, at −80 °C, as described in Urbano PCM et al. [6].

24.4 Organoid Culturing

For intestinal crypt isolation, samples must be devoid of underlying muscle tissue. This can be achieved with a surgical blade or with surgical scissors [7]. All processing steps in the organoid generation protocols are to be performed at low temperatures, using cold phosphate buffered saline (PBS) and ethylenediaminetetraacetic acid (EDTA) chelation buffers. Typically, this refers to refrigerator temperatures (2–8 °C).

Tissue fragments should be about 5 mm in size [8]. After fragmenting the tissue into small pieces with a surgical blade, the fragments are washed in cold PBS, and then incubated with EDTA chelation buffer. In order to best separate the crypts from the fragments, several steps of resuspension followed by sedimentation are required. Sato et al. recommend 6–8 resuspension/sedimentation cycles [8]. However, depending on the sample, the number of crypts isolated in the supernatant can be assessed microscopically and the number of cycles adjusted.

The supernatant containing the crypts is centrifuged in order to pellet the crypts and separate them from single cells. After discarding the supernatant, the pelleted crypts are resuspended in extracellular matrix extract (ECM). Table 24.1 presents a

Table 24.1 Extracellular matrices used in intestinal organoid culture

Extracellular matrix type	Reference article
Matrigel (basement membrane extract)	Sato, T., et al. (2009). *Nature*, 459(7244), 262–265. https://doi.org/10.1038/nature07935 [2]
Cultrex (basement membrane extract)	Co, J. Y., et al. (2019). *Cell Reports*, 26(9), 2509–2520. e4. https://doi.org/10.1016/j.celrep.2019.01.108 [9]
Collagen I hydrogels	Peng, H., et al. (2015). *ACS Biomaterials Science & Engineering*, 1(1), 37–42. https://doi.org/10.1021/ab500041d [10]
Matrigel (basement membrane extract)	Watson, C. L., et al. (2014). *Nature Medicine*, 20(11), 1310–1314. https://doi.org/10.1038/nm.3737 [11]
Polyethylene glycol hydrogels (PEG RGD)	Gjorevski, N., et al. (2016). *Nature*, 539(7630), 560–564. https://doi.org/.1038/nature20168 [12]
PEG-4MAL	Cruz-Acuña, R., et al. (2017). *Nature Cell Biology*, 19(11), 1326–1335. https://doi.org/10.1038/ncb3632 [13]
Decellularized human intestinal scaffolds/Cultrex (basement membrane extract)	Meran, L., et al. (2020). *Nature Medicine*, 26(10), 1593–1601. https://doi.org/10.1038/s41596-022-00751-1
Matrigel (basement membrane extract)	Lei, N. Y., et al. (2014). *PLOS ONE*, 9(1), e84651. https://doi.org/10.1371/journal.pone.0084651 [14]
PEG RGD with laminin-111	Gjorevski, N., & Lutolf, M. P. (2017). *Nature Protocols*, 12(11), 2263–2274. https://doi.org/10.1038/nprot.2017.095 [15]
Matrigel (basement membrane extract)	Spence, J. R., et al. (2011). *Nature*, 470(7332), 105–109. https://doi.org/10.1038/nature09691 [16]
Type I collagen–Matrigel mix	Nikolaev, M., et al. (2020). *Nature*, 585(7826), 574–578. https://doi.org/10.1038/s41586-020-2724-8 [17]

PEG RGD polyethylene glycol with arginine-glycine-aspartic acid peptide, *PEG-4MAL* polyethylene glycol with 4 maleimide functional groups, *ECM* extracellular matrix, *DMEM/F12* Dulbecco's modified eagle medium/nutrient mixture F-12, *RGD* arginine-glycine-aspartic acid (a cell adhesion peptide)

list of extracellular matrices that have been used in several articles employing intestinal organoid culturing in their experiments. As a general laboratory good practice rule, when developing cultures that need very specific growth factors to thrive, it is adamant to use growth factor reduced ECMs.

After resuspending the crypts in ECM, small domes of the mixture are pipetted into the culture plates. The size of the culture plate used should be determined by the amount of sample available—small samples should be plated in smaller wells (e.g., 48 or 24 wells) so that the crypts would not be too sparsely distributed. Depending on the type of ECM used, the domes containing the crypts polymerize and solidify (manufacturers' instructions should be followed) (Table 24.1).

After the ECM is fully polymerized, growth medium is added to each well, and the plate is incubated at 37 °C, in 5% carbon dioxide atmosphere. Table 24.2 presents a list of culture media that have been used in several articles employing intestinal organoid culturing in their experiments.

Table 24.2 Culture media used in intestinal organoid culture

Culture media type	Reference article
Advanced DMEM/F12, HEPES, Glutamax, B27, NACC, Gastrin, EGF, Nicotinamide, A83-01, Wnt3a, RSPO, Noggin, antibiotic	Sato, T., et al. (2009). *Nature*, 459(7244), 262–265. https://doi.org/10.1038/nature07935 [2]
Advanced DMEM/F12, HEPES, Glutamax, B27, NACC, Gastrin, EGF, Nicotinamide, A83-01, Wnt3a, RSPO, Noggin, antibiotic	Co, J. Y., et al. (2019). *Cell Reports*, 26(9), 2509–2520.e4. https://doi.org/10.1016/j.celrep.2019.01.108 [9]
Advanced DMEM/F12, HEPES, Glutamax, B27, NACC, Gastrin, EGF, Nicotinamide, RSPO, Noggin, N2, antibiotic	Peng, H., et al. (2015). *ACS Biomaterials Science & Engineering*, 1(1), 37–42. https://doi.org/10.1021/ab500041d [10]
Advanced DMEM/F12, HEPES, Glutamax, B27, EGF, Noggin, antibiotic	Watson, C. L., et al. (2014). *Nature Medicine*, 20(11), 1310–1314. https://doi.org/10.1038/nm.3737 [11]
Advanced DMEM/F12, HEPES, Glutamax, B27, NACC, Gastrin, EGF, Nicotinamide, RSPO, Noggin, N2, CHIR99021, valproic acid, antibiotic	Gjorevski, N., et al. (2016). Nature, 539(7630), 560–564. https://doi.org/10.1038/nature20168 [12]
Advanced DMEM/F12, HEPES, Glutamax, B27, EGF, RSPO, Noggin, antibiotic	Cruz-Acuña, R., et al. (2017). *Nature Cell Biology*, 19(11), 1326–1335. https://doi.org/10.1038/ncb3632 [13]
Advanced DMEM/F12, HEPES, Glutamax, B27, NACC, Gastrin, EGF, Nicotinamide, A83-01, Wnt3a, RSPO, Noggin, SB202190, CHIR99021, antibiotic	Meran, L., et al. (2020). *Nature Medicine*, 26(10), 1593–1601. https://doi.org/10.1038/s41596-022-00751-1
Advanced DMEM/F12, HEPES, Glutamax, B27, NACC, EGF, RSPO, Noggin, antibiotic	Lei, N. Y., et al. (2014). *PLOS ONE*, 9(1), e84651. https://doi.org/10.1371/journal.pone.0084651 [14]
Advanced DMEM/F12, HEPES, Glutamax, B27, EGF, RSPO, Noggin, N2, CHIR99021, valproic acid, antibiotic	Gjorevski, N., & Lutolf, M. P. (2017). *Nature Protocols*, 12(11), 2263–2274. https://doi.org/10.1038/nprot.2017.095 [15]
mTesR1 medium (before differentiation); after differentiation: Advanced DMEM/F12, HEPES, L-Glutamine, B27, EGF, RSPO, Noggin, N2, antibiotic	Spence, J. R., et al. (2011). *Nature*, 470(7332), 105–109. https://doi.org/10.1038/nature09691 [16]
Advanced DMEM/F12, HEPES, Glutamax, B27, NACC, EGF, RSPO, Noggin, N2, CHIR99021, valproic acid, antibiotic	Nikolaev, M., et al. (2020). *Nature*, 585(7826), 574–578. https://doi.org/10.1038/s41586-020-2724-8 [17]

DMEM/F12 Dulbecco's modified eagle medium/nutrient mixture F-12, *HEPES* 4-(2-hydroxyethyl)-1-piperazineethanesulfonic acid (a buffering agent), *B27* B27 supplement (a serum-free additive for neural/epithelial cultures), *NACC* N-acetylcysteine, *EGF* epidermal growth factor, *RSPO* R-spondin (a Wnt signaling activator), *Noggin* bone morphogenetic protein inhibitor, *N2* N2 supplement (a nutrient mix for neuronal and epithelial cultures), *CHIR99021* GSK-3β inhibitor (activates Wnt/β-catenin signaling), *A83-01* TGF-β type I receptor inhibitor, *SB202190* p38 MAP kinase inhibitor, *mTeSR1* maintenance medium for human pluripotent stem cells

During the first few days, the cultures should be followed closely for potential signs of infection. After that, culture media is changed according to each sample's growth rate.

24.5 Alternative Scaffolding and the Perspective of Xenotransplantation

A protocol published in 2023 has engineered human mucosal grafts from PDOs. The novelty presented in the study is that the intestinal PDOs derived from intestinal crypts were co-cultured with fibroblasts and embedded in a natural scaffold derived from resected human intestine [8] (Table 24.2).

The decellularized human intestine scaffold is obtained from fresh surgically resected human intestine. The cells go through a process of osmotic shock disintegration, followed by several steps of enzymatic treatment, using a detergent (in order to successfully remove lipids).

Removal of residual cells is performed with a mild detergent (Na deoxycholate) followed by Dnase-I (an endonuclease that is active against both packaged and unpackaged DNA).

According to the authors, the scaffold thus obtained may have a stability of months, but may be preserved for up to several years. Another study on human tissue derived scaffold (oesophagus-derived) has reported a stability of 6 months in liquid nitrogen [18]. The intestinal scaffold was recellularized at the luminal pole, in a bioreactor, first with the fibroblasts and then with the intestinal organoids.

Intestinal grafts obtained from both patient-derived scaffolding and patient-derived organoids represent a promising technology for xenotransplantation. Furthermore, a study published in 2022 reports developing a xenotransplantation system that embeds human intestinal organoids in decellularized mouse intestines. The authors have reported successfully repopulating scaffolds with both wild-type and tumoral organoids, and obtaining intestinal crypts and tumoral tissue resembling the tissue of origin, respectively [19].

Organoids and organoid co-culture systems have emerged as crucial scientific tools in basic science. Their potential applications range from disease modeling and drug discovery and testing, to personalized regenerative medicine and tissue engineering. The development of new scaffolding materials and the automation of organoid generation represent a promising avenue for bioengineering patient-derived tissue and xenotransplantation, with the potential to bypass the shortcomings of transplantation and offer short bowel syndrome patients more effective therapies in the future.

References

1. Neelis EG, Olieman JF, Hulst JM, de Koning BA, Wijnen RM, Rings EH. Promoting intestinal adaptation by nutrition and medication. Best Pract Res Clin Gastroenterol. 2016;30(2):249–61. https://doi.org/10.1016/j.bpg.2016.03.002. Epub 2016 Mar 8. PMID: 27086889.

2. Sato T, Vries RG, Snippert HJ, van de Wetering M, Barker N, Stange DE, van Es JH, Abo A, Kujala P, Peters PJ, Clevers H. Single Lgr5 stem cells build crypt-villus structures in vitro without a mesenchymal niche. Nature. 2009;459(7244):262–5. https://doi.org/10.1038/nature07935. Epub 2009 Mar 29. PMID: 19329995.
3. Fujii M, Sato T. Somatic cell-derived organoids as prototypes of human epithelial tissues and diseases. Nat Mater. 2021;20(2):156–69. Epub 2020 Aug 17. PMID: 32807924. https://doi.org/10.1038/s41563-020-0754-0.
4. Grützmeier SE, Kovacevic B, Vilmann P, Rift CV, Melchior LC, Holmström MO, Brink L, Hassan H, Karstensen JG, Grossjohann H, Chiranth D, Toxværd A, Hansen CP, Høgdall E, Hasselby JP, Klausen P. Validation of a novel EUS-FNB-derived organoid co-culture system for drug screening in patients with pancreatic cancer. Cancers (Basel). 2023;15(14):3677. https://doi.org/10.3390/cancers15143677. PMID: 37509338; PMCID: PMC10377599.
5. Driehuis E, Gracanin A, Vries RGJ, Clevers H, Boj SF. Establishment of pancreatic organoids from normal tissue and tumors. STAR Protoc. 2020;1(3):100192. https://doi.org/10.1016/j.xpro.2020.100192. PMID: 33377086; PMCID: PMC7757566.
6. Urbano PCM, Angus HCK, Gadeock S, Schultz M, Kemp RA. Assessment of source material for human intestinal organoid culture for research and clinical use. BMC Res Notes. 2022;15(1):35. https://doi.org/10.1186/s13104-022-05925-4. PMID: 35144661; PMCID: PMC8830126.
7. Sato T, Stange DE, Ferrante M, Vries RG, Van Es JH, Van den Brink S, Van Houdt WJ, Pronk A, Van Gorp J, Siersema PD, Clevers H. Long-term expansion of epithelial organoids from human colon, adenoma, adenocarcinoma, and Barrett's epithelium. Gastroenterology. 2011;141(5):1762–72. https://doi.org/10.1053/j.gastro.2011.07.050. Epub 2011 Sep 2. PMID: 21889923.
8. Meran L, Tullie L, Eaton S, De Coppi P, Li VSW. Bioengineering human intestinal mucosal grafts using patient-derived organoids, fibroblasts and scaffolds. Nat Protoc. 2023;18(1):108–35. https://doi.org/10.1038/s41596-022-00751-1. Epub 2022 Oct 19. PMID: 36261633.
9. Co JY, Margalef-Català M, Li X, Mah AT, Kuo CJ, Monack DM, Amieva MR. Controlling epithelial polarity: a human enteroid model for host-pathogen interactions. Cell Rep. 2019;26(9):2509–20.e4. https://doi.org/10.1016/j.celrep.2019.01.108. PMID: 30811997; PMCID: PMC6391775.
10. Peng H, Poovaiah N, Forrester M, Cochran E, Wang Q. Ex vivo culture of primary intestinal stem cells in collagen gels and foams. ACS Biomater Sci Eng. 2015;1(1):37–42. https://doi.org/10.1021/ab500041d. Epub 2014 Dec 8. PMID: 33435081.
11. Watson CL, Mahe MM, Múnera J, Howell JC, Sundaram N, Poling HM, Schweitzer JI, Vallance JE, Mayhew CN, Sun Y, Grabowski G, Finkbeiner SR, Spence JR, Shroyer NF, Wells JM, Helmrath MA. An in vivo model of human small intestine using pluripotent stem cells. Nat Med. 2014;20(11):1310–4. https://doi.org/10.1038/nm.3737. Epub 2014 Oct 19. PMID: 25326803; PMCID: PMC4408376.
12. Gjorevski N, Sachs N, Manfrin A, Giger S, Bragina ME, Ordóñez-Morán P, Clevers H, Lutolf MP. Designer matrices for intestinal stem cell and organoid culture. Nature. 2016;539(7630):560–4. https://doi.org/10.1038/nature20168. Epub 2016 Nov 16. PMID: 27851739.
13. Cruz-Acuña R, Quirós M, Farkas AE, Dedhia PH, Huang S, Siuda D, García-Hernández V, Miller AJ, Spence JR, Nusrat A, García AJ. Synthetic hydrogels for human intestinal organoid generation and colonic wound repair. Nat Cell Biol. 2017;19(11):1326–35. https://doi.org/10.1038/ncb3632. Epub 2017 Oct 23. PMID: 29058719; PMCID: PMC5664213.
14. Lei NY, Jabaji Z, Wang J, Joshi VS, Brinkley GJ, Khalil H, Wang F, Jaroszewicz A, Pellegrini M, Li L, Lewis M, Stelzner M, Dunn JC, Martín MG. Intestinal subepithelial myofibroblasts support the growth of intestinal epithelial stem cells. PLoS One. 2014;9(1):e84651. https://doi.org/10.1371/journal.pone.0084651. PMID: 24400106; PMCID: PMC3882257.
15. Gjorevski N, Lutolf MP. Synthesis and characterization of well-defined hydrogel matrices and their application to intestinal stem cell and organoid culture. Nat Protoc. 2017;12(11):2263–74. https://doi.org/10.1038/nprot.2017.095. Epub 2017 Oct 5. PMID: 28981121.

16. Spence JR, Mayhew CN, Rankin SA, Kuhar MF, Vallance JE, Tolle K, Hoskins EE, Kalinichenko VV, Wells SI, Zorn AM, Shroyer NF, Wells JM. Directed differentiation of human pluripotent stem cells into intestinal tissue in vitro. Nature. 2011;470(7332):105–9. https://doi.org/10.1038/nature09691. Epub 2010 Dec 12. PMID: 21151107; PMCID: PMC3033971.
17. Nikolaev M, Mitrofanova O, Broguiere N, Geraldo S, Dutta D, Tabata Y, Elci B, Brandenberg N, Kolotuev I, Gjorevski N, Clevers H, Lutolf MP. Homeostatic mini-intestines through scaffold-guided organoid morphogenesis. Nature. 2020;585(7826):574–8. https://doi.org/10.1038/s41586-020-2724-8. Epub 2020 Sep 16. PMID: 32939089.
18. Urbani L, Maghsoudlou P, Milan A, Menikou M, Hagen CK, Totonelli G, Camilli C, Eaton S, Burns A, Olivo A, De Coppi P. Long-term cryopreservation of decellularised oesophagi for tissue engineering clinical application. PLoS One. 2017;12(6):e0179341. https://doi.org/10.1371/journal.pone.0179341. PMID: 28599006; PMCID: PMC5466304.
19. Sugimoto S, Kobayashi E, Kanai T, Sato T. In vivo intestinal research using organoid transplantation. Keio J Med. 2022;71(4):73–81. https://doi.org/10.2302/kjm.2022-0019-IR. Epub 2022 Dec 1. PMID: 36450523.

MIX
Papier aus verantwortungsvollen Quellen
Paper from responsible sources
FSC® C105338

If you have any concerns about our products,
you can contact us on
ProductSafety@springernature.com

In case Publisher is established outside the EU,
the EU authorized representative is:
Springer Nature Customer Service Center GmbH
Europaplatz 3, 69115 Heidelberg, Germany

Printed by Libri Plureos GmbH
in Hamburg, Germany